Culture and Well-Being

Melissa)

Be happy and prosper!

E. Diener

Social Indicators Research Series

Volume 38

This new series aims to provide a public forum for single treatises and collections of papers on social indicators research that are too long to be published in our journal Social Indicators Research. Like the journal, the book series deals with statistical assessments of the quality of life from a broad perspective. It welcomes the research on a wide variety of substantive areas, including health, crime, housing, education, family life, leisure activities, transportation, mobility, economics, work, religion and environmental issues. These areas of research will focus on the impact of key issues such as health on the overall quality of life and vice versa. An international review board, consisting of Ruut Veenhoven, Joachim Vogel, Ed Diener, Torbjorn Moum, Mirjam A.G. Sprangers and Wolfgang Glatzer, will ensure the high quality of the series as a whole.

For futher volumes:
http://www.springer.com/series/6548

Ed Diener
Editor

Culture and Well-Being

The Collected Works of Ed Diener

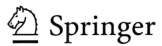 Springer

Editor
Prof. Ed Diener
University of Illinois
Dept. Psychology
603 E. Daniel St.
Champaign IL 61820
USA
ediener@uiuc.edu

ISSN 1387-6570
ISBN 978-90-481-2351-3   e-ISBN 978-90-481-2352-0
DOI 10.1007/978-90-481-2352-0
Springer Dordrecht Heidelberg London New York

Library of Congress Control Number: 2009926877

Cover design: Boekhorst Design BV

Printed on acid-free paper

Springer is part of Springer Science+Business Media (www.springer.com)

Contents

Contributors

Dong-Won Choi
Department of Psychology, California State University, East Bay, USA, dong-won.choi@csueastbay.edu

Incheol Choi
Department of Psychology, Seoul National University, Korea

Ed Diener
Department of Psychology, University of Illinois, Urbana-Champaign, IL 61820, USA, ediener@uiuc.edu

Carol Diener
Department of Psychology, University of Illinois, Urbana-Champaign, IL, USA, cdiener@uiuc.edu

Marissa Diener
Department of Family and Consumer Studies, University of Utah, Salt Lake City, UT 84112, USA, marissa.diener@fcs.utah.edu

Robert Biswas-Diener
Center for Applied Positive Psychology, robert@cappeu.org

Vivian Dzokoto
Department of African American Studies, Virginia Commonwealth University, Richmond, VA 23284, USA, vdzokoto@vcu.edu

Michael Eid
Freie Universität Berlin, eid@zedat.fu-berlin.de

Richard E. Lucas
Department of Psychology, Michigan State University, East Lansing, MI 48824, USA, lucasri@msu.edu

Shigehiro Oishi
Department of Psychology, University of Virginia, Charlottesville, VA 22904, USA, soishi@virginia.edu

Chu Kim-Prieto
Department of Psychology, The College of New Jersey, Ewing, NJ 08628-
0718, USA, kim@tcnj.edu

Christie Napa Scollon
School of Social Sciences, Singapore Management University, Singapore 178903,
cscollon@smu.edu.sg

Eunkook M. Suh
Department of Psychology, Yonsei University, Shinchon-dong, Seoul, Korea,
esuh@yonsei.ac.kr

William Tov
School of Social Sciences, Singapore Management University, Singapore 178903,
williamtov@smu.edu.sg

John A. Updegraff
Department of Psychology, Kent State University, Ohio, USA, jupdegr1@kent.edu

Joar Vittersø
Department of Psychology, University of Tromsø, Norway, joarv@psyk.uit.no

Endorsements

Over the past several decades Professor Diener has contributed more than any other psychologist to the rigorous research of subjective well-being. The collection of this work in this series is going to be of invaluable help to anyone interested in the study of happiness, life-satisfaction, and the emerging discipline of positive psychology.

Mihaly Csikszentmihalyi, Professor of Psychology and Management, Claremont Graduate University

---

Ed Diener, the Jedi Master of the world's happiness researchers, has inspired and informed all of us who have studied and written about happiness. His life's work epitomizes a humanly significant psychological science. How wonderful to have his pioneering writings collected and preserved for future students of human well-being, and for practitioners and social policy makers who are working to promote human flourishing.

David G. Myers, Hope College, and author, *The Pursuit of Happiness*

Ed Diener's work on life satisfaction – theory and research – has been ground-breaking. Having his collected works available will be a great boon to psychologists and policy-makers alike.

Christopher Peterson, Professor of Psychology, University of Michigan

---

By looking at happiness and well-being in many different cultures and societies, from East to West, from New York City to Calcutta slums, and beyond, Ed Diener has forever transformed the field of culture in psychology. Filled with bold theoretical insights and rigorous and, yet, imaginative empirical studies, this volume will be absolutely indispensable for all social and behavioral scientists interested in transformative power of culture on human psychology.

Shinobu Kitayama, Professor and Director of the Culture and Cognition Program, University of Michigan

---

Ed Diener is one of the most productive psychologists in the world working in the field of perceived quality of life or, as he prefers, subjective wellbeing. He has served the profession as a researcher, writer, teacher, officer in professional organizations, editor of leading journals, a member of the editorial board of still more journals as well as a member of the board of the Social Indicators Research Book Series. As an admirer of his work and a good friend, I have learned a lot from him, from his students, his relatives and collaborators. The idea of producing a collection of his works came to me as a result of spending a great deal of time trying to keep up with his work. What a wonderful public and professional service it would be, I thought, as well as a time-saver for me, if we could get a substantial number of his works assembled in one collection. In these three volumes we have not only a fine selection of past works but a good number of new ones as well. So, it is with considerable delight that I write these lines to thank Ed and to lend my support to this important publication.

Alex C. Michalos, Ph.D., F.R.S.C., Chancellor, Director, Institute for Social Research and Evaluation; Professor Emeritus, Political Science, University of Northern British Columbia

Editor's note concerning source publications

Tov & Diener: Culture and Subjective Well-Being, (S. Kitayama, D. Cohen) *Handbook of Cultural Psychology*, 2007, Guilford Press

Diener, Diener & Diener: Factors Predicting the Subjective Well-Being of Nations, *Journal of Personality and Social Psychology*, 69/5 (1995), American Psychological Association

Diener & Diener: Cross-Cultural Correlates of Life Satisfaction and Self Esteem, *Journal of Personality and Social Psychology*, 68/4 (1995), American Psychological Association

Oishi & Diener: Goals, Culture, and Subjective Well-Being, *Personality and Social Psychology Bulletin*, 27/12 (2001), SAGE

Oishi, Diener, Lucas, & Suh: Cross-Cultural Variations in Predictors of Life Satisfaction: Perspectives from Needs and Values, *Personality and Social Psychology Bulletin*, 25/8 (1999), SAGE

Suh, Diener, & Updegraff: From Culture To Priming Conditions: Self-Construal Influences on Life Satisfaction Judgments, *Journal of Cross-Cultural Psychology*, 39/1 (2008), SAGE

Oishi, Diener, Choi, Kim-Prieto, & Choi: The Dynamics of Daily Events and Well-Being Across Cultures: When Less is More, *Journal of Personality and Social Psychology*, 93/4 (2007), American Psychological Association

Eid & Diener: Norms for Experiencing Emotions in Different Cultures: Inter- and intranational differences, *Journal of Personality and Social Psychology*, 81/5 (2001), American Psychological Association

Scollon, Diener, Oishi, & Biswas-Diener: Emotions Across Cultures and Methods, *Journal of Cross-Cultural Psychology*, 35/3 (2004), SAGE

Diener, Scollon, Oishi, Dzokoto, & Suh: Positivity and the Construction of Life Satisfaction Judgments: Global Happiness Is Not Sum of Its Parts, *Journal of Happiness Studies*, 1/2 (2000), Springer SBM

Biswas-Diener, Vitterso, & Diener: Most People are Pretty Happy, but There is Cultural Variation: The Inughuit, The Amish, and The Maasai, *Journal of Happiness Studies*, 6/3 (2005), Springer SBM

Biswas-Diener & Diener: Making the Best of a Bad Situation: Satisfaction in the Slums of Calcutta, *Social Indicators Research*, 55/3 (2001), Springer SBM

Introduction – Culture and Well-Being Works by Ed Diener

Ed Diener

Cultural Differences

A central issue in the study of well-being is cultural differences. Do cultures have an effect on well-being? Do people in different cultures have different conceptions of well-being that, in turn, influence the feelings they deem most desirable? Are the causes of well-being similar or distinct in different cultures? These questions speak to the fundamental nature of subjective well-being; and, therefore, under-standing in this field cannot proceed without first acknowledging the influence of culture.

One would think that the well-being of people around the world would have been assessed by anthropologists, given that they have studied various cultural groups in such depth. However, anthropologists studied values, practices, and beliefs, but rarely intensively studied emotions, and even more rarely mentioned well-being. For one thing, cultural anthropologists might have considered the discussion of the well-being of other groups to be inappropriate because that could mean judging these groups using western values rather than the values unique to each culture. In addition, anthropologists usually believed that it would be impossible to compare groups' well-being because the concept of quality of life would be idiosyncratic to each culture. It was considered taboo to evaluate societies (Shweder, 2000). Robert Edgerton (1992) broke with this tradition when he wrote of assessing the quality of life of cultures by comparing them as to whether they provided good health and met human needs. However, the direct study of well-being among anthropologists has been rare.

Large scale studies of subjective well-being by survey researchers, both psychologists and sociologists, moved into the cross-cultural tradition when they began to collect data across a number of nations. For example, George Gallup (1976) and Hadley Cantril (1965) both collected well-being data from a number of nations and world regions. Easterlin (1974), working from the early world surveys, concluded

E. Diener (✉)
Department of Psychology, University of Illinois, Champaign, IL 61820, USA
e-mail: ediener@uiuc.edu

E. Diener (ed.), *Culture and Well-Being: The Collected Works of Ed Diener*, Social Indicators Research Series 38, DOI 10.1007/978-90-481-2352-0_1,
© Springer Science+Business Media B.V. 2009

that well-being was not substantially related to the income of nations. The surveys examined the well-being of nations primarily with regard to the impact of factors such as income.

In 1993, Ruut Veenhoven published his comprehensive analysis of the well-being of nations: *Happiness in nations: Subjective appreciation of life in 56 nations 1946–1992*. This work was a major advance for the field in that a larger number of nations were analyzed, and many predictor variables were considered. Veenhoven discussed his results within the framework of "livability," conditions of quality of life in societies that meet human needs, and, therefore, cause those within these societies to experience higher subjective well-being. The livability concept suggests that there are certain universal human conditions that will lead to well-being and that cultural variability will be a relatively minor factor, except insofar as it relates to creating objectively better living conditions.

In 1995, Diener, Diener, and Diener compared a relatively large number of nations on well-being and used the cultural variable of individualism as one of its predictors. We found that individualism was highly predictive of the mean levels of subjective well-being in nations, although individualism was very highly correlated with national income, and, therefore, the results might have been due to economic development rather than to other aspects of culture. This study was a first attempt at examining culture vis-à-vis well-being beyond the effects of objective characteristics such as national income. In that same year, Diener and Diener asked whether the predictors of well-being within cultures might differ. In this study of 31 nations, we found that the correlates of well-being, not just mean levels, varied across societies. Both of these papers, reprinted in this volume, represent the approach of studying cultural effects by examining many nations and aligning well-being with cultural dimensions. These studies went beyond the examination of the impact of income and other objective conditions to consider whether traditional cultural dimensions might relate to the levels and causes of well-being. Thus, by the mid-1990s, a beginning had been made in better analyzing the well-being of societies and cultures, and this volume represents our advances from 1995 to the present.

When considering well-being across cultures, there are many important questions: (1) Are there mean level differences between different types of well-being across cultures, and, if so, what are the predictors of these differences? (2) Do cultures differ in well-being primarily because of objective conditions such as income, or do they differ because of cultural factors such as norms, values, and the form of social relationships? (3) Are there differences in the structure and composition of well-being across cultures—for example, in which emotions are considered pleasant and desirable? (4) Is subjective well-being valued differently in different cultures? (5) Do different measurement methods provide converging answers about which cultures have high compared with low well-being? (6) Do the correlates and causes of well-being differ within cultures? (7) Do certain personality characteristics correlate with well-being consistently across cultures, and are cultural differences in personality related to mean differences in well-being? (8) Do the outcomes or behaviors following from high well-being differ across cultures? (9) To what extent do material boundaries capture cultural effects? The articles contained in this volume offer initial answers to most of these questions.

The culture and well-being questions are of fundamental importance to understanding in the entire field and to scientific knowledge in the behavioral sciences as a whole. Unless we understand what is universal and what is specific, we cannot hope to understand the processes governing well-being. Unfortunately, our scientific knowledge in most behavioral science fields, including the study of well-being, has been built on a narrow database drawn from westernized, industrialized nations. This means that we have only a little knowledge of whether our findings are generalizable to all peoples of the globe and to universal human psychological processes. Fortunately, during the last decade my students and I, as well as others working in this area, have rapidly expanded our knowledge of well-being vis-à-vis culture. The first attempt to summarize the findings in this area came in 1999 with *Culture and Subjective Well-Being*, a book edited by Eunkook Suh and Diener. The current volume represents a renewed effort to give a broad overview of major findings in this area and to point to the important directions for future research.

Composition of This Volume

I am very pleased with the articles presented in this volume because I believe that they represent true advances in our fundamental understanding of subjective well-being. I am very grateful to my respective co-authors because without their efforts and creativity none of these articles would exist. I believe the articles here are important because they begin to show what is universal as opposed to culture-specific about well-being, and, in so doing, they give important clues to the processes that create subjective well-being.

The first chapter reprinted here is a 2007 review paper by myself and William Tov, which reviews many of the important advances in our knowledge of culture vis-à-vis well-being. This paper documents several of the major themes of this volume. Although there are universal causes of well-being across cultures and nations, there are also unique influences as well. Similarly, the experience of well-being has certain pancultural aspects, and yet, there are also specific ways that well-being is experienced in various cultures as well.

The next two papers in the volume, authored together with my wife Carol and daughter Marissa in 1995, included several new findings. The Diener, Diener, and Diener (1995) article focused on predictors of mean levels of well-being across 55 nations. At the time this was considered to be a very large number of nations, and the article reviewed a more diverse set of cultures than had been examined in previous studies. We found that rich, individualistic nations tended to have higher subjective well-being, but also that factors such as human rights were related to the average well-being experienced in nations. However, even with the larger number of countries, it was difficult to separate the effects of the predictors because they were so highly correlated with one another. This article showed clearly that, contrary to Easterlin's (1974) conjecture, the wealth of nations was associated with the well-being experienced in them, and strongly so.

The Ed Diener and Marissa Diener article represents the initial demonstration that the correlates of subjective well-being (SWB) vary across cultures. Indeed, the degree to which self-esteem was correlated with life satisfaction varied dramatically across cultures and showed a much stronger association in individualistic societies. This finding gave support to two important conclusions. First, it confirmed that the predictors of SWB vary substantially across cultures; and second, it revealed that feeling good about oneself carries more weight in individualistic nations. In this paper, we also found that financial satisfaction showed a stronger association with life satisfaction in poorer nations than in richer nations. Therefore, the findings clearly indicated that cultures vary in terms of what is most relevant to life satisfaction. Moreover, the study was an advance in that it had a larger number of societies, 31, than most previous cross-cultural studies, and a more diverse set of nations. Many of the previous cross-cultural studies of well-being had relied on comparisons between only two nations, or had analyzed several nations that were very similar to one another.

In the article that I authored with Shigehiro Oishi in 2001, we discovered that achieving goals can vary in relation to well-being across cultures depending on the degree to which the goals are valued in the cultures. We found that the attainment of certain goals is more related to well-being in collectivist cultures, and that the attainment of other types of goals is more relevant to well-being in individualistic cultures. When participants pursued goals for fun and enjoyment, this increased satisfaction more among individualists than among collectivists, whereas pursuing goals to please others increased SWB more among collectivists.

The Oishi, Diener, Lucas, and Suh (1999) article drives home the point that there are different predictors of well-being in different cultures and situations, and it replicated several of the findings of Diener and Diener (1995). For example, financial satisfaction was a better predictor of life satisfaction among the poor, whereas, among the wealthy, home life was a better predictor of life satisfaction. In the second study, we found, also supporting the conclusions of Diener and Diener, that self-esteem and freedom were better predictors of life satisfaction in individualistic nations than in collectivist ones.

Eunkook Suh, Diener, and John Updegraff (2008) go even farther in suggesting that the correlates of well-being differ across cultures, showing in both correlational and experimental studies that collectivists use their emotions less as information that is relevant in reporting their life satisfaction. In other words, not only do the predictors of well-being vary across cultures, but the associations among various forms of subjective well-being also vary. In this paper, we were able to establish causal direction because we used an experimental priming methodology in addition to simple correlations. We found that collectivists relied more on social appraisals of their lives in computing life satisfaction than do individualists. Thus, some factors that might be considered as universals in causing well-being—the appraisal of others and our own emotional feelings—vary in their strength of association with life satisfaction across cultures.

The next paper, with Shigehiro Oishi as lead author (2007), furthered our understanding of cultural differences in the causes of well-being to an even greater degree. In this paper, Oishi, myself, and our colleagues found that the degree to which positive events stimulated positive feelings varied across cultures. Paradoxically, positive events stimulate less within-person change among persons and in cultures characterized by high life satisfaction. It appeared that people low in satisfaction experienced fewer good events, and consequentially, these events had more impact when they did occur. Although European-Americans had more good events and higher life satisfaction, over time they reacted less strongly to each good event. This finding suggests that a series of good events would raise one's long-term moods so that simple good events produce less change.

Taken together, our studies demonstrate that the causes of well-being differ in predictable ways across cultures. The values of people in a particular culture, as well as the nature of their everyday experience, influence the factors that most strongly affect their well-being. This does not mean, of course, that there are no universals, but it certainly places boundaries on the idea that the causes of well-being are completely pancultural.

The article by Michael Eid and Diener (2001) revealed that whether various emotions are seen as desirable varies to some degree across cultures. There are universals in that some emotions are generally seen as desirable and others as undesirable. But certain self-conscious emotions such as guilt and pride vary in how they are valued and how much they are experienced. Norms for positive emotions such as pride and contentment were more associated with reports of experiencing them than were the norms for negative emotions. This suggests that emotion norms do not merely reflect the types of affect experienced in a culture because the relation is asymmetrical for positive and negative emotions. Instead, it may be that situational and personality factors more strongly influence the experience of negative emotions, whereas positive emotions are more under people's control and are more highly subject to the effects of socialization. An unexpected finding from the Eid and Diener study is that there is more variability within collectivist nations than individualistic societies in terms of the norms governing emotions.

The next two papers in the volume concern conceptual issues related to the assessment of emotions. We were concerned with the issue of the psychological processes influencing various types of measures of well-being. In the Scollon, Diener, Oishi, and Biswas-Diener (2004) paper, we examined several different types of measures, assessing a variety of emotions across five cultural groups. Indigenous emotions that were particular to specific cultures clustered with other similar positive or negative emotions rather than being in a space by themselves, suggesting that they might differ from other emotions but are not so different that they fall outside the common space of emotions across cultures.

The relative position of cultural groups was consistent across the various types of measures of well-being, with Hispanics always ranking at the top. However, cultures differed most on certain emotions such as pride. Furthermore, cultures varied substantially with regard to the positioning of some emotions; pride clustered more closely with the positive emotions in some cultures and with the negative emotions in other cultures, for example. Love was closer or farther from sadness depending on the culture. Thus, although there is a core of pleasant versus unpleasant feelings across cultures, the way certain emotions are experienced can differ.

An interesting finding in the Scollon et al. study was that the memory for one's emotions was biased by one's global self-perceptions differentially across cultures. In some cultures, a person's general emotional self-perception colored the memory they had of the week's emotions and added substantially to the memory prediction from actual on-line emotion reports, whereas in other cultures, the memories were more accurate.

In the article I published in 2000 with Scollon, Oishi, Dzokoto, and Suh, we studied the propensity toward positivity in responding in 41 societies. We proposed that people might across cultures differ in their propensity to be generally positive about the world. Naturally, people in all cultures would be unlikely to be positive about something that is clearly negative, such as pain. However, when conditions are ambiguous, or so complex that they defy ready categorization, people might differ in their judgments of positivity simply because the judgment is less about the world and more about their own personality, feelings, and cultural attitudes toward the world.

We assessed positivity by comparing people's ratings of global topics, such as education, with more concrete and specific topics, such as professors or textbooks, the idea being that people would be grounded in the concrete judgments but could express their predispositions more readily when broad categories were judged. We found that our measure of positivity, the difference in people's ratings of broad areas of their lives versus the specific components of those areas, predicted life satisfaction and was related to norms for positive emotions. Although preliminary, these findings suggest that while some part of life satisfaction depends on circumstances, part also depends on people's propensities to judge things in a positive light if they have some freedom to do so. The findings also suggest that the magnitude of cultural differences in well-being will to some extent depend on the concreteness and specificity of the measure.

These studies have implications both for the theoretical understanding of emotional well-being across cultures and for the cross-cultural measurement of well-being. We now know, for instance, that cultural groups might differ more on memories of emotions than they do on actual emotional experience, and we know that people's positive predispositions can color reports of well-being even beyond influencing how they react to the concrete elements of their circumstances. Although these differences across cultures might be labeled as "biases," they are also substantive in that they reflect people's actual reactions and might influence future behavior. Obviously much more work in this area is needed, and I will describe some essential future directions in the concluding chapter of this volume.

Importantly, not all emotions that are considered positive in western cultures are necessarily evaluated or experienced as positive in all cultures—pride, for instance. Thus, we must be careful in assessing people's emotional well-being across cultures to make sure that we are aggregating emotions that are actually of the same valence.

The final two articles reprinted in this volume describe the well-being of "exotic," or smaller groups, rather than large societies. My son, Robert Biswas-Diener, published with Joar Vitterso and Diener (2005) an article that describes self-reports of well-being among three groups: the Amish in the USA, the Inughuit (and Inuit people in Northern Greenland), and the Maasai (a herding people living in the Serengeti of Africa). Although all three groups were "happy" in that they were generally above neutral, the Maasai showed the highest life satisfaction of the three groups. Their scores suggest that material luxuries are not necessary for high well-being in all cultures because the Maasai lead a very simple life that in western cultures would be considered to be desperately impoverished.

There were also differences in the specific patterns of well-being, for example with the Maasai reporting very high levels of pride, the Amish being unsatisfied with self-related domains, and both the Amish and Inughuit being relatively dissatisfied with the material domains of their lives. Thus, cultures do not simply differ in a general way on "happiness"; asking which cultures are happiest is bound to over-simplify matters to some extent. Cultures will differ in some forms of well-being and not in others; it is important, therefore, to assess a variety of types of SWB to fully capture the well-being of a society.

Robert Biswas-Diener and Diener (2001) examined another "exotic" group in our study in the slums of Calcutta. We studied those living in a shanty-town, pavement dwellers (homeless), and sex workers. The life satisfaction scores were slightly below neutral in the groups we studied, but not as low as one might expect given the difficult conditions. Surprisingly, people were positive about many domains of their lives, including the social domain. An interesting feature of this study is that we used an unusual measure of SWB beyond the typical self-report scales, and that was to ask people to list positive and negative events from their lives during the past day and past year. We used the difference in number of good versus bad events recalled as an assessment of well-being. In this case, the slum dwellers were able to list slightly more positive than negative events, supporting the conclusion that they find rewards in life despite their dire circumstances.

The papers collected in this volume do not represent the entirety of my works in the area of culture and well-being. For example, in 2000 Eunkook Suh and Diener edited a book entitled *Culture and Subjective Well-Being*, and we have published many more articles in this area, as have others. Hopefully the articles reprinted in this book, however, will give readers a good overview of the questions being asked and some of the answers that have been found.

References

Biswas-Diener, R., & Diener, E. (2001). Making the best of a bad situation: Satisfaction in the slums of Calcutta. *Social Indicators Research, 55,* 329–352.

Biswas-Diener, R., Vitterso, J., & Diener, E. (2005). Most people are pretty happy, but there is cultural variation: The Inughuit, the Amish, and the Maasai. *Journal of Happiness Studies: An Interdisciplinary Periodical on Subjective Well-Being, 6,* 205–226.

Cantril, H. (1965). *Pattern of human concerns.* New Brunswick: Rutgers University Press.

Diener, E., & Diener, M. (1995). Cross-cultural correlates of life satisfaction and self-esteem. *Journal of Personality and Social Psychology, 68,* 653–663.

Diener, E., Diener, M., & Diener, C. (1995). Factors predicting the subjective well-being of nations. *Journal of Personality and Social Psychology, 69,* 851–864.

Diener, E., Scollon, C. K. N., Oishi, S., Dzokoto, V., & Suh, E. M. (2000). Positivity and the construction of life satisfaction judgments: Global happiness is not the sum of its parts. *Journal of Happiness Studies: An Interdisciplinary Periodical on Subjective Well-Being, 1,* 159–176.

Diener, E., & Tov, W. (2007). Culture and subjective well-being. In S. Kitayama & D. Cohen (Eds.), *Handbook of cultural psychology.* New York: Guilford.

Diener, E., & Suh, E. M. (Eds.) (2000). *Culture and subjective well-being.* Cambridge, MA: MIT Press.

Easterlin, R. A. (1974). Does economic growth improve the human lot? In P. A. David and M. W. Reder (Eds.), *Nations and households in economic growth: Essays in honor of Moses Abramovitz.* New York: Academic Press, Inc.

Edgerton, R. B. (1992). *Sick societies: Challenging the myth of primitive harmony.* New York: Free Press.

Eid, M., & Diener, E. (2001). Norms for experiencing emotions in different cultures: Inter-and intranational differences. *Journal of Personality and Social Psychology, 81,* 869–885.

Gallup, G. (1976). Human needs and satisfactions: A global survey. *Public Opinion Quarterly, 40,* 459–467.

Oishi, S., & Diener, E. (2001). Goals, culture, and subjective well-being. *Personality and Social Psychology Bulletin, 27,* 1674–1682.

Oishi, S., Diener, E., Choi, D. W., Kim-Prieto, C., & Choi, I. (2007). The dynamics of daily events and well-being across cultures: When less is more. *Journal of Personality and Social Psychology, 93,* 685–698.

Oishi, S., Diener, E., Lucas, R. E., & Suh, E. (1999). Cross-cultural variations in predictors of life satisfaction: Perspectives from needs and values. *Personality and Social Psychology Bulletin, 25,* 980–990.

Scollon, C. N., Diener, E., Oishi, S, & Biswas-Diener, R. (2004). Emotions across cultures and methods. *Journal of Cross-Cultural Psychology, 35,* 304–326.

Suh, E. M., Diener, E., & Updegraff, J. A. (2008). From culture to priming conditions – Self-construal influences on life satisfaction judgments. *Journal of Cross-Cultural Psychology. 39,* 3–15.

Shweder, R. A. (2000). Moral maps, "First World" conceits, and the new evangelists. In L. E. Harrison & S. P. Huntington (Eds.), *Culture matters: How values shape human progress* (pp. 158–172). New York: Basic Books.

Veenhoven, R. (1993). *Happiness in nations: Subjective appreciation of life in 56 nations 1946–1992.* Rotterdam, The Netherlands: Risbo.

Culture and Subjective Well-Being

William Tov and Ed Diener

Abstract Subjective well-being (SWB) is composed of people's evaluations of their lives, including pleasant affect, infrequent unpleasant affect, life satisfaction (LS). We review the research literature concerning the influence of culture on SWB. We argue that some types of well-being, as well as their causes, are consistent across cultures, whereas there are also unique patterns of well-being in societies that are not comparable across cultures. Thus, well-being can be understood to some degree in universal terms, but must also be understood within the framework of each culture. We review the methodological challenges to assessing SWB in different cultures. One important question for future research is the degree to which feelings of well-being lead to the same outcomes in different cultures. The overarching theme of the paper is that there are pancultural experiences of SWB that can be compared across cultures, but that there are also culture-specific patterns that make cultures unique in their experience of well-being.

Introduction

> With great perseverance
> He meditates, seeking
> Freedom and happiness.
> —from THE BUDDHA, Chapter 2, *The Dhammapada*

Over two thousand years ago, the Buddha perceived suffering to be the nature of existence. But for him, the attainment of nirvana was not simply a break from this cycle of suffering, it was also a return to true bliss. Although it was not the direct purpose of meditation, happiness was certainly an important consequence, and a critical topic in Buddhist philosophy (Gaskins, 1999). Across time and cultures, generations of people have in their own way reflected upon the question of happiness. As long as it has been pondered, it may come as a surprise that the scientific

W. Tov (✉)
School of Social Sciences, Singapore Management University, 90 Stamford Road, Level 4, Singapore 178903
e-mail: williamtov@smu.edu.sg

E. Diener (ed.), *Culture and Well-Being: The Collected Works of Ed Diener*, Social Indicators Research Series 38, DOI 10.1007/978-90-481-2352-0_2,
© Springer Science+Business Media B.V. 2009

study of happiness, or subjective well-being (SWB; Diener, 1984) has advanced only recently.

One of the challenges has been defining happiness in a way that enables it to be measured. Given that conceptions of happiness may vary across different societies, a number of questions arises regarding *how* culture influences the idea and experience of happiness. Does the structure and content of SWB differ? Do certain cultures emphasize some components more than others? Are the correlates and causes of happiness similar across cultures? Do people react differently to the experience of well-being (e.g., when they feel pleasant affect)?

As it has been studied over the past two decades, SWB involves frequent pleasant emotion, infrequent unpleasant emotion, and life satisfaction (LS). The first two components are affective; the last is a cognitive evaluation. These three components are not the only elements of SWB. Happiness also can be said to consist of other dimensions such as meaning and purpose in life. However, in this review we focus on LS, pleasant affect, and unpleasant affect in part because these constructs have been researched more frequently across cultures. Furthermore, these components of SWB are major focal points that allow for a certain degree of precision in measuring the fuzzier, folk concept of happiness.

Why Study SWB Across Cultures?

The cross-cultural study of SWB is one indicator of the quality of life in a society. It was once considered taboo to suggest that societies could be evaluated at all (Shweder, 2000). To appraise *any* aspect of a culture was to ignore its worth and integrity. However, this extreme form of cultural relativism has given way to the view that, though one must be careful in comparing and evaluating societies, they may differ in variables such as health and satisfaction that are desirable in most cultures. It is true that some indicators of life quality may impose values about the good life that are not shared by all people. However, even if SWB is internally framed with respect to each culture, societies could still be evaluated in terms of how well they succeed according to these internal criteria.

Culture and SWB research can also shed light on basic emotional processes. In measuring SWB across various societies, researchers have confronted issues regarding the universality of emotions, and how the representation of emotions in memory are influenced by cultural norms. The field can also add to our understanding of culture. For example, how do cultures differ in their socialization of pleasant and unpleasant affect, and how do emotions contribute to the reinforcement of cultural values and practices? These questions reflect a cultural psychological perspective. Thus, the topic is of both applied and theoretical importance.

History of This Field of Inquiry

Anthropologists adopted cultural relativity as a way of avoiding a Western, ethnocentric bias in observing other cultures. They made the important observation that values and practices might vary across cultures, but this need not imply that some cultures were necessarily better than others. In particular, we should avoid judging other cultures by the standards of our own. However, taken to extremes, cultural relativism would prevent one from saying that Nazi Germany, or Cambodia under the Khmer Rouge, were in many respects undesirable cultures (Edgerton, 1992). This level of extreme value relativity would make cultural psychology irrelevant to public discourse. According to Edgerton (1992), not all practices in a culture are adaptive; some may even be harmful. He defined maladaptive cultures as those in which there was rampant dissatisfaction or impaired physical and mental health. Thus, there are certain criteria by which we can judge the success of a culture. As one such criterion, SWB is important because a society functions poorly when a majority of its people are discontent and depressed.

It should be noted that very little quantitative work has examined the well-being of small cultures (e.g., Biswas-Diener, Vittersø, & Diener, 2005), although a number of international surveys of SWB in modern nations have been conducted (e.g., Cantril, 1965; Inglehart, 1990; see Table 1). Only recently has research examined the structure and causes of SWB in different cultures. In 1995, for example, E. Diener and M.L. Diener found that self-esteem correlated more strongly with LS in individualist than in collectivist cultures, and that financial satisfaction more strongly predicted LS in poor than in rich nations. Since then, there has been a rapid growth in the field of culture and well-being, and both universal and unique correlates of SWB have been documented. We foresee further growth in this research area in the decade to come.

General Approaches to Cross-Cultural Comparisons of SWB

The comparisons that researchers make across cultures are guided by their assumptions about the interplay between culture and SWB. We review some of these approaches below.

Dimensional Approach

Some theorists hold that the causes of well-being are fundamentally the same for all people. Ryff and Singer (1998) posited that purpose in life, quality relationships, self-regard, and a sense of mastery were universal features of well-being. Self-determination theorists (Deci & Ryan, 1985; Ryan & Deci, 2000) maintain that well-being hinges on the fulfillment of *innate* psychological needs such as autonomy, competence, and relatedness. If these sources of well-being are universal, they provide dimensions along which we can compare societies. Cultures should differ in SWB to the extent that they provide people with different levels autonomy, meaning, and relationships.

A related perspective is the universalist position on emotions. Drawing on diverse findings, some researchers propose that there are discrete, basic emotions that appear in all cultures (Ekman & Friesen, 1971; Izard & Malatesta, 1987;

Table 1 Life satisfaction in various nations (1999–2002)*

Nation	Year	LS	SD
Puerto Rico	2001	8.49	1.97
Denmark	1999	8.24	1.82
Malta	1999	8.21	1.62
Ireland	1999	8.20	1.83
Mexico	2000	8.14	2.35
Iceland	1999	8.05	1.59
Austria	1999	8.03	1.92
Northern Ireland	1999	8.00	1.75
Finland	2000	7.87	1.65
Netherlands	1999	7.85	1.34
Canada	2000	7.85	1.88
Luxembourg	1999	7.81	1.87
USA	1999	7.66	1.82
Sweden	1999	7.64	1.86
Venezuela	2000	7.52	2.50
El Salvador	1999	7.50	2.43
Belgium	1999	7.43	2.13
Germany	1999	7.42	1.96
Great Britain	1999	7.40	1.94
Argentina	1999	7.30	2.26
Singapore	2002	7.24	1.80
Italy	1999	7.17	2.11
Chile	2000	7.12	2.16
Spain	1999	7.09	1.92
Czech Republic	1999	7.06	1.97
Portugal	1999	7.04	1.96
Israel	2001	7.03	2.17
France	1999	7.01	1.99
Indonesia	2001	6.96	2.06
Nigeria	2000	6.87	2.32
Croatia	1999	6.68	2.30
Greece	1999	6.67	2.19
Philippines	2001	6.65	2.53
China	2001	6.53	2.47
Vietnam	2001	6.52	2.06
Japan	2000	6.48	1.97
Peru	2001	6.44	2.40
Iran	2000	6.38	2.41
South Africa	2001	6.31	2.69
South Korea	2001	6.21	2.32
Poland	1999	6.20	2.53
Morocco	2001	6.06	2.54
Slovakia	1999	6.03	2.22
Estonia	1999	5.93	2.18
Hungary	1999	5.80	2.42
Bosnia-Herzegovina	2001	5.77	2.39
Bangladesh	2002	5.77	2.18
Algeria	2002	5.67	2.86
Uganda	2001	5.65	2.47
Montenegro	2001	5.64	2.38
Turkey	2000	5.62	2.79

Table 1 (continued)

Nation	Year	LS	SD
Serbia	2001	5.62	2.47
Jordan	2001	5.60	2.50
Bulgaria	1999	5.50	2.65
Egypt	2000	5.36	3.35
Latvia	1999	5.27	2.39
Romania	1999	5.23	2.77
Lithuania	1999	5.20	2.66
Albania	2002	5.17	2.25
India	2001	5.14	2.23
Macedonia	2001	5.12	2.72
Pakistan	2001	4.85	1.46
Belarus	2000	4.81	2.21
Russia	1999	4.56	2.57
Ukraine	1999	4.56	2.59
Moldova	2000	4.56	2.32
Zimbabwe	2001	3.95	2.79
Tanzania	2001	3.87	3.22

Note: Life satisfaction scores are based on responses to the question "All things considered, how satisfied are you with your life as-a-whole now?" on a 10-pt scale from 1 (*dissatisfied*) to 10 (*satisfied*).
Source. Veenhoven (n.d.).

Plutchik, 1980; Tomkins, 1962, 1963). For example, facial expressions of anger, sadness, and joy appear early in infancy (Izard & Malatesta, 1987), and are easily recognized in many different cultures (Ekman & Friesen, 1971; Ekman et al., 1987). Facial expressions of laughing and crying among congenitally blind infants (Thompson, 1941) suggest that there may be genetic programs directing the expression of emotions. The possibility of biologically based, basic emotions is important for it implies that we can compare people across societies on these emotions (however, see Ortony & Turner, 1990 for a critique of the basic emotions concept).

Uniqueness Approach

In contrast to the universalist approach, some ethnographers emphasize emotions as social constructions. According to these researchers, the very concept of emotion may differ across cultures. Lutz (1988) noted that Western ethnopsychologies often view emotions as hidden and private. In contrast, her work in Micronesia revealed that Ifalukian concepts of emotions were more public and relational. Cultures may also differ in their labeling of specific feelings. For example, according to Wierzbicka (1986) there is no word for disgust in Polish. Extreme versions of the uniqueness approach hold that emotions are purely a Western idea, and that internal experiences can be represented in countless ways across cultures. More moderate formulations, on the other hand, maintain that biologically based emotions may be universal, but that culture can significantly alter their development and labelling. Thus, although sadness is often considered a basic emotion with recognizable antecedents, the Tahitians do not appear to have such a label for it (Levy, 1982). Instead, they often refer to feelings of sickness or exhaustion, for which the causes are nonspecific. Although the uniqueness approach does not preclude the possibility of making comparisons across cultures (e.g., Wierzbicka, 1986), it takes as its starting point the culturally patterned subtleties of emotional experience.

Identity Approach

Another perspective on universality is that regardless of the specific elements, all cultures enjoy *identical levels* of SWB. Cultures may differ in their values and in the needs they fulfill, but people eventually adapt leading all societies to be relatively happy. The identity approach likens well-being to a "hedonic treadmill" upon which people run but never change position. Only when cultures are severely disrupted or experiencing trauma (e.g., warfare or famine) will adaptation be impossible, resulting in widespread unhappiness. This position may sound absurd, but in Table 2, diverse groups appear enjoy somewhat comparable levels of LS. For instance, the Amish, Inughuit, and Maasai all report LS that is not significantly different from the richest Americans, suggesting that material luxury is not necessary for well-being. All these groups may be meeting needs such as social relationships, which are critical for SWB. Thus, there may be important conditions for happiness that are met in non-industrial societies such as the Maasai. In contrast, the LS of the homeless indicates that not all groups are happy, and that people do not fully adapt to all conditions.

Table 2 Life satisfaction of selected groups

Positive groups	Life satisfaction
Forbes Richest Americans[a]	5.8
Pennsylvania Amish[b]	5.8
Inughuit (Inuit Group from Northern Greenland)[c]	5.8
East African Maasai[c]	5.4
International College Students (47 nations)[b]	4.9
Calcutta Slum Dwellers[d]	4.6
Neutral point of scale=4.0	
Groups below neutral (below neutral)	
Calcutta Sex Workers[d]	3.6
Calcutta Homeless[d]	3.2
California Homeless[b]	2.9

Note: Life satisfaction scores are based on responses to the statement "You are satisfied with your life," on a 7-point scale from 1 (*strongly disagree*) to 7 (*strongly agree*).
[a]Diener Horwitz, and Emmons (1985).
[b]Diener and Seligman (2005).
[c]Biswas-Diener et al. (2005).
[d]Diener and Biswas-Diener (2000).

The Middle Path

In this chapter, we take a middle path. We argue that there are some universals, such as the tendency for people to be *slightly* happy unless they are exposed to harsh conditions. Some variables influence SWB in all cultures such as temperament and positive relationships. There may also be common goals, such as the need for respect, that characterize people in all cultures. Furthermore, because cultural influences often permeate national boundaries, cultures are not completely independent of one another. However, each culture also retains unique qualities and should not be compared with others in a careless way. Not all comparisons of SWB are meaningful because the value placed on certain subjective states and the labels for them, often differ. The patterning of well-being may also vary across cultures, making it dangerous to compare variables at a high level of abstraction. Thus, although comparisons are possible, they should only be made with due care to the unique factors present in various societies.

Cultural differences in SWB can be likened to differences between individuals. People can be compared on certain universal features such as height and weight. They can also be compared on factors such as health, but health is made up of many lower-order concepts that may relate to each other differently across individuals. Although societies can be compared on longevity, the patterns of illness differ across cultures. In a similar way, cultures can be compared on SWB, but there are also unique facets of well-being in each society that are best captured by specific descriptions of the local culture.

In the sections that follow, we cover several major topics in culture and SWB research. We begin with the issue of patterning and structure, examining how the elements of SWB cohere across societies. Next, we consider whether cultures differ in mean levels of SWB where the structures can be compared, and what factors might contribute to these differences. We then review various correlates and causes of SWB, showing both similarities and differences in cultural recipes for happiness. Following this discussion, we ask whether SWB leads to the same outcomes in different cultures, or whether there are unique effects that depend on the role of emotions in a culture. Finally, we assess the various challenges involved in measuring SWB across cultures, and the impact that measurement artifacts may have on the findings.

Patterning and Structure

The validity of cross-cultural comparisons of SWB depends on how it is structured in different societies. If there are both universal and culture-specific emotions, are aggregates like pleasant and unpleasant affect applicable in all cultures? Is the concept of LS understood by people in all societies? Also, do the three components of SWB relate to each other similarly across cultures? We review the research bearing on these issues below.

Levels of Analyses

As discussed earlier, the existence of universal emotions has been debated for some time. Researchers have used a number of methodologies to answer the question of universality including ethnography, facial expression recognition, and emotion taxonomies. After conducting cross-cultural research on facial expression recognition, Ekman and his colleagues (Ekman & Friesen, 1971; Ekman et al., 1987) suggested that happiness, anger, fear, sadness, and disgust were universal. However, there are also emotions that appear in some cultures, but not others. Some appear to be labeling of specific situation-outcome pairings in relation to feelings. In Japan, for example, the term *kanashii* refers specifically to sadness arising from personal loss (Mesquita & Frijda, 1992). Other indigenous emotions seem to be complex blends such as *aviman* in India, which has been described as "prideful, loving anger" (Scollon, Diener, Oishi, & Biswas-Diener, 2004).

According to Mesquita, Fridja, and Scherer (1997), the debate over universality has hindered culture and emotion research by focusing on the mere presence of certain emotions in a culture rather than on how emotions are "practiced." They argued that emotional experience is a process that includes appraisal of a situation, physiological reactions, overt behaviors and other components. What distinguishes one emotion from another is the *pattern* of components. At a general level, universal patterns of emotional experience may exist, due to innate, neurophysiological programs. For example, joy may inherently feel pleasant and evoke the urge to laugh or smile. However, at the level of specific components, cultural differences may abound. The *type* of events that elicit joy, or attempts to regulate it may vary across societies.

The perspective provided by Mesquita et al. resonates with several lines of research on well-being. In assessing the cross-cultural applicability of pleasant and unpleasant affect, SWB researchers have not only been interested in *which* emotions are present, but also in how frequently they are experienced, how they are patterned, and how norms can shape the structure and composition of pleasant and unpleasant affect. In short, the field of culture and SWB has been concerned as much with the ecology or practice of emotions (Mesquita et al., 1997), as it has with the comparability of SWB across cultures. We will see that the distinction between pleasant and unpleasant affect can be made at a general level, and that there are both similarities and differences in the specific aspects of these emotions.

Structural Evidence

In an early study, Watson, Clark, and Tellegen (1984) found that the mood structure of Japanese participants formed two factors identifiable as positive and negative affect. This two-factor structure was very similar to that of American participants. Hierarchical cluster analyses of emotion words from the U.S., Italy, and China also revealed superordinate groupings of positive and negative emotions (Shaver, Wu, & Schwartz, 1992). Pleasant and unpleasant emotion clusters were also observed in experience sampling data provided by Japanese, Indian, and two American samples (Scollon et al., 2004). Moreover, indigenous emotions that were included in the Japanese and Indian samples did not form separate clusters, but grouped together with the pleasant and unpleasant emotions.

M.L. Diener, Fujita, Kim-Prieto, and E. Diener (2004) studied the frequency of twelve emotions and found that they formed positive and negative clusters in seven regions of the world (Africa, Latin America, East Asia, Southeast Asia, West Asia, Eastern Europe, and Western Europe). Moreover, in virtually all of these regions, a core group of emotions consistently loaded onto either positive or negative clusters. That is, positive emotions consisted of *pleasant*, *cheerful*, and *happy*, whereas negative emotions consisted of *unpleasant*, *sad*, and *angry*. Similarly, Shaver et al. (1992) found that one positive (*joy*) and three negative emotions (*anger, sadness*, and *fear*) formed basic level categories in all three cultures they studied. Finally, Kuppens, Ceulemans, Timmerman, Diener, and Kim-Prieto (2006) found that positive affect and negative affect emerged as strong universal intracultural dimensions, as well as smaller but significant nation-level dimensions on which nations could be discriminated.

Thus, when speaking of emotion aggregates, there is compelling evidence that pleasant and unpleasant affect are perceived in all cultures. There is also support for the universality of particular emotions such as joy, anger, and sadness. However, cultural differences may arise regarding more specific emotions. For instance, outside of the core emotions, M.L. Diener et al. (2004) observed differences in how other emotions clustered. *Pride* clustered with positive emotions in Latin America, Western Europe, and East Asia, but with the negative emotions in Africa, Southeast Asia, Eastern Europe, and West Asia. *Pride* also aligned with the negative emotions among smaller samples in India and Italy (Scollon et al., 2004; Shaver et al., 1992). These findings should be interpreted cautiously. The simple fact that pride clusters with negative emotions in a culture does not necessarily mean that it is experienced as a negative emotion. In the case of M.L. Diener et al.'s data, the cluster analyses were based on the frequency of experience and included weights for means, standard deviations, and correlations—any of which could have affected how emotion terms clustered. In those regions where *pride* was experienced less frequently, it clustered with the negative emotions, which were generally experienced less often than the positive emotions. In contrast, *worry* and *stress* clustered with the positive emotions in Western Europe and East Asia primarily because they were frequently experienced in those areas. Thus, emotional experience may be universal in some ways, but culturally varied in other ways. Recently, Kuppens et al. (in press) found that although positive affect and negative affect emerged as strong universal intracultural dimensions, there were also smaller but significant nation-level dimensions of emotional experience on which nations could be discriminated.

Differences in the frequency of emotions may be related to cultural norms. For example, cultural norms might make some situations more common than others. Thus, the American cultural environment might afford more opportunities for self-enhancement (and the experience of pride), whereas the Japanese cultural environment might be more conducive to self-criticism (Kitayama, Markus, Matsumoto, & Norasakkunkit, 1997). According to Markus & Kitayama (1994), normative social behavior and cultural models of the self might also shape the desirability of certain emotions. In individualist cultures, pride is an enjoyable emotion that highlights individual achievement as well as success in meeting the cultural goals of autonomy and independence. However, in collectivist cultures, emotions resulting from sympathy and humility may feel good because they are consistent with the cultural goals of interdependence. Emotions that conflict with these norms may be de-emphasized and less frequently experienced. Thus, pride may not be as valued in some collectivist Asian cultures because it is self-focusing and separates the individual from the group (Kitayama & Markus, 2000; Markus & Kitayama, 1994; Scollon et al., 2004). In a similar way, the Oriyas in India devalue anger because it is regarded as socially destructive (Menon & Shweder, 1994). On the other hand, shame[1] is viewed as a good emotion for *women* to have because it is integral to sustaining the patriarchal order of society.

The Oriya case draws attention to *intra*cultural variation in emotion norms. That is, norms may not apply or be uniformly perceived across all individuals within a culture. Eid and Diener (2001) investigated this issue by examining the desirability and appropriateness of pleasant and unpleasant affect in the U.S., Australia, China, and Taiwan. They found that norms for pleasant emotions (e.g., joy, affection, pride, and contentment) were more heterogeneous in China and Taiwan than in the U.S. and Australia. For instance, the vast majority (83%) of Australians and Americans regarded all four pleasant emotions as appropriate. In contrast, only 9% of Chinese and 32% of Taiwanese felt this way. A majority of the Taiwanese (57%) had mixed feelings about pride, although joy, affection, and contentment were appropriate. A plurality of the Chinese (32%) felt that joy and affection were appropriate, but that pride was clearly inappropriate. Another class of individuals found only among the Chinese (16%), regarded all pleasant emotions as *inappropriate*. These findings suggest that culture may influence emotion norms in two ways. First, cultures may foster unique normative patterns, as was observed in the Chinese sample. Second, some patterns may be pancultural, but their relative frequency within cultures may differ. All pleasant emotions are clearly favored in the U.S. and Australia. The ambivalence towards pride in China and Taiwan is consistent with previous research on collectivist Asian cultures.

However, the relation between emotion norms and emotional experience may not always be direct. Recent work by Tsai, Knutson, and Fung (2006) suggests that the emotions that people value (ideal affect) are not necessarily the ones they experience most frequently (real affect), although the correlations are moderate.

---

[1] The Oriya emotion *lajya* or *lajja* was translated by Menon and Shweder (1994) as shame. However, a less negative, alternative translation is "feeling shy." These two emotions are related but not the same. We thank Vijay Kumar Shrotryia for this observation. Our point is simply that, the meaning of an emotion (and hence its value) can shift in different cultural contexts in ways that are not obvious from its valence alone.

These researchers found that although cultural values predicted the *preference* for high versus low arousal pleasant emotions, the reported *frequency* of these emotions was better predicted by personality traits. Furthermore, norms may influence some emotions more than others. M.L. Diener et al. (2004) found that the correlation between the appropriateness and frequency of an emotion was larger for "secondary" emotions like pride, guilt, gratitude, and jealousy, than it was for the core emotions. That is, norms appear to predict the experience of secondary emotions more than the experience of core emotions. Indeed, the main cultural differences in structure were due to how the secondary emotions clustered, and the various geopolitical regions diverged most in the frequency of these emotions. For example, people from Southeast Asia reported more frequent experience of guilt and shame, whereas those from Latin America registered more pride than people from other areas. Also, norms for pride and guilt were more variable across cultures than norms for other emotions (Eid & Diener, 2001). Differences in the experience of peripheral emotions such as pride may reflect cultural ideologies regarding attribution styles, such as whether success should be attributed to the self or to the situation (Heine, Lehman, Markus, & Kitayama, 1999). In contrast, a core emotion like happiness is much broader and may tend to follow from outcomes that are considered good in each culture, so that valuing general happiness is likely to be more common across cultures.

In addition to emotions, there is also support for similarity in the structure of LS across cultures. Vitterso, Roysamb, and Diener (2002) carried out confirmatory factor analyses on the five items of the Satisfaction With Life Scale (SWLS; Diener, Emmons, Larsen, & Gribbin, 1985) and found that a one-factor model fit the data reasonably well in forty-one nations. In all nations, the comparative fit index was above 0.90. This finding suggests that the SWLS measures a single construct and that the concept of "life satisfaction" may be similarly understood across a wide range of cultures. That is not to say that the *criteria* for LS are universal, but rather that people in a number of diverse cultures appear to react to queries about LS in a consistent way.

The Relation Between Emotions and Life Satisfaction (LS)

Although the structure of emotions is somewhat consistent across cultures, and the items of the SWLS also seem to cohere reliably, the relation between emotions and LS may vary across cultures (Schimmack, Radhakrishnan, Oishi, Dzokoto & Ahadi, 2002; Suh, Diener, Oishi, & Triandis, 1998). Suh et al. (1998) examined the relation between LS and affect balance (the difference in frequency of pleasant and unpleasant affect). They found that LS and affect balance correlated positively across forty nations; thus, experiencing more pleasant than unpleasant affect predicted greater LS across cultures. However, the correlations were stronger in more individualist countries. Suh et al. (Study 2) also assessed cultural norms for LS by asking participants what they perceived to be the ideal level of LS in their culture. When LS was predicted from both emotions and perceived norms for LS, the former was highly predictive among individualist cultures, accounting for 76% of the variance in LS. In contrast, norms and emotions were equally predictive of LS in collectivist cultures, accounting for 39 and 40% of the variance, respectively. A possible explanation is that in individualist cultures, where personal goals and preferences are emphasized, emotions may be important because one's own feelings are often a relevant factor in one's judgments. However, in collectivist cultures, there may be a greater tendency to use norms as a guide for one's attitudes and behavior and not be the "nail that stands out". Thus, when judging their LS, people from collectivist cultures might weigh norms at least as much as their own emotions. This raises the possibility that collectivists are simply responding in a normatively appropriate manner. Though it is difficult to rule out this alternative explanation, other data suggest that this is not invariably the case. For example, perceived norms for negative emotions were not reliably related to self-reported frequency of these emotions among Chinese and Taiwanese respondents (Eid & Diener, 2001; we discuss further methodological issues later in the chapter).

Conclusions

There are universals in the structure of SWB that make some comparisons possible. Pleasant affect, unpleasant affect, and LS are not concepts that are unfamiliar to most of the world's people. Nevertheless, to some degree, cultural norms shape which emotions are pleasant and unpleasant to feel. Therefore, when using aggregates such as pleasant and unpleasant affect, one must be careful because specific emotions may cohere differently with the larger aggregate. The comparison of emotion aggregates should only be made with emotions that cohere similarly in each culture. Finally, emotions may be more relevant to global LS in individualist cultures, where internal experience is highly valued. This difference highlights the importance of measuring emotions and LS as separate components of SWB. That is affective and cognitive evaluations of well-being reflect different aspects of the superordinate construct of SWB.

Comparing the Mean Levels of SWB of Cultures

In discussing the happiness of societies, it may seem surprising that a majority of people in the world report being happy. That is not to say that all of humanity is in state of elation or jubilance, or that there is no variation across cultures in overall levels of well-being. There may be a wide range of economic, sociocultural, and biological factors that affect the mean level of subjective well-being in a society, but in most cultures the mean level is above neutral.

Most People Are Happy

A study involving 31 nations ($N = 13,118$) revealed that 63% of men and 70% of women reported positive levels of LS (E. Diener & M. Diener, 1995). These findings could be limited in that many of the nations that were studied were fairly industrialized, and most of the participants were college students. However, E. Diener and C. Diener (1996) plotted the distribution of mean SWB responses from nationally representative samples from 43 nations and found that 86% were above the neutral point (see Table 1 for more data based on representative, probability samples). Furthermore, positive levels of well-being appear to be fairly stable over time. National levels of SWB in the U.S., Japan, and France fluctuated over a 46-year period, but never dipped below neutral (Veenhoven, 1993). Positive levels of well-being have also been observed among smaller, non-industrialized societies such as the Maasai in Kenya, the Inughuit in Greenland, and the Amish in the U.S. (Biswas-Diener, Vittersø, & Diener, 2005).

The claim that "most people are happy" is not meant to deny that there remains significant ill-being and suffering in the world. It is important to note that data from the poorest nations of the world—e.g., Rwanda, Mozambique, and Afghanistan—are often lacking (see Table 1). Moreover, although most people report levels of SWB above the midpoint, very few report being extremely happy. Only 4% of E. Diener and M. Diener's (1995) sample were at the top of the scale in LS. Similarly, although the Maasai, Inughuit, and Amish were all significantly above neutral on several measures of SWB, a very small minority reported perfect LS, or *always* experiencing pleasant affect (Biswas-Diener et al., 2005). Thus, the skew in well-being seems to reflect a moderate form of happiness. Although measurement artifacts are an important concern (see Methodological Issues), the replicability of these findings across numerous societies, and over a number of different methods is impressive.

Perhaps it should not seem so shocking that most people are at least mildly happy with their lives. Some researchers argue that a disposition toward pleasant affect facilitates exploratory behavior, which could have conferred evolutionary advantages (E. Diener & C. Diener, 1996; Fredrickson, 1998; Ito & Cacioppo, 1999). According to Ito and Cacioppo (1999), the motivational system is slightly biased toward approach behavior, even in the absence of stimuli – a phenomenon called "positivity offset." Such a bias would be more advantageous than a purely neutral disposition because, in the absence of danger, it would help humans learn more about their environment. As a consequence of broadening behavioral and attentional foci, positive emotions might also have helped humans to build social relationships and other resources important for survival (Fredrickson, 1998). The connection between pleasant affect and approach tendencies receives some support from a 27-nation study by Wallbott and Scherer (1988). With few cultural differences, participants reported that "moving toward" was an action tendency most characteristic of joy, whereas "withdrawing" was more typical of unpleasant emotions.

In light of the above research, it becomes important to ask when and why a society falls below the midpoint of SWB. One trend that has been observed is that people living in severe destitution often report being unhappy. Prostitutes and home-less people living in Calcutta, India, reported negative levels of LS (Biswas-Diener & Diener, 2001). The LS of Malaysian farmers living below the poverty line also fell below the midpoint (Howell, Howell, & Schwabe, 2006). Difficulty in meeting basic needs, or other circumstances such as lack of respect, might have decreased the well-being of these groups. In the next section, we consider how economic factors might influence the SWB of a society.

Economic Development and Related Variables

The wealth of a nation frequently correlates with its level of SWB. Depending on whether one looks at purchasing power or per capita gross domestic product, the correlation between economic wealth and the SWB of a nation ranges from 0.58 to 0.84 (E. Diener, M. Diener, & C. Diener, 1995; Inglehart & Klingemann, 2000; Veenhoven, 1991). As robust as this finding is, the exact process by which economic development increases happiness remains unclear.

Wealthier societies are better able to meet the basic needs of their citizens and this contributes to SWB (E. Diener & M. Diener, et al., 1995). We will consider the role of basic need fulfillment in a later section. For now, it is also worth noting that economic development is often associated with many other social conditions. For example, wealth correlates with greater human rights, as well as greater equality (in income, access to education, and between the sexes; E. Diener & M. Diener, et al., 1995). Rights and equality also correlate with each other. Further still, people in wealthier nations are often more satisfied with friends and home life (Diener & Suh, 1999). A possible explanation proposed by Ahuvia (2002) is that rising wealth alters the cultural environment by freeing the individual from economic dependence on his or her family. This independence could attenuate norms for reciprocity while facil-itating the pursuit of individual happiness (e.g., by allowing more choice in friends and lifestyle). Thus, several mechanisms are possible and the various correlates of wealth make it difficult to isolate the unique contribution of wealth to SWB. The relation between economic development and SWB is thus entangled in a causal web of several factors, and future researchers need to separate their causal influences on SWB.

Aside from economic development, Inglehart and Klingemann (2000) suggested that national levels of SWB might also reflect historical factors. In 1997, the former communist states of Eastern Europe and the U.S.S.R. had among the lowest levels of well-being—lower than nations with less wealth, but without a history of com-munism. Even after controlling for wealth, rights, and other variables, the number of years under communist rule negatively predicted a nation's mean level of SWB. However, Inglehart and Klingemann (2000) warn against hasty praise for capitalistic or democratic societies. Although the collapse of communism in the Soviet Union was preceded by relatively low levels of SWB, it was followed by *even lower* levels of SWB (see also Veenhoven, 2001). Political instability and economic decline after the fall of communism may have created conditions that were inimical to SWB. These ideas require further research, especially as conditions change in the region.

Norms for Emotions

As mentioned earlier, the experience of well-being can be shaped by cultural norms regarding the desirability of LS or certain emotions (M.L. Diener et al., 2004; Suh et al., 1998). Emotions that are desirable might be experienced more frequently than those that are seen as inappropriate (M.L. Diener et al., 2004) or they may correlate more with general happiness (Markus & Kitayama, 1994). Norms for emotions may explain why Asian—especially East Asian—samples often report lower SWB than those from Europe and the Americas (E. Diener & M. Diener, 1995; Kang, Shaver, Sue, Min, & Jing, 2003; Sheldon et al., 2004; Suh, 2002). Economic development may be a factor, but it cannot completely account for the lower SWB of East Asians. For example, Japan has greater purchasing power than many Latin American nations (E. Diener, M. Diener, et al., 1995), yet it reports lower SWB than do the latter (Diener & Suh, 1999; Diener & Oishi, 2000). This could be because Japanese and other Asians show a greater acceptance of unpleasant emotions than people in the Americas (Diener & Suh, 1999). Moreover, East Asians may also value low activation positive affect (e.g., serene) more than high activation positive affect (e.g., excited) because these emotions facilitate collectivist goals of attending to the social context (Tsai et al., 2006).

How might emotion norms translate into experience? One pathway is through the socialization of emotions in children (M.L. Diener & Lucas, 2004), through the willingness to report specific emotions, or through recall of which emotions are experienced (Oishi, 2002). Wirtz (2004) asked participants to report how they felt about past events, both currently and at the time of the event. Whether the emotions were pleasant or unpleasant, Japanese participants' current feelings were less intense than they were remembered to be in the past. In contrast, European Americans reported significant decay for unpleasant but not pleasant emotions. Thus, cultural norms might also shape the relation between recalled emotions and current feelings, which might also influence judgments about current LS.

Schimmack, Oishi, and Diener (2002) suggested that East Asian views of pleasant and unpleasant emotions might be rooted in the dialecticism of Asian philosophies (e.g., Buddhism and Daoism) that have historically shaped these cultures. For example, in Chinese folk wisdom, both sides of a contradiction are equally likely, and a compromise between the two is preferable (Peng & Nisbett, 1999). East Asian emotion norms may be dialectical in the sense that a middle way between extreme pleasant and extreme unpleasant affect is considered desirable. In contrast, many Western European and Latin American cultures prefer pleasant over unpleasant affect. These cultural differences are reflected in emotion reports. Among participants from Western Europe and the Americas, the frequency of pleasant affect was inversely related to the frequency of unpleasant affect (Schimmack et al., 2002). Among Asian participants, however, this negative correlation was weak (see also Bagozzi, Wong, & Yi, 1999). Kitayama et al. (2000) actually observed a *positive* correlation between pleasant and unpleasant affect in Japan. Finally, over a one-week period of experience sampling, Scollon et al. (2004) found that European- and Hispanic Americans experienced more pleasant affect than Asians and Asian Americans. Moreover, there were no differences in unpleasant emotions. Asians and

Asian Americans did not experience as much pleasant affect as the other groups, but they were not biased in the direction of greater unpleasant affect either.

Are East Asians simply unhappy at worst and apathetic at best? Caution must be taken not to equate lower levels of well-being as *ill-being*. First, the SWB of East Asians is lower *in comparison to* Latin Americans and Western Europeans. Although mean levels of SWB are often lower among Asian samples, they are rarely below the neutral midpoint. Second, Kitayama and Markus (2000) note that balance and moderation are central to East Asian concepts of health. A preference for low rather than high activation positive affect may be consistent with this perspective (Tsai et al., 2006).

Another source of cultural variation in emotion norms may be religious doctrine. Across 40 nations, Kim-Prieto and Diener (2004) found that Christians reported a greater frequency of happiness and less shame than Muslims, even after controlling for the effect of nations. A subsequent analysis of the emotion content of religious texts revealed that joy and love were most frequently mentioned in the New Testament whereas shame and guilt were most frequently mentioned in the Quran. Thus, differences in norms or the socialization of emotions may be rooted in religious doctrine. An important implication of these findings is that the cultural forces that impinge on SWB may extend beyond ethnic and geographic delineations.

Genetic Differences

Might cultural differences in well-being be due to genetic differences between groups? Although much more research is needed, some individual differences in SWB may be related to genetics. Polymorphisms in the serotonin-related 5-HTT gene have been linked to individual differences in anxiety (Lesch et al., 1996), as well as susceptibility to depression (Caspi et al., 2003). Lykken and Tellegen (1996) maintain that roughly half of the individual variance in SWB is related to genetic variation.

A limitation of the above research is that it has been carried out within single societies, and effects *within* a sample may not necessarily be driven by the same causal forces as those *between* samples. Although there are ethnic and cultural differences in gene frequencies (Cavalli-Sforza, 1991), direct links between such differences and SWB have not yet been made. However, studies of infant temperament reinforce the possibility of genetic effects. Freedman and Freedman (1969) found ethnic differences in infants less than four days old. Compared to European American infants, Chinese American infants were calmer and less reactive to a cloth placed on their face. Similarly, four-month old infants in China exhibited less behavioral arousal than European American and Irish infants (Kagan et al., 1994). Nevertheless, the role of socialization practices cannot be overlooked. In contrast to the above findings, Ahadi, Rothbart, and Ye (1993) found that six-year old Chinese children exhibited relatively more negative affectivity than their European American peers. The authors suggested that strict Chinese socialization practices might foster a greater sensitivity to punishment, leading to more frequent negative affect. Thus, genetic influences do not rule out the impact that life circumstances can have on the various components of SWB. Recently, Diener and colleagues (Diener, Lucas, & Scollon, 2005; Fujita & Diener, 2005) argued for a "soft set point" conception of SWB. People can adapt to many situations and genes may account for some of the stability in SWB. However, life events and social conditions (e.g., widowhood or poverty) can still have a substantial impact on happiness at both, the individual and group levels. Much more research on culture, genetics, and SWB is required before firm conclusions can be made.

Conclusion

In many societies, a majority of the people report being happy, but very few report extreme happiness. Although there are biological and evolutionary accounts for why this is so, other factors are likely to influence mean levels of well-being. These factors include economic development and cultural norms for emotions. However, much more research is needed before we can understand exactly how and why societal levels of SWB differ across cultures. Specifically, the exact process underlying the relation between economic development and SWB remains unclear, as well as how such development affects cultural values related to well-being.

Correlates and Causes of SWB

Not only might cultures differ in the experience of emotions and their frequency, they might also differ in the causes of SWB. Often the evidence is in terms of cross-sectional correlations, however, and so we mostly review what covaries with pleasant and unpleasant affect, and LS in different cultures. Further, Kitayama and Markus (2000) suggested that SWB is not just personal happiness, but includes one's relations with others. Thus, happiness might take different forms across cultures, with different factors causing it.

The Self and SWB

To the extent that self-concepts vary across cultures (Markus & Kitayama, 1991), one might expect the relation between self and SWB to vary as well. For instance, although self-esteem is often a strong correlate of LS, Heine et al. (1999) questioned the need for positive self-views in collectivist cultures. In Japan, where interdependence is emphasized, a self-critical tendency may be valued as a way of improving one's ability to meet social obligations (but see Brown & Kobayashi, 2002, 2003, for evidence of self-enhancement in Japan, and Heine's, 2003 response). Miller, Wang, Sandel, and Cho (2002) found that rural Taiwanese mothers also placed little emphasis on developing their children's self-esteem and some worried that high self-esteem would impair their child's capacity to take criticism. Thus, in collectivist cultures, self-esteem may be viewed as unimportant, or even *undesirable* for achieving cultural goals. In contrast, a primary concern for European American mothers was to help their children develop and maintain a strong sense of self-esteem (Miller et al., 2002).

If high self-esteem is de-emphasized in collectivist cultures, then one might expect self-esteem to relate less strongly to LS than it would in more individualist cultures. This is exactly what a number of researchers have found (E. Diener & M. Diener, 1995; Oishi, Diener, Lucas & Suh, 1999; Park & Huebner, 2005). Although self-esteem correlated with LS across most countries, the strength of association could be predicted by the individualism of a country. For example, self-esteem and LS correlated 0.60 in the U.S., but only 0.08 among women in more collectivist India (E. Diener & M. Diener, 1995). Similarly, Park and Huebner (2005) found that satisfaction with self was a much stronger predictor of LS for U.S. adolescents than it was for Korean adolescents. As with emotions (Suh et al., 1998), people in collectivist cultures may be guided by norms downplaying the importance of self-esteem when they make life satisfaction judgments. Alternatively, people with high self-esteem may be frowned upon in collectivist cultures for holding or expressing attitudes that violate norms. Of course, norms should also influence the factors that *do* correlate with LS. For example, Park and Huebner suggested that the heavy emphasis on academic achievement in Korea might explain why school satisfaction predicted LS for Korean adolescents but not for American adolescents.

Another characteristic that may be less socially valued in collectivist cultures and less important for SWB is identity consistency. In traditional Western psychology, self-consistency across situations implies a coherent self-identity and good mental health. However, in East Asian cultures, where individuals are expected to adjust themselves to the social situation, identity consistency might be taken as a sign of immaturity. Suh (2002) found that Americans evinced greater consistency across social roles than Koreans. For example, if Americans were talkative with their friends, they were also more likely to be talkative with parents, siblings, and strangers than were Koreans. Furthermore, identity consistency was a much stronger predictor of SWB for Americans than Koreans. Not only were self-consistent individuals happier in the American sample, but they were also rated by informants as more likable and socially skilled than less consistent individuals. In contrast, Korean informants showed no such preference for consistent targets (Suh, 2002).

Culture may also affect the relation between personality and LS. On the one hand, research suggests that the influence of personality on emotional experience may be pancultural (Lucas, Diener, Grob, Suh, & Shao, 2000; Tsai et al., 2006). In five countries, Schimmack et al. (2002) found that extraversion correlated positively with affect balance, whereas neuroticism was negatively correlated. Moreover, the relation between personality and LS was mediated by affect balance. Thus, extraverts enjoy greater LS in part because they experience frequent pleasant affect. However, because the relation between *emotions* and LS was stronger in individualist cultures (see Patterning and Structure), the relation between personality and LS was also moderated by culture. Thus, extraversion and neuroticism were more predictive of LS in individualist cultures (Germany and the U.S.) than in collectivist cultures (Ghana, Japan, Mexico). Extraverts everywhere may experience more pleasant affect than neurotics, but how much this contributes to LS may depend on the cultural value of emotional experience. Alternatively, Benet-Martínez and Karakitapoglu-Aygun (2003) proposed that cultures favor the development of some personality traits over others. They found that individualism predicted both extraversion and neuroticism, and that the relationship between personality and LS was mediated by self-esteem and friendship satisfaction.

An important issue concerns the role of autonomy in SWB. Self-determination theorists (SDT; Deci & Ryan, 1985; Ryan & Deci, 2000) contend that autonomy is a basic human need that, if not fulfilled, will lead to lower levels of well-being. One source of the debate may be the very definition of autonomy. For example, Oishi (2000) operationalized autonomy as horizontal individualism (i.e., an emphasis on independence and individual self-worth). He found that the positive association between autonomy and LS was stronger in more individualist nations like Australia and Denmark, than it was in more collectivist nations like China, Korea, and Bahrain. However, Chirkov, Ryan, Kim, and Kaplan (2003) argued that the construct of autonomy must be distinguished from independence and individualism (see also Ryan & Deci, 2000). In the framework of SDT, autonomy is the sense that one has willingly engaged in and fully endorses an act. Individuals may be dependent on others and still experience autonomy if they find value in that dependence and engage in it of their own volition. What is of importance is the *internalization* of the values that one is exercising. Thus, although Koreans viewed their culture as more collectivist and less individualist than Americans viewed their own culture, the internalization of *both* types of values predicted SWB in both countries, as well as in Russia and Turkey (Chirkov et al., 2003). Using a similar definition of autonomy, Sheldon et al. (2004) found that self-concordant individuals (i.e., those who pursued goals they perceived as freely chosen) tended to report higher levels of SWB in the U.S., South Korea, Taiwan, and China. Thus, autonomy as independence is not universal, whereas autonomy as feeling that one's behavior is freely chosen and not coerced may be universal.

These views are not contrary to the goal-as-moderator model advanced by Oishi (2000). This model posits that the relation between culture and SWB is moderated by personal goals. Culture may influence one's goals, but individuals do not always pursue culturally endorsed goals. For example, a Chinese student who values personal success may be happier studying alone than offering help to his fellow classmates, although the latter better reflects the cultural goal of interdependence. However, although attaining personal goals may bring emotional well-being, it may not always yield a sense of meaning in life. Ideally, personal goals that are aligned with cultural values lead to both happiness and meaning (Oishi, 2000). Thus, the role of personal goals is similar to the importance of internalization proposed by self-determination theory. Thus, although independence of others might not predict happiness equally across cultures, acting from one's volition is predicted by both self-determination and Oishi's theory to lead to happiness universally.

Both perspectives suggest that the distinction between personal and collective goals may often be blurred. For example, the SWB of Asians and Asian Americans is better predicted by satisfaction with goals involving family and friends than with goals concerned mainly with the self (Oishi & Diener, 2001; Radhakrishnan & Chan, 1997). However, among collectivist cultures, the goals of one's group may also be experienced as one's own (Markus & Kitayama, 1994), making them both collective and personal. In contrast, only personal goals were predictive of European American's SWB (Oishi & Diener, 2001; Radhakrishnan & Chan, 1997). Taken together, the findings suggest that there may be motives that correlate universally with well-being, and other motives or goals that are culture-specific correlates of well-being.

Relationships with Others and SWB

The above research implies that social relationships may influence SWB differently across cultures. For instance, although emotional experience is often considered private and internal, Kitayama and Markus (2000) suggested that the Japanese may experience good feelings *intersubjectively*, as features of an interpersonal situation that dissipate once the individual is out of that context. Consistent with this idea, Oishi, Diener, Scollon, and Biswas-Diener (2003) found that Japanese reported less pleasant affect when alone than did Americans. Further, although both groups experienced more pleasant affect when with friends than when alone, the effect was greater for the Japanese (as well as for Hispanic Americans; Oishi et al., 2003).

In general, East Asians may be more other-focused in their emotional experience than North Americans (Cohen & Gunz, 2002; Kitayama, Markus, & Kurokawa, 2000). Kitayama et al. (2000) compared how *engaged* (relationship focused) and *disengaged* (self focused) emotions relate to general good feelings (e.g., happiness) among Japanese and American participants. For Japanese, positive engaged emotions (e.g., friendly feelings) correlated more strongly with general good feelings than did positive disengaged emotions (e.g., pride). The reverse was true for American participants. However, a recent priming study by No and Hong (2004) suggests that the influence of culture on emotional experience is dynamic. Compared to baseline, Korean American biculturals who were primed with Korean cultural icons became more relational and less egocentric in their projection of emotions onto others. Similar effects may be observed in the experience of SWB. That is, what makes an individual happy may shift as the salience of cultural frames shifts, as when living in another culture for an extended period of time.

The relative importance of relationships across cultures also influences LS. Among Hong Kong Chinese, for example, relationship harmony was just as important as self-esteem in predicting LS (Kwan, Bond, & Singelis, 1997). In contrast, self-esteem was a stronger predictor of LS for Americans. Interestingly, relationship quality may have both, direct and indirect effects on LS. Kang et al. (2003) not only replicated Kwan et al.'s (1997) findings in the U.S., Korea, and mainland China, but they also showed that relationship quality was positively associated with self-esteem in the latter two groups. Relationship quality was also predictive of Asian Americans' self-esteem, but *not* of European Americans' self-esteem (Kang et al., 2003).

A relationship of particular relevance to SWB is marriage. Across 42 societies, married people reported more pleasant and less unpleasant affect than the divorced (Diener, Gohm, Suh, & Oishi, 2000). However, small cultural effects were observed. Divorce seems to reduce pleasant affect to a lesser extent in collectivist than in individualist cultures. Gohm, Oishi, Darlington, and Diener (1998) also found that in collectivist cultures, the offspring of divorced parents reported greater LS than those whose parents remained in high-conflict marriages. These groups did not differ in individualist cultures. Both findings could be related to greater social support in collectivist cultures, which would help sustain well-being after divorce. Alternatively, the pressure to stay together may be greater in these societies so that couples divorce only after severe marital conflict. In this case, the decision to divorce might offer greater relief to spouses and their offspring. More research is needed to test these hypotheses.

Income and SWB

According to Veenhoven (1991), income contributes to SWB only insofar as it allows one to fulfill basic needs. Beyond the level needed to satisfy physical needs, income has less of an impact on SWB. Veenhoven's theory resembles Maslow's (1954), which posits that lower order needs (e.g., physical and security needs) must be gratified before higher order needs (i.e., belongingness, esteem, and self-actualization) become salient. However, some scholars have questioned whether the fulfillment of needs follows a linear hierarchy (Yang, 2003). Moreover, diminishing returns on the effects of material goods do not always imply that higher order needs have been prioritized. An implication drawn from both theories, however, is that income has a greater impact on SWB in poor societies because physical needs like having adequate food, water and housing are highly salient, and the effects of income on meeting these needs are direct. Indeed, researchers have found that financial satisfaction predicts LS more strongly in poorer than in wealthier countries (E. Diener & M. Diener, 1995; Oishi et al., 1999).

Although the relation between income and happiness is reduced among the wealthier nations, it is worth noting that income still contributes to SWB *beyond* the basic subsistence level (E. Diener, M. Diener, et al., 1995; E. Diener, Sandvik, Seidlitz, & M. Diener, 1993). Perhaps greater amounts of income facilitate the pursuit of other goals (e.g., relationships or philanthropy) that add to one's level of SWB, though little is known about *how* money is spent across cultures.

Although Maslow's needs hierarchy provides some understanding of the link between income and SWB, it is important to consider recent revisions of and critiques on the cross-cultural applicability of this model. Yang (2003) argued that Maslow's higher order needs (belongingness, esteem, and self-actualization) were framed within an individualist context. He suggested that in collectivist societies, these needs are framed in ways that reaffirm social relationships and group identity. Moreover, he proposed (after Yu, 1992; cited in Yang, 2003) that bearing and rearing children be considered needs that were present in all societies because they ensured the transmission of genes to the next generation. Unlike the strictly hierarchical nature of Maslow's model, Yang suggested that needs can be experienced and fulfilled simultaneously. For example, raising children may fulfill both belongingness and esteem needs. Furthermore, individuals may emphasize or de-emphasize transmission needs throughout the life course. The relative importance of child rearing versus esteem needs might also differ across cultures, and the role that income plays in satisfying these needs could likewise vary.

Conclusion

A number of correlates of SWB are strikingly different across cultures, and yet some correlates appear to be universal. Variations in the cognitive and affective experience of happiness correspond with cultural differences in self-definition and the importance of social relationships. Income also contributes to SWB, though the relation is stronger among poorer than wealthier societies. Thus cultural psychological differences are not only rooted in values, but in the material world as well. However, because culture is dynamic, what makes people happy may change across generations, as well as within the individual as different aspects of a culture become salient. Nevertheless, there may be some universal correlates of SWB even in the face of cultural variations, such as autonomous internalization of cultural values.

Outcomes of SWB

Research on SWB has traditionally been a search for the who, what, and how of happiness. That is, who is happy, what makes people happy, and how the various components of happiness relate to each other. Because happiness has historically been thought of as an end in itself, these were the first questions to be asked, and the field of SWB advanced greatly as these issues began to be studied more rigorously. However, the question of *why* happiness is important has only recently come under more serious attention.

Lyubomirsky, King, and Diener (2005) proposed that although success may produce happiness, it may also be the case that happiness leads to success. They reviewed several experimental and longitudinal studies suggesting that many outcomes of pleasant affect are desirable (e.g., prosocial behavior, self-esteem, likeability, creativity, and longevity). These characteristics, in turn, lead to success in many life domains such as marriage, work, and health. The framework developed by Lyubomirsky et al. is an intriguing area that requires much more research. Not only does the direction of causality await further clarification in some domains, but the benefits and *costs* of pleasant affect must be investigated in a wider range of cultures.

The studies reviewed by Lyubomirsky et al. were conducted primarily in North America, Europe, and Australia. Whether or not pleasant affect is similarly beneficial in, for example, East Asia is certainly open for analyses. Would pleasant emotions produce similar outcomes in Japan where self-criticism and self-improvement are seen as important for success (Heine et al., 1999)? Heine et al. (2001) observed that North Americans were more likely to persist on a task after receiving success feedback, whereas Japanese were motivated to persist if they received failure feedback. The facilitative effect of pleasant affect among Westerners may be related to the general desirability of these emotions in their cultures (Eid & Diener, 2001). However, East Asian cultures do not devalue all pleasant emotions (e.g., Tsai et al., 2006). An important topic for future investigations is whether specific pleasant emotions are beneficial whereas others (e.g., pride; Eid & Diener, 2001; Scollon et al., 2004) are detrimental for success in certain cultures.

At a societal level, Inglehart and Klingemann (2000) suggested that rising levels of SWB might help legitimize and stabilize newly formed governments. They point out that major political changes in Belgium and the former U.S.S.R. in the early 1990s were *preceded* by decreasing levels of SWB. Furthermore, although many democratic societies had high levels of well-being, democracy did not predict SWB after controlling for GNP (Inglehart & Klingemann, 2000). Thus democratic institutions may increase SWB through rising wealth, but greater SWB might also help to sustain these institutions. These propositions are preliminary and more research is required to understand the causal process. Measuring national levels of SWB consistently and over a broad period of time could shed light on how fluctuations in well-being relate to sociopolitical developments.

Methodological Issues

A critical question is whether measures of SWB are valid and reliable across cultures. Even within cultures, Schwarz and Strack (1999) pointed out several potential threats to the validity of self-reported SWB. They warned that self-reports are vulnerable to contextual factors (e.g., question wording and order effects) that can change the standards by which people evaluate their lives. However, Schimmack, Oishi and their colleagues (Schimmack, Diener, & Oishi, 2002; Oishi, Schimmack, & Colcombe, 2003) showed that the information that people use to make life satisfaction judgments is largely systematic and personally relevant. Thus, although self-reports of SWB may be open to momentary influences, more often than not, they convey meaningful information about an individual's evaluation of his or her life.

Nevertheless, there are additional challenges when SWB research is conducted across cultures. A basic issue is the adequate translation of written materials. Poor translations could alter the intended meaning of SWB measures, leading to spurious cultural differences. A number of studies, however, suggest that translation effects are unlikely to explain the substantial cultural differences that have been observed. For example, bilingual Chinese reported lower life satisfaction than bilingual European Americans, whether they completed the SWLS in Chinese or in English (Shao, 1993). Similarly, M.L. Diener et al. (2004) gathered reports of emotional experience from multiple locations in China, Singapore, and India. Within the same country, some subsamples completed the survey in the local language, whereas others completed an English version. Results indicated that subsamples *within* a nation were more similar in emotional experience, regardless of the language that was used. Cultural differences obtained with translated measures of SWB have also been substantiated by *non*-self-report measures (Balatsky & Diener, 1993; Biswas-Diener et al., 2005). For instance, not only did Russians report lower SWB than Americans, they also recalled proportionately less positive events than did the latter (Balatsky & Diener, 1993).

Another issue is whether the use of numbers, or unfamiliarity with Likert scales could affect findings. In the slums of Calcutta, Biswas-Diener and Diener (2001) supplemented their seven-point Likert scales with a gradient of frowning and smiling faces. Some respondents were still confused by the task, forcing the researchers to reduce their measures to a three-point scale. Despite these initial difficulties, they obtained an alpha of 0.80 for the SWLS. Still, when conducting research in certain cultures, the novelty of psychological testing can result in lower reliabilities (e.g., Biswas-Diener et al., 2005). Moreover, the reliability of the SWLS was found to correlate positively with the GNP of a nation (Vitterso et al., 2002). Higher reliabilities do not completely account for the greater LS found in wealthier nations, but they do appear to influence results and may be due to greater familiarity with psychological testing in those countries. Nevertheless, measures of life satisfaction and happiness are predictive of social integration and elderly suicide rates across nations (Wu & Bond, 2006), providing some evidence that these measures are capturing important aspects of people's life experiences.

Different response styles have occasionally been proposed as an explanation for cultural differences in well-being, especially with regard to the lower SWB found among Asian samples. One hypothesis is that due to humility norms, Asian respondents tend toward neutrality by over-selecting responses at the midpoint of the scale. Diener, Suh, Smith, and Shao (1995) examined this possibility among Chinese, Japanese, Korean, and American samples, but did not find such a tendency. East Asians showed as much variation as Americans in their satisfaction with various domains. The former even reported a greater range of emotional intensity than the latter. Similarly, Veenhoven (2001) showed that negative response tendencies were unlikely to explain the lower levels of SWB among Russians. Interestingly, the lower scores on SWB run counter to the finding that acquiescence bias (the tendency to respond in agreement with items) tends to be higher in collectivistic nations (Johnson, Kulesa, Cho, & Shavitt, 2005; Smith, 2004). If acquiescence influenced responses on SWB measures, one would expect to see higher means in East Asia, but this is clearly not the case.

On the other hand, social desirability may underlie some differences in reported SWB. In cultures where LS and pleasant affect are considered desirable, there may be a tendency to project higher SWB. People in some cultures appear to have a "positivity bias" in which satisfaction with global domains (e.g., education) are high even though satisfaction with more specific domains (e.g., textbooks, professors, and lectures) are *lower* on average (Diener, Scollon, Oishi, Dzokoto, & Suh, 2000). Diener et al. (2000) found that this positivity bias predicted LS beyond objective measures like income, and that it correlated positively with norms for LS. This finding may explain the discrepant relation between wealth and happiness in Japan and Latin America. Latin Americans exhibited high desirability for LS, as well as a strong positivity bias. In contrast, Japan and other East Asians reported lower desirability for LS and a corresponding *negativity* bias, such that global satisfaction was lower than would be expected from specific domain satisfactions (Diener et al., 2000). These biases could be considered artifacts, but they may also represent interesting cultural phenomena in and of themselves. Furthermore, it is worth reiterating that cultural differences in satisfaction judgments and emotional experience have been observed using other methodologies. For instance, a one-week daily diary study showed that European Americans' global past-week satisfaction was more positive than their average satisfaction for *each day* of that week (Oishi, 2002). In contrast, Asian American participants did not exhibit a significant bias in global versus daily satisfaction ratings. Similarly, Kim-Prieto (2005) found that European-Americans and Asians were similar in happiness reported "now," but that Asians reporting feeling less during the past year and "in general." Finally, the recall of *pleasant* but not unpleasant emotions during a vacation predicted the desire of European Americans to repeat the trip, whereas for Asian Americans the reverse was true (Wirtz, 2004). Interestingly, experience-sampling data revealed that the two groups did not differ in their *online* experience of pleasant and unpleasant emotions. Thus, the global judgment and not the specific reports influenced participants' decisions. Instead of dismissing global judgments altogether, Diener et al. (2000) suggested that global and domain-specific judgments are both distinctly informative aspects of SWB. Nevertheless, cross-cultural researchers should continue to use multiple methods (e.g., memory measures, informant reports, etc.), whenever possible.

Perhaps a fundamental concern is whether it is appropriate to use nations as a proxy for studying culture. Researchers often define groups by their countries of origin and attribute any differences among these groups to culture. However, culture is not necessarily confined to geopolitical boundaries (Hermans & Kempen, 1998; Hong & Chiu, 2001). By equating entire nations with single cultures, we risk overlooking important differences within nations, as well as similarities that extend beyond national borders. In the case of emotion norms, many different norm patterns for pleasant and unpleasant affect may co-exist within a nation (Eid & Diener, 2001). At the same time, however, nations within a certain *region* (e.g., East Asia or Latin America) appear to have similar patterns of emotional experience (M.L. Diener et al., 2004).

It is not entirely meaningless to group samples by nation. People living within a country are likely to have shared experiences and common histories, which are crucial in the formation of a common culture. Still, cultural entities may be defined at different levels, in any number of ways. It is important to realize the tradeoffs inherent at a given level of analysis. Speaking of "regional cultures" allows us to make generalizations, but at the sacrifice of specificity. A focus on subcultural grouping may provide rich, nuanced data, but at the cost of generalizability. A further point is that culture is dynamic. The penetration of Western media and popular culture into other parts of the world can stimulate cultural change, leading to generational differences within nations. Thus, different age groups within a nation might differ in their attitudes and experience of SWB. More longitudinal research is needed to disentangle cohort effects from developmental effects.

Finally, group differences in SWB might be related to socioeconomic status (SES), not just cultural beliefs and values per se. Income and education levels can determine the quality of life for people in a society, which in turn could lower or raise SWB. However, SES may sometimes be confounded with cultural groupings, especially when a history of discrimination has prevented certain groups from attaining higher status (Betancourt & López, 1993). Apart from discrimination, people from high versus low SES groups may face different realities and prioritize different values and beliefs (e.g., Snibbe & Markus, 2005). In either case, controlling for SES would result in a removal of cultural effects as well. Thus, separating SES from culture may not always be a straightforward task. On the other hand, cultural effects that persist even after controlling for socioeconomic variables pose interesting questions for future research and theory (see Rice & Steele, 2004) concerning the nature of culture and how it should be operationalized.

Future Directions

Although cultural variations in SWB have been replicated across self-report and memory measures, an important agenda for future research is to determine the extent to which these differences are reflected in the actual experience of well-being. More frequent applications of the experience sampling method across cultures will provide further clarification of such differences. In one of the few such studies, Scollon et al. (2004) found that cultural differences in reports of past emotional experience do have some basis in on-line experience, but they also reflect aspects of the self-concept that independently influence the recall of emotions. These findings are provocative, but must be replicated across more cultures. Other methods of assessing SWB, such as Kim's (2004) implicit association measure of life satisfaction, have only recently been developed and could provide further insights. Also critical will be the further development and integration of biological markers of well-being. For example, a predisposition toward positive affectivity has been linked to individual differences in chronic left brain activation (Ito & Cacioppo, 1999). The immune system and neurotransmitter systems (e.g., serotonin and dopamine) may also play a role in well-being. These and other types of measures will help us know whether differences in SWB lie in actual experience or in self-reports.

There is also a continuing need for theory on the functioning of SWB in culture— how it is defined in each culture, how it supports culture, and the types of outcomes associated with SWB in various societies. SWB is an important criterion for evaluating the success of a society, but by itself is insufficient. To just be happy in the face of starvation or inequality would seem preposterous to most people. Happiness and cultural conceptions of the good life are often tied to the sociomoral fabric of a society. As Markus and Kitayama (1994) suggested, being a competent member of one's culture typically "feels good" or "right." Thus, in some ways, LS may involve an implicit moral judgment on one's life, or on oneself as a person. Future studies of indigenous concepts of well-being, as well as the relation of SWB to the moral structures of a society will help researchers to further contextualize their interpretations of SWB.

Finally, viewing culture dynamically will enhance our understanding of cultural variation in SWB. Dynamic constructionists (e.g., Hong & Chiu, 2001) suggest that the influence of culture is not rigid and sweeping, but that it can fluctuate with the social context. Particularly among immigrants and other individuals who have been exposed to multiple cultures, *which* culture is influential may depend on cues in the environment (e.g., at home versus at school) that activate different sets of cultural knowledge. An intriguing issue is how such cultural frame-switching might mediate or moderate the relation between LS and correlates such as self-esteem. How bicultural individuals feel about and integrate their cultural identities (Haritatos & Benet-Martínez, 2002; Kim, B.R. Sarason, & I.G. Sarason, 2006) might also influence their well-being as they navigate between different cultural contexts. A related topic is how the causes of SWB change across the life span, or across different cohorts within the same culture. Thus, dynamic cultural perspectives contribute to a more fluid notion of SWB, raising new questions about the structure of well-being and its outcomes.

Conclusions

We have learned that comparisons of well-being are possible for some variables, and that there are probably some universal causes of well-being and ill-being. At the same time, we have learned that there are fascinating differences between cultures in the patterning and content of SWB variables, as well as in the causes and correlates of SWB. These differences should guide us in our attempts to make valid comparisons. For instance, some emotions may be understood similarly across cultures, whereas others have different connotative meanings. Direct comparisons, then, should be made with the former and not the latter. Even where SWB components are different, cultures could be compared according to their own criteria by measuring the attainment of culturally valued goals and experiences. Such an approach to well-being still allows success to be assessed in different cultural contexts.

The effect size of culture can vary depending on the specific component of SWB under study. Cultures perhaps vary more in frequency and perceived norms for pleasant emotions than for unpleasant emotions (Eid & Diener, 2001; Scollon et al., 2004). In the case of unpleasant emotions, there is a stronger trend toward much larger differences within than between cultures. The uneven effects of culture on

SWB not only resonate with dynamic views of culture, but they also call for circumspection in the type of inferences we draw from societal levels of SWB.

Much has been learned in the past decade of research in culture and SWB. Researchers began by making simple comparisons of nations on life satisfaction and happiness. Next they began to ask questions about the validity of measures across cultures, and about the causes and correlates of SWB in different societies. The field continues to advance with more sharply focused research questions concerning *when* cultural influences come into play, *which* aspects of well-being are affected, and *what* the outcomes of SWB are across cultures. We are also entering an era in which research will treat culture as more dynamic, and individuals as bearers of more than one cultural tradition. These issues will continue to require multimeasure strategies, and hopefully stimulate the development of new methodologies. In this regard, progress in the various areas of cultural psychology and SWB, as well as more interdisciplinary work with the other social and biological sciences will benefit both perspectives greatly.

Acknowledgments We would like to thank Sumie Okazaki for her helpful and insightful comments on an earlier draft of this paper. This work was supported by a National Science Foundation Graduate Fellowship awarded to William Tov.

References

Ahadi, S. A., Rothbart, M. K., & Ye, R. (1993). Children's temperament in the US and China: Similarities and differences. *European Journal of Personality, 7*, 359–377.

Ahuvia, A. C. (2002). Individualism/collectivism and cultures of happiness: A theoretical conjecture on the relationship between consumption, culture and subjective well-being at the national level. *Journal of Happiness Studies, 3*, 23–36.

Bagozzi, R. P., Wong, N., & Yi, Y. (1999). The role of culture and gender in the relationship between positive and negative affect. *Cognition and Emotion, 13*, 641–672.

Balatsky, G., & Diener, E. (1993). Subjective well-being among Russian students. *Social Indicators Research, 28*, 225–243.

Benet-Martínez, V., & Karakitapoglu-Aygun, Z. (2003). The interplay of cultural syndromes and personality in predicting life satisfaction: Comparing Asian Americans and European Americans. *Journal of Cross-Cultural Psychology, 34*, 38–60.

Betancourt, H., & López, S. R. (1993). The study of culture, ethnicity, and race in American psychology. *American Psychologist, 48*, 629–637.

Biswas-Diener, R., & Diener, E. (2001). Making the best of a bad situation: Satisfaction in the slums of Calcutta. *Social Indicators Research, 55*, 329–352.

Biswas-Diener, R., Vittersø, J., & Diener, E. (2005). Most people are pretty happy, but there is cultural variation: The Inughuit, the Amish, and the Maasai. *Journal of Happiness Studies: An Interdisciplinary Periodical on Subjective Well-Being, 6*, 205–226.

Brown, J. D., & Kobayashi, C. (2002). Self-enhancement in Japan and America. *Asian Journal of Social Psychology, 5*, 145–168.

Brown, J. D., & Kobayashi, C. (2003). Motivation and manifestation: Cross-cultural expression of the self-enhancement motive. *Asian Journal of Social Psychology, 6*, 85–88.

Cantril, H. (1965). *The pattern of human concerns*. New Brunswick, NJ: Rutgers University Press.

Caspi, A., Sugden, K., Moffitt, T. E., Taylor, A., Craig, I. W., Harrington, H., et al. (2003). Influence of life stress on depression: Moderation by a polymorphism in the 5-HTT gene. *Science, 301*, 386–389.

Cavalli-Sforza, L. L. (1991). Genes, peoples, and languages. *Scientific American, 256*(5), 104–110.

Chirkov, V., Ryan, R. M., Kim, Y., & Kaplan, U. (2003). Differentiating autonomy from individualism and independence: A self-determination theory perspective on internalization of cultural orientations and well-being. *Journal of Personality and Social Psychology, 84*, 97–110.

Cohen, D., & Gunz, A. (2002). As seen by the other: Perspective on the self in the memories and emotional perceptions of Easterners and Westerners. *Psychological Science, 13*, 55–59.

Deci, E. L., & Ryan, R. M. (1985). *Intrinsic motivation and self-determination in human behavior.* New York: Plenum.

The Dhammapada: The sayings of the Buddha. (1976). (T. Byron, Trans.). New York: Random House.

Diener, E. (1984). Subjective well-being. *Psychological Bulletin, 95*, 542–575.

Diener, E., & Biswas-Diener, R. (2000). New directions in subjective well-being research: The cutting edge. *Indian Journal of Clinical Psychology, 27*, 21–33.

Diener, E., & Diener, M. (1995). Cross-cultural correlates of life satisfaction and self-esteem. *Journal of Personality and Social Psychology, 68*, 653–663.

Diener, E., & Diener, C. (1996). Most people are happy. *Psychological Science, 7*, 181–185.

Diener, E., Diener, M., & Diener, C. (1995). Factors predicting the subjective well-being of nations. *Journal of Personality and Social Psychology, 69*, 851–864.

Diener, E., Emmons, R. A., Larsen, R. J., & Griffin, S. (1985). The Satisfaction With Life Scale. *Journal of Personality Assessment, 49*, 71–75.

Diener, M. L., Fujita, F., Kim-Prieto, C., & Diener, E. (2004). Culture and emotional experience. *Manuscript submitted for publication.*

Diener, E., Gohm, C. L., Suh, E., & Oishi, S. (2000). Similarity of the relations between marital status and subjective well-being across cultures. *Journal of Cross-Cultural Psychology, 31*, 419–436.

Diener, E., Horwitz, J., & Emmons, R. (1985). Happiness of the very wealthy. *Social Indicators Research, 16*, 263–274.

Diener, M. L., & Lucas, R. E. (2004). Adult's desires for children's emotions across 48 countries: Associations with individual and national characteristics. *Journal of Cross-Cultural Psychology, 35*, 525–547.

Diener, E., Lucas, R., & Scollon, C. N. (2005). Beyond the hedonic treadmill: Revisions to the adaptation theory of well-being. *Manuscript submitted for publication.*

Diener, E. & Oishi, S. (2000). Money and happiness. In E. Diener and E. M. Suh (Eds.), *Culture and subjective well-being* (pp. 185–218). Cambridge, MA: MIT Press.

Diener, E., Sandvik, E., Seidlitz, L., & Diener, M. (1993). The relationship between income and subjective well-being: Relative or absolute? *Social Indicators Research, 28*, 195–223.

Diener, E., Scollon, C. K. N., Oishi, S., Dzokoto, V., & Suh, E. M. (2000). Positivity and the construction of life satisfaction judgments: Global happiness is not the sum of its parts. *Journal of Happiness Studies, 1*, 159–176.

Diener, E., & Seligman, M. E. P. (2004). Beyond money: Toward an economy of well-being. *Psychological Science in the Public Interest, 5*, 1–31.

Diener, E., & Suh, E. M. (1999). National differences in subjective well-being. In D. Kahneman, E. Diener, & N. Schwarz (Eds.), *Well-being: The foundations of hedonic psychology* (pp. 434–450). New York: Russell Sage Foundation.

Diener, E., Suh, E. M., Smith, H., & Shao, L. (1995). National differences in reported subjective well-being: Why do they occur? *Social Indicators Research, 34*, 7–32.

Edgerton, R. B. (1992). *Sick societies: Challenging the myth of primitive harmony.* New York: Free Press.

Eid, M., & Diener, E. (2001). Norms for experiencing emotions in different cultures: Inter- and intranational differences. *Journal of Social and Personality Psychology, 81*, 869–885.

38   W. Tov and E. Diener

Ekman, P., & Friesen, W. V. (1971). Constants across cultures in the face and emotion. *Journal of Social and Personality Psychology, 17*, 124–129.
Ekman, P., Friesen, W. V., O'Sullivan, M., Chan, A., Diacoyanni-Tarlatzis, I., Heider, K., et al. (1987). Universals and cultural differences in the judgments of facial expressions of emotion. *Journal of Social and Personality Psychology, 53*, 712–717.
Fredrickson, B. L. (1998). What good are positive emotions? *Review of General Psychology, 2*, 300–319.
Freedman, D. G., & Freedman, N. C. (1969). Behavioural differences between Chinese-American and European-American newborns. *Nature, 224*, 1227.
Fujita, F., & Diener, E. (2005). Life satisfaction set point: Stability and change. *Journal of Personality and Social Psychology, 88*, 158–164.
Gaskins, R. W. (1999). "Adding legs to a snake": A reanalysis of motivation and the pursuit of happiness from a Zen Buddhist perspective. *Journal of Educational Psychology, 91*, 204–215.
Gohm, C. L., Oishi, S., Darlington, J., & Diener, E. (1998). Culture, parental conflict, parental marital status, and the subjective well-being of young adults. *Journal of Marriage and the Family, 60*, 319–334.
Haritatos, J., & Benet-Martínez, V. (2002). Bicultural identities: The interface of cultural, personality, and socio-cognitive processes. *Journal of Research in Personality, 36*, 598–606.
Heine, S. J. (2003). Self-enhancement in Japan? A reply to Brown & Kobayashi. *Asian Journal of Social Psychology, 6*, 75–84.
Heine, S. J., Kitayama, S., Lehman, D. R., Takata, T., Ide, E., Leung, C., et al. (2001). Divergent consequences of success and failure in Japan and North America: An investigation of self-improving motivations and malleable selves. *Journal of Personality and Social Psychology, 81*, 599–615.
Heine, S. J., Lehman, D. R., Markus, H. R., & Kitayama, S. (1999). Is there a universal need for positive self-regard? *Psychological Review, 106*, 766–794.
Hermans, H. J. M., & Kempen, H. J. G. (1998). Moving cultures: The perilous problems of cultural dichotomies in a globalizing society. *American Psychologist, 53*, 1111–1120.
Hong, Y., & Chiu, C. (2001). Toward a paradigm shift: From cross-cultural differences in social cognition to social-cognitive mediation of cultural differences. *Social Cognition, 19*, 181–196.
Howell, C. J., Howell, R. T., & Schwabe, K. A. (2006). Does wealth enhance life satisfaction for people who are materially deprived? Exploring the association among the *Orang Asli* of Peninsular Malaysia. *Social Indicators Research, 76*, 499–524.
Inglehart, R. (1990). *Culture shift in advanced industrial society*. Princeton, NJ: Princeton University Press.
Inglehart, R., & Klingemann, H.-D. (2000). Genes, culture, democracy, and happiness. In E. Diener & E. M. Suh (Eds.), *Culture and subjective well-being* (pp. 185–218). Cambridge, MA: MIT Press.
Ito, T. A., & Cacioppo, J. T. (1999). The psychophysiology of utility appraisals. In D. Kahneman, E. Diener, & N. Schwartz (Eds.), *Well-being: The foundations of hedonic psychology* (pp. 470–488). New York: Russell Sage Foundation.
Izard, C. E., & Malatesta, C. Z. (1987). Perspectives on emotional development I: Differential emotions theory of early emotional development. In J. D. Osofsky (Ed.), *Handbook of infant development* (2nd ed., pp. 494–554). New York: John Wiley & Sons.
Johnson, T., Kulesa, P., Cho, Y. I., & Shavitt, S. (2005). The relation between culture and response styles: Evidence from 19 countries. *Journal of Cross-Cultural Psychology, 36*, 264–277.
Kagan, J., Arcus, D., Snidman, N., Feng, W. Y., Hendler, J., & Greene, S. (1994). Reactivity in infants: A cross-national comparison. *Developmental Psychology, 30*, 342–345.
Kang, S.-M., Shaver, P. R., Sue, S., Min, K.-H., & Jing, H. (2003). Culture-specific patterns in the prediction of life satisfaction: Roles of emotion, relationship quality, and self-esteem. *Personality & Social Psychology Bulletin, 29*, 1596–1608.
Kim, D.-Y. (2004). The implicit life satisfaction measure. *Asian Journal of Social Psychology, 7*, 236–262.

Kim, D.-Y., Sarason, B. R., & Sarason, I. G. (2006). Implicit social cognition and culture: Parent-child relations and traditional cultural values, explicit and implicit psychological acculturation, and distress of Korean-American young adults. *Journal of Social and Clinical Psychology, 25,* 1–32.

Kim-Prieto, C. Y. (2005). *Culture's influence on experienced and remembered emotions.* Unpublished doctoral dissertation, University of Illinois, Urbana-Champaign.

Kim-Prieto, C. & Diener, E. (2004). *Religion's role in cultural differences in emotional experiences.* Unpublished manuscript, University of Illinois, Urbana-Champaign.

Kitayama, S., & Markus, H. R. (2000). The pursuit of happiness and the realization of sympathy: Cultural patterns of self, social relations, and well-being. In E. Diener & E. M. Suh (Eds.), *Culture and subjective well-being* (pp. 113–161). Cambridge, MA: MIT Press.

Kitayama, S., Markus, H. R., & Kurokawa, M. (2000). Culture, emotion, and well-being: Good feelings in Japan and the United States. *Cognition and Emotion, 14,* 93–124.

Kitayama, S., Markus, H. R., Matsumoto, H., & Norasakkunkit, V. (1997). Individual and collective processes in the construction of the self: Self-enhancement in the United States and self-criticism in Japan. *Journal of Personality and Social Psychology, 72,* 1245–1267.

Kuppens, P., Ceulemans, E., Timmerman, M. E., Diener, E., & Kim-Prieto, C. (2006). Universal intracultural and intercultural dimensions of the recalled frequency of emotional experience. *Journal of Cross-Cultural Psychology, 37,* 491–515.

Kwan, V. S. Y., Bond, M. H.., & Singelis, T. M. (1997). Pancultural explanations for life satisfaction: Adding relationship harmony to self-esteem. *Journal of Personality and Social Psychology, 73,* 1038–1051.

Lesch, K.-P., Bengel, D., Heils, A., Sabol, S. Z., Greenberg, B. D., Petri, S., et al. (1996). Association of anxiety-related traits with a polymorphism in the serotonin transporter gene regulatory region. *Science, 274,* 1527–1531.

Levy, R. I. (1982). On the nature and functions of the emotions: An anthropological perspective. *Social Science Information, 21,* 511–528.

Lucas, R. E., Diener, E., Grob, A., Suh, E. M., & Shao, L. (2000). Cross-cultural evidence for the fundamental features of extraversion. *Journal of Personality and Social Psychology, 79,* 452–468.

Lutz, C. A. (1988). *Unnatural emotions: Everyday sentiments on a Micronesian atoll and their challenge to Western theory.* Chicago: University of Chicago Press.

Lykken, D., & Tellegen, A. (1996). Happiness is a stochastic phenomenon. *Psychological Science, 7,* 186–188.

Lyubomirsky, S., King, L., & Diener, E. (2005). Is happiness a strength? An examination of the benefits and costs of frequent positive affect. *Psychological Bulletin, 131,* 803–855.

Markus, H. R., & Kitayama, S. (1991). Culture and the self: Implications for cognition, emotion, and motivation. *Psychological Review, 98,* 224–253.

Markus, H. R., & Kitayama, S. (1994). The cultural construction of self and emotion: Implications for social behavior. In S. Kitayama & H. R. Markus (Eds.), *Emotion and culture: Empirical studies of mutual influence* (pp. 89–130). Washington, DC: American Psychological Association.

Maslow, A. H. (1954). *Motivation and personality.* New York: Harper & Row.

Menon, U., & Shweder, R. A. (1994). Kali's tongue: Cultural psychology and the power of shame in Orissa, India. In S. Kitayama & H. R. Markus (Eds.), *Emotion and culture: Empirical studies of mutual influence* (pp. 241–284). Washington, DC: American Psychological Association.

Mesquita, B., & Frijda, N. H. (1992). Cultural variations in emotions: A review. *Psychological Bulletin, 112,* 179–204.

Mesquita, B., Fridja, N. H., & Scherer, K. R. (1997). Culture and emotion. In J. W. Berry, P. Dasen, & Saraswath (Eds.), *Handbook of cross-cultural psychology* (2nd ed., Vol. 2,pp. 255– 297). Boston: Allyn & Bacon.

Miller, P. J., Wang, S., Sandel, T., & Cho, G. E. (2002). Self-esteem as folk theory: A comparison of European American and Taiwanese mother's beliefs. *Parenting, Science and Practice, 2,* 209–239.

No, S., & Hong, Y.-y. (2004). Negotiating bicultural identity: Contrast and assimilation effects in cultural frame switching. Poster presented at the 2004 annual meeting of the Society for Personality and Social Psychology, Austin, TX, January, 2004.

Oishi, S. (2000). Goals as cornerstones of subjective well-being. In E. Diener & E. M. Suh (Eds.), *Culture and subjective well-being* (pp. 87–112). Cambridge, MA: MIT Press.

Oishi, S. (2002). The experience and remembering of well-being: A cross-cultural analysis. *Personality and Social Psychology Bulletin, 28*, 1398–1406.

Oishi, S., & Diener, E. (2001). Goals, culture, and subjective well-being. *Personality and Social Psychology Bulletin, 27*, 1674–1682.

Oishi, S., Diener, E. F., Lucas, R. E., & Suh, E. M. (1999). Cross-cultural variations in predictors of life satisfaction: Perspectives from needs and values. *Personality and Social Psychology Bulletin, 25*, 980–990.

Oishi, S., Diener, E., Scollon, C. N., & Biswas-Diener, R. (2003). Cross-situational consistency of affective experiences across cultures. *Journal of Personality and Social Psychology, 86*, 460–472.

Oishi, S., Schimmack, U., & Colcombe, S. J. (2003). The contextual and systematic nature of life satisfaction judgments. *Journal of Experimental Social Psychology, 39*, 232–247.

Ortony, A., & Turner, T. J. (1990). What's basic about basic emotions? *Psychological Review, 97*, 315–331.

Park, N., & Huebner, E. S. (2005). A cross-cultural study of the levels and correlates of life satisfaction among adolescents. *Journal of Cross-Cultural Psychology, 36*, 444–456.

Peng, K., & Nisbett, R. E. (1999). Culture, dialectics, and reasoning about contradiction. *American Psychologist, 54*, 741–754.

Plutchik, R. (1980). *Emotion: A psychoevolutionary synthesis*. New York: Harper & Row.

Radhakrishnan, P., Chan, D.K.-S. (1997). Cultural differences in the relation between self-discrepancy and life satisfaction. *International Journal of Psychology, 32*, 387–398.

Rice, T. W., & Steele, B. J. (2004). Subjective well-being and culture across time and space. *Journal of Cross-Cultural Psychology, 35*, 633–647.

Ryan, R. M., & Deci, E. L. (2000). Self-determination theory and the facilitation of intrinsic motivation, social development, and well-being. *American Psychologist, 55*, 68–78.

Ryff, C. D., & Singer, B. (1998). The contours of positive human health. *Psychological Inquiry, 9*, 1–28.

Schimmack, U., Diener, E., & Oishi, S. (2002). Life-satisfaction is a momentary judgment and a stable personality characteristic: The use of chronically accessible and stable sources. *Journal of Personality, 70*, p. 345–384.

Schimmack, U., Oishi, S., & Diener, E. (2002). Cultural influences on the relation between pleasant emotions and unpleasant emotions: Asian dialectic philosophies or individualism-collectivism? *Cognition and Emotion, 16*, 705–719.

Schimmack, U., Radhakrishnan, P., Oishi, S., Dzokoto, V., & Ahadi, S. (2002). Culture, personality, and subjective well-being: Integrating process models of life satisfaction. *Journal of Personality and Social Psychology, 82*, 582–593.

Schwarz, N., & Strack, F. (1999). Reports of subjective well-being: Judgmental processes and their methodological implications. In D. Kahneman, E. Diener, & N. Schwarz (Eds.), *Well-being: The foundations of hedonic psychology* (pp. 61–84). New York: Russell Sage Foundation.

Scollon, C. N., Diener, E., Oishi, S., Biswas-Diener, R. (2004). Emotions across cultures and methods. *Journal of Cross-Cultural Psychology, 35*, 304–326.

Shao, L. (1993). *Multilanguage comparability of life satisfaction and happiness measures in mainland Chinese and American students*. Unpublished master's thesis, University of Illinois, Urbana-Champaign.

Shaver, P. R., Wu, S., & Schwartz, J. C. (1992). Cross-cultural similarities and differences in emotion and its representation: A prototype approach. In M. S. Clark (Ed.), *Emotion. Review of personality and social psychology* (Vol. 13, pp. 175–212). Newbury Park, CA: Sage.

Sheldon, K. M., Elliot, A. J., Ryan, R. M., Chirkov, V., Kim, Y., Wu, C., et al. (2004). Self-concordance and subjective well-being in four cultures. *Journal of Cross-Cultural Psychology*, 35, 209–223.

Shweder, R. A. (2000). Moral maps, "First World" conceits, and the new evangelists. In L. E. Harrison & S. P. Huntington (Eds.), *Culture matters: How values shape human progress* (pp. 158–172). New York: Basic Books.

Smith, P. B. (2004). Acquiescent response bias as an aspect of cultural communication style. *Journal of Cross-Cultural Psychology, 35*, 50–61.

Snibbe, A. C., & Markus, H. R. (2005). You can't always get what you want: Educational attainment, agency, and choice. *Journal of Personality and Social Psychology, 88*, 703–720.

Suh, E. M. (2002). Culture, identity consistency, and subjective well-being. *Journal of Personality and Social Psychology, 83*, 1378–1391.

Suh, E., Diener, E., Oishi, S., & Triandis, H. C. (1998). The shifting basis of life satisfaction judgments across cultures: Emotions versus norms. *Journal of Personality and Social Psychology, 74*, 482–493.

Thompson, J. (1941). Development of facial expression of emotion in blind and seeing children. *Archives of Psychology, 264*.

Tomkins, S. S. (1962). *Affect, imagery, and consciousness: Vol.1. The positive affects*. New York: Springer.

Tomkins, S. S. (1963). *Affect, imagery, and consciousness: Vol.2. The negative affects*. New York: Springer.

Tsai, J., Knutson, B., & Fung, H. H. (2006). Cultural variation in affect valuation. *Journal of Personality and Social Psychology*, 90, 228–307.

Veenhoven, R. (n.d.). Distributional findings in nations. *World database of happiness*. Retrieved September 5, 2004, from www.eur.nl/fsw/research/happiness

Veenhoven, R. (1991). Is happiness relative? *Social Indicators Research*, 24, 1–34.

Veenhoven, R. (1993). *Happiness in nations*. Rotterdam, The Netherlands: Risbo.

Veenhoven, R. (2001). Are the Russians as unhappy as they say they are? Comparability of self-reports across nations. *Journal of Happiness Studies, 2*, 111–136.

Vittersø, J., Røysamb, E., & Diener, E. (2002). The concept of life satisfaction across cultures: Exploring its diverse meaning and relation to economic wealth. In E. Gullone & R. A. Cummins (Eds.), *The universality of subjective wellbeing indicators* (pp. 81–103). Dordrecht, The Netherlands: Kluwer Academic Publishers.

Wallbott, H. G., & Scherer, K. (1988). How universal and specific is emotional experience? Evidence from 27 countries on five continents. In K. R. Scherer (Ed.), *Facets of emotion: Recent research* (pp. 31–56). Hillsdale, NJ: Lawrence Erlbaum.

Watson, D., Clark, L. A., & Tellegen, A. (1984). Cross-cultural convergence in the structure of mood:: A Japanese replication and a comparison with U.S. findings. *Journal of Social and Personality Psychology, 47*, 127–144.

Wierzbicka, A. (1986). Human emotions: Universal or culture-specific? *American Anthropologist*, 88, 584–594.

Wirtz, D. (2004). *Focusing on the good versus focusing on the bad: An analysis of East-West differences in subjective well-being*. Unpublished doctoral dissertation, University of Illinois, Urbana-Champaign.

Wu, W. C. H., & Bond, M. H. (2006). National differences in predictors of suicide among young and elderly citizens: Linking societal predictors to psychological factors. *Archives of Suicide Research, 10*, 45–60.

Yang, K. S. (2003). Beyond Maslow's culture-bound linear theory: A preliminary statement of the double-Y model of basic human needs. In V. Murphy-Berman & J. J. Berman (Eds.), *Nebraska symposium on motivation, 2002* (Vol. 49, pp. 176–255). Lincoln, NE: University of Nebraska Press.

Factors Predicting the Subjective Well-Being of Nations

Ed Diener, Marissa Diener and Carol Diener

Abstract Subjective well-being (SWB) in 55 nations, reported in probability surveys and a large college student sample, was correlated with social, economic, and cultural characteristics of the nations. The SWB surveys, representing nations that include three fourths of the earth's population, showed strong convergence. Separate measures of the predictor variables also converged and formed scales with high reliability, with the exception of the comparison variables. High income, individualism, human rights, and societal equality correlated strongly with each other, and with SWB across surveys. Income correlated with SWB even after basic need fulfillment was controlled. Only individualism persistently correlated with SWB when other predictors were controlled. Cultural homogeneity, income growth, and income comparison showed either low or inconsistent relations with SWB.

Subjective well-being (SWB), people's cognitive and affective evaluations of their lives, is an emerging research area in the social sciences. Reviews of this field are available from Diener (1984; Diener & Larsen, 1993), Myers and Diener (1995), and Veenhoven (1984), and a discussion of the definition and measurement of SWB can be obtained from Diener (1994). In the present study, we examined the degree to which a number of national characteristics correlate with reports of well-being in order to shed light on the macrosocial variables that influence mean levels of SWB.

The guiding framework of this study was that variables influence SWB if they affect people's ability to achieve their goals (Emmons, 1986). Societal resources that allow people to make progress in achieving their goals should lead to life satisfaction and affective well-being. Thus, we hypothesized that income and human rights should correlate strongly with SWB because they are likely to influence one's ability to reach diverse goals. A second set of variables was used to examine the relativistic approach to SWB: the idea that happiness depends on one's position relative to variable standards. The relativistic model suggests that SWB depends not on one's absolute level of resources, but on how one's resources compared to

E. Diener (✉)
Department of Psychology, University of Illinois Champaign, IL 61820, USA
e-mail: ediener@uiuc.edu

E. Diener (ed.), *Culture and Well-Being: The Collected Works of Ed Diener*, Social
Indicators Research Series 38, DOI 10.1007/978-90-481-2352-0_3,
© Springer Science+Business Media B.V. 2009

relevant comparison standards such as one's past level or the level of others. In this study we examined the effect of income growth on SWB in order to test the relative-standards idea that SWB depends on comparison to one's past income rather than on one's absolute level of income. Similarly, we examined the effects of social comparison of income on SWB in order to test the hypothesis that the effects of income on SWB depend on a comparison of one's wealth to that of others. Finally, we explored the effects of three other important sociocultural variables—cultural heterogeneity, equality, and individualism—on SWB.

Material Well-Being

At a theoretical level, wealth should predict higher SWB because greater resources allow people a greater ability to achieve some of their goals and also because high income confers higher status. In terms of the goals provided by Maslow's (1954) hierarchy of needs, income confers advantages in terms of basic physical needs, security, and the actualization of one's abilities (due to the greater freedom of action afforded by increased income). It appears that possessing a high income is the goal of a large number of people throughout the world. Because goal success is a predictor of SWB (Emmons, 1986), it seems likely that those with greater incomes will possess greater SWB.

It might be argued based on the relativistic model of SWB, however, that people adapt to their incomes so that wealth makes little long-term difference to SWB. Thus, we examined whether income levels relate to SWB even when income growth is controlled. Furthermore, Easterlin (1974) argued that people compare their incomes to those around them, and therefore differences between nations in income do not produce differences in SWB. He reasoned that income only makes a difference relative to what nearby others have. Because people tend to compare their incomes to the wealth of their neighbors, Easterlin argued that national differences in wealth should not produce differences in SWB. Thus, although there are psychological arguments as to why income should increase SWB, relativistic models predict that income should not be related to SWB.

Although income is not usually a strong predictor of individual well-being (e.g., E. Diener, Sandvik, Seidlitz, & M. Diener, 1993), in past research it has been a highly replicable predictor of SWB within countries (e.g., Easterlin, 1974; Veenhoven, 1991). Similarly, at the national level, poorer countries appear to possess lower SWB than richer ones (e.g., E. Diener et al., 1993; Veenhoven, 1991). Nevertheless, cross-national work in the past was based on a very small number of nations (e.g., Easterlin, 1974; Veenhoven, 1991) and heavily weighted toward European states (e.g., Inglehart and Rabier, 1986). In the present study, we examined the relation between wealth and SWB in 55 diverse countries, using both a college student survey and also broad, representative samples from most countries. Unlike several past studies, we included relatively fewer industrialized, westernized nations. There were several communist countries (at the time of the surveys) which included: Cuba, the United Soviet Socialist Republic, East Germany, Yugoslavia, and Poland. Levels of income varied from a low of $120 per person per year in Tanzania to $32,790 per person per year in Switzerland. Based on past research findings, and the idea that adequate resources cause positive moods because they allow one to achieve one's goals (Diener & Fujita, 1995), we hypothesized that national wealth would covary with SWB. Furthermore, we hypothesized that income would have an effect on SWB even when past income (as indexed by income growth) was controlled. We reasoned that higher income would help one achieve goals, regardless of one's past income.

In addition to the simple question of whether income correlates with SWB, we also examined whether this relation is curvilinear (with decreasing marginal utility for higher incomes). Veenhoven (1991) suggested that increasing wealth may have a diminishing effect, so that one sees its influence primarily in poorer countries. He hypothesized that differences in wealth have little influence at higher levels of income because wealth contributes to SWB primarily in meeting basic physical needs.

Because nations tend to vary in the meeting of basic physical needs mainly across the lower distribution of wealth, whereas wealthier nations tend to uniformly meet the physical needs of virtually all of their citizens, Veenhoven maintained that wealth should correlate weakly with income in the richer nations. If so, this ought to manifest itself in a curvilinear rather than linear relation between wealth and SWB. The relation between basic needs, income, and SWB is theoretically significant because it is related to whether well-being depends on meeting universal biological needs, or whether it hinges on having resources to reach a broader set of cultural goals.

Veenhoven's (1991) line of reasoning raises several important issues: (a) What is the relation between income and basic need fulfillment across nations?, (b) Is the level of fulfillment of basic needs correlated with SWB across countries?, and (c) Does income have any influence beyond the effects of basic needs? We measured the fulfillment of basic physical needs in nations with five variables (life expectancy, average calories available per person, percent of the population with safe drinking water, the percent of people with access to sanitary facilities, and the rate of infant mortality). Longevity, health, food, and water are among the most basic ingredients of physical well-being and, thus, should correlate with the well-being of nations if Veenhoven is correct. The nations we examined differed greatly in their ability to meet basic needs, and therefore there was an adequate range on this variable to explore its covariation with SWB.

Political and Civil Rights

Nations differ markedly in the liberties they afford their citizens (Gupta, Jongman, & Schmid, 1994). In some there are few civil or political rights, and individuals are at the mercy of the desires of those in power. In others, individuals are largely protected by laws and possess extensive civil rights and freedoms. Based on a number of psychological theories, we hypothesized that nations with greater rights would have greater SWB. First, self-efficacy should be greater in nations in which individuals feel that they have more control over their individual and collective destiny. Second, people are more likely to experience the second of Maslow's needs—security—in nations where individuals have more rights. In such countries, people are less likely to disappear, to be tortured, or to be arrested without charges. Finally, individuals in nations with more rights ought to be better able to meet their needs because they are better able to use diverse behaviors to pursue various courses of action. For example, in order to increase their incomes, people in nations with many rights may move to a new job, go on strike, or organize a boycott. Possessing civil and political rights is thus likely to help individuals to achieve diverse goals, and therefore we hypothesized that it would correlate with SWB.

Income Growth

E. Diener et al. (1993) found that high economic growth was correlated with low SWB. They hypothesized that a rapid rise in income led to lower SWB because rapid growth is likely to be accompanied by high aspirations and also by dislocations such as employment moves and family separation. The Diener et al. sample, however, was limited to college students. Furthermore, the high growth countries in their study were virtually all located on the Pacific Rim of Asia. In the present research, we examined the correlation between the growth of per capita gross domestic product (GDP) of nations and SWB, using broad national samples and a larger and more diverse selection of nations. The relation between income growth and SWB will help shed light on relativistic models that maintain that SWB is due to change in resources rather than to the absolute level of resources. Headey and Wearing (1992) found that recent changes in events led to changes in SWB, and Suh, Diener, and Fujita (1996) replicated this finding. Thus, it may be that changes in people's income are more important to happiness than is the absolute level of income.

Social Comparison

The second relative-standards variable we assessed was the influence of income social comparison on SWB. The idea is that individuals will be happier if their income is higher than a reference standard set by the income of others, but will be less happy if they are below that standard. We previously found that social comparison influences satisfaction in laboratory situations (Smith, Diener, & Wedell, 1989), but did not find these effects in natural situations (E. Diener et al., 1993; Fujita, Diener, & Gallagher, 1994). Although it seems plausible that the effects of one's income on one's SWB will depend on the income of salient others, our past findings indicate that it is difficult to predict when this will occur in natural situations. We tested three different possible manifestations of social comparison effects.

First, we examined the effects of having wealthy versus poor neighboring countries on the SWB of a society. People may set their economic aspirations based on those around them. If the citizens of neighboring countries possess a high standard of living, this may raise people's aspirations. If social comparison across neighboring borders influences SWB, we should find that nations with poorer neighbors have higher well-being, whereas nations with richer neighboring countries should have lower SWB. Michalos (1991) hypothesized that individual social comparisons influence the SWB of people. It may be that the wealth of neighboring countries has an analogous influence on the average SWB within a country. The nations we studied varied from those whose neighbors were on average richer (e.g., Belgium) to those whose neighbors were on average poorer (e.g., Singapore).

The second social comparison measure was based on the skewing of income within nations. Parducci (1984) has argued that negatively skewed distributions will produce more happiness, and positively skewed distributions will produce less happiness. Smith et al. (1989) extended Parducci's argument to the case of social comparison and showed in a laboratory study that positively skewed distributions led to less satisfaction. In a highly positively skewed situation, a few individuals score very high and the rest score lower than this elite group. Therefore, satisfaction is lessened because most individuals have poor outcomes relative to the privileged group. In order to test this approach across nations, income skewing for nations was correlated with average SWB. We hypothesized that nations with more positively skewed income distributions (a few individuals making much more money than everyone else) would report lower mean SWB.

In the third approach to social comparison effects, we correlated the income standard deviations within countries with the standard deviations of SWB within nations. The idea was that, to the extent that comparison of one's income with the income of others in the same nation influences SWB, there should be more spread in SWB in nations in which there is more variability in income. If poor individuals are further from the mean income within their nation, their SWB should also be further from the mean. Based on the same reasoning, if wealthier individuals are only slightly richer than the mean in their country, their happiness ought to be only slightly above average. Thus, we predicted, based on social comparison effects for income, that nations with more spread in income ought to have more spread in SWB.

Equality

Equality among individuals is a major way that societies differ from one another. We examined equality of length of life, equality of income, and equal access of the sexes to education in terms of their ability to predict SWB. We hypothesized that equality would predict SWB for several reasons. First, it seems likely that a greater percentage of individuals will be able to achieve their goals in nations where there is relatively more equality. Second, where inequalities are great, issues of equity and social justice are likely to arise.

Independence-Interdependence

A broad cultural variable that may potentially influence SWB is individualism–collectivism (I–C; Triandis, 1989), which is also labeled independence–interdependence (Hofstede, 1980, 1991; Markus & Kitayama, 1991). In individualistic societies, people are oriented toward their personal goals and desires, and they perceive the individual as the basic unit. In contrast, collectivists view the group as of primary importance and focus their attention on achieving group goals. Although the I–C dimension is one of the most pervasive ways that cultures differ, its effects on SWB cannot be predicted with certainty. In collectivist cultures, there might be greater feelings of social support, which ought to enhance SWB. In individualistic cultures, however, there is more personal freedom, and individuals have more ability to pursue their individual goals. Furthermore, individualists are likely to place more value on personal well-being and thus seek SWB to a greater extent. However, because of high internality, individuals in individualistic cultures might feel more responsible for both their failures and successes. Thus, we examined the correlation between the I–C dimension and SWB but did not make firm predictions about the direction of this relation. The countries we examined varied from quite collectivist (e.g., Bangladesh and Cameroon) to very individualistic (e.g., the United States and Australia), with all levels in between. Therefore, there was sufficient range to uncover a relation between SWB and individualism.

Cultural Homogeneity

A variable that has not yet been studied in reference to SWB is the cultural homogeneity of countries. In recent years divisions between diverse cultural groups led to intense conflict in a number of nations. Indeed, internal differences led to the breakup of several of the nations we studied. It may be that countries which are more homogeneous in terms of ethnicity, religion, language, and culture will suffer from less internal strife and have greater political unity. Interpersonal relationships may be more harmonious in culturally homogeneous countries where social expectations are more uniform. Individuals in homogeneous countries possess similar norms for behavior and thus are less likely to experience conflicts based on differences in values and beliefs. Therefore, we predicted a positive correlation between the homogeneity of people within a country and their aggregate level of SWB. Again, we were in the position to give this hypothesis a strong test because our sample of countries included many nations in both the homogeneous (e.g., Denmark) and heterogeneous (e.g., Tanzania) categories.

Conclusion

We examined four SWB surveys in a total of 55 countries, with a combined population of 4.1 billion people. These surveys included a total sample of over 100,000 respondents. The results of these surveys were correlated with objective nation-descriptive variables. Because our sample of countries was much larger and much more diverse than those included in previous studies, and because we included a number of predictor variables that were each assessed through multiple measures, we expected to reach firm conclusions on several correlates of the subjective well-being of nations. Furthermore, because we analyzed a number of surveys for each country, we could examine the convergence between SWB surveys and examine the replicability of findings.

Method

National Surveys

Veenhoven (1993) compiled the results of national SWB surveys. We used data from these surveys in this study. For example, one survey asked respondents how happy they were and gave three response options varying from *very happy* to *not too happy*. In another survey people were asked how satisfied they were with their lives, and the 11 response options varied from *very satisfied* to *not satisfied*. For each country, we used the last survey that was reported by Veenhoven. In the case in which there was only one survey in a country, that survey was used. In order to calibrate different surveys, Veenhoven carried out a procedure of assigning a value from 0 to 10 for each response option in each survey. These values were derived from 10 expert ratings of how positive each response option appeared to be. Thus, the response options from every survey were given a calibrated value varying continuously from 0 to 10. The expert raters were persons working on the World Database of Happiness (Veenhoven, 1993) and were therefore individuals who were well acquainted with the different SWB scales. Thereafter, the scale values were multiplied by the number of respondents with each response in each survey. An average SWB value was then computed for each survey for each nation, and this value could vary from 0 to 10. Thus, even though different surveys with different response formats were involved, the results were all weighted so as to achieve a Thurstone SWB scale for each survey. In summary, the Last National Survey variable represents Veenhoven's 0 to 10 Thurstone value for each country for the last (or only) survey conducted in that nation.

For countries in which more than one survey was conducted, we separately calculated the value for "happiness" surveys and surveys of "life satisfaction." In this case, rather than use Veenhoven's weights, we standardized each survey (with a mean of 0 and *SD* of 1.0) across all nations using that instrument. Where there were multiple types of surveys using the same basic question (but different response formats), we computed separate means for surveys involving the root term *happiness* and for surveys querying *satisfaction*. This allowed an alternative method of comparing surveys when they involved different response formats. When identical survey instruments were administered a number of times within a country, data from the last administration (not counting the "Last Survey") were used. The standardization and averaging procedure allowed us to achieve an average across surveys using a method very different from that used by Veenhoven. In this case, we did not prejudge the value of the responses, but used standardization against all nations using that survey instrument. Thus, we calibrated surveys with different response formats by giving them all a standardized score. Although there are pros and cons to the procedures used by Veenhoven and by us, the strength is that we can compare the results of two very different procedures of averaging survey instruments to examine the convergence of the results. Unfortunately, the data were not reported by Veenhoven by sex, so gender analyses could not be performed.

Sampling within nations. National probability samples of each country where SWB was measured were summarized by Veenhoven (1993; e.g., Eurobarometer, 1991; Gallup, 1976). Data on convenience samples (e.g., high school students) or limited populations (e.g., young adults) were summarized separately and were not included in this study. Examples of the probability surveys used in our analyses were: the UNESCO's Tension Study, the German Welfare Survey, the Korean survey by the Institute for Social Sciences, Seoul National University, the Eurobarometer annual survey conducted by the Commission of the European Community, and Gallup's Public Opinion Survey. Most national surveys included adults over the age of 17 and were based on a multistage sampling procedure. The first stages included selecting representative samples of large geographical areas (e.g., standard metropolitan statistical areas) and then smaller geographical areas (e.g., census tracts, neighborhoods, or blocks). These geographical areas were typically selected on a stratified random basis to represent key demographic features of the nation. In the final stages, dwelling units were randomly selected, and then the respondent was systematically selected from each housing unit, usually based on procedures described by Kish (1965). Although dwelling units were selected based on probability, the response rates of the selected individuals often varied slightly by groups (e.g., men vs. women) and the number of adults living in dwellings also varied. Thus, many studies included weighting procedures to recognize these factors in the final statistics. Furthermore, some studies under-sampled in certain geographical areas and used weighting procedures to compensate for this. Occasionally, exemplary groups were selected to sample hard to reach populations (e.g., Black South Africans living in remote tribal homelands). Because the dwelling unit was used as the preliminary sampling unit, certain groups were underrepresented in most surveys: people living on military reservations, prison inmates, transients, and hospitalized individuals. The percent of respondents not answering the SWB question (given by Veenhoven, 1993) was typically quite small, in the 1 or 2% range. The sampling procedures were always of sufficient quality to yield a broad and heterogeneous participant sample which represented the vast majority of individuals of each nation. Most of the samples contained a margin of error of approximately 2–5%. The mean size of the national samples was 1,406, and the smallest sample included 300 respondents.

College Student Survey

During 1984–1986, colleagues of Alex Michalos from around the world collected data from college students in their respective countries. The measures asked the students to report how happy they were and how satisfied they were with their lives on 7-point delighted-terrible scales. When more than one university was involved in a country, the data were aggregated so as to achieve an overall happiness and life satisfaction score for that nation. The data, which included 18,032 student respondents, were compiled by Michalos and made available to the collaborators on the project (in this case, to Ed Diener). The Michalos data on Taiwan were excluded from the present analyses because of the lack of information on this nation in many sources (because it is not a member of the United Nations). Although we reported partially on SWB and income and income growth in E. Diener et al. (1993), it was deemed important to include these data in the present article because more predictor variables were included here, and an analysis of the convergence of the student results with the findings from national samples could be examined. Furthermore, Diener et al., working from the raw data rather than means provided by Michalos, did not include exactly the same countries or participants as are covered here. The Michalos data were averaged across the happiness and life satisfaction questions. We have used a question which is virtually identical to the Michalos satisfaction question with college students in both the USSR and the People's Republic of China (Balatsky & Diener, 1993; Shao, 1993). Therefore, we included these surveys with the Michalos survey. The mean sample size from 40 nations was approximately 390 per nation, and the smallest sample included 91 respondents.

The Sample of Nations

The 55 nations we studied are those included in the review by Veenhoven (1993) and in the study organized by Michalos. Of the 55 nations, data on 43 came from national surveys. The Michalos data and our data included 12 additional nations as well as data that overlapped with the national surveys for 28 countries. Although not sovereign nations, Northern Ireland and Puerto Rico provided data, and so they were included as 2 of the 55 societies studied. Although several of the nations have changed form since the data were collected (e.g., Yugoslavia and the USSR), we used earlier data, and the nations are therefore referred to by their names at the time the data were collected. The sample of nations was not only much larger than that included in past research but was also more diverse in that many past studies focused almost exclusively on highly industrialized countries such as the United States and Western Europe. In addition to the traditional European and North American nations, the present study included six nations from Africa, eight nations from Asia, seven nations from Latin America, three nations from the Middle East, four Pacific countries, as well as several additional scattered countries such as Iceland and the Dominican Republic.

Although the sample sizes are not given for all of the national surveys, it is estimated that about 120,000 individuals in all took part in the surveys we report. The total population represented by the nations included in this study is about 4.1 billion, or almost 75% of the world's 1990 population. Thus, the sample is much more representative of the world than past studies, although extremely poor countries and small nations are still underrepresented, and European societies are overrepresented.

Summary of Surveys

To summarize, we used four measures of SWB. One of these measures was from the same large-scale survey of college students organized by Michalos (1991) and involved the average of a life satisfaction and a happiness question. Three additional measures were generated from separate national probability surveys. One was the last survey reported for each country by Veenhoven, with the results being the Thurstone scale he calculated. The other two measures were separately derived for life satisfaction and happiness when additional surveys that covered these terms were conducted in a country. If more than one of these surveys was conducted, the latest survey using each response format was used. If more than one response format was used per term in different surveys, we averaged across the response formats by first standardizing each survey type across countries. Thus, the measures of SWB we examined included two types of samples—national and college student—and different years, response formats, and methods of calibrating across surveys. By this use of multiple methods, we explored the replicability of our findings.

Predictor Variables

For each predictor concept, three measures were obtained that represented differing manifestations of the construct in question.

Wealth. Measure 1: Figures for per capita wealth of most nations were obtained from Wright (1992) and Hoffman (1991), and from references on specific countries. The figures represent the gross domestic product (GDP) of the country divided by the population, or GDP per person. When GDP figures were not available, gross national product (GNP) was used. Our sample of nations included some of the poorest in the world (Tanzania, Bangladesh, and India) and most of the wealthiest nations in the world (e.g., Switzerland, Luxembourg, Finland, and Japan).

Measure 2: A second measure of income was the per capita income of nations in terms of the purchasing power of individuals (World Development Report, 1994). Purchasing income across nations was computed by taking a standard basket of market goods and computing how much of this could be purchased with the mean per capita income in each nation. Thus, this index considers income in light of consumer price information in each nation. The U.S. value is set at 100 because it has the highest per capita purchasing power, and other nations are expressed as a percent of this. Thus, purchasing power is defined as how much the per capita GNP of a nation would buy (the amount of a fixed basket of products in the domestic market) as one dollar would buy in the United States. For example, India scored 5 on this index, Poland scored 33, and Switzerland scored 96. Scores varied from 3 for Tanzania to 100 for the United States (see Table 1).

Measure 3: The fulfillment of basic physiological needs was indexed in each nation by five variables: the percent of the population having safe drinking water in 1986–1987, the rate of infant mortality rate per 1,000 in 1990, the mean life expectancy in the nation in 1990, the percent of people having sanitary toilet facilities in 1986–1987, and the average daily calorie supply per person in 1989. These figures were obtained from Wright (1992). The mean correlations of these variables with each other (with infant mortality reversed to the positive direction by computing the inverse value) was 0.74. The five variables were standardized and averaged to create a composite basic need fulfillment score for each nation. The Cronbach's alpha for the combined Basic Needs score, when all five components were available, was 0.93.

Rights. Gupta et al. (1994) assigned each nation a score on the degree to which they possessed 40 different human rights. A discriminant function across countries revealed that these rights fell onto three related dimensions: Measure 1. Gross human rights violations (e.g., disappearances, extra judicial killings, detention without charge, and torture); Measure 2. Civil rights (e.g., no searches without warrant, independent courts, innocent until proven guilty, no secret trials, freedom to teach ideas, and no arbitrary seizure of property). This figure is given in Table 1; and Measure 3. Political rights (e.g., freedom of the press, freedom to peacefully assemble, multiparty elections by secret ballot, and independent trade unions allowed). Based on a weighting of these 40 indicators, Gupta et al. computed the three rights scores for each nation. A low score represents more rights on all three scales.

Growth of wealth. The growth of wealth statistics were obtained primarily from data contained in the *Universal Almanac* (Wright, 1992) or from the *International Monetary Fund* (1992). These figures, shown in Table 1, are 1-year growth figures of GNP per person. The growth of real wealth (adjusted for inflation) covered a large range varying from −3.0 to 9.5.

Income social comparison. Measure 1: First, the average income per capita of neighboring nations was computed for each country. The GDP per capita of each nation bordering the target country was determined, and a mean value for all bordering nations was computed for every society. In the case of island nations such as Iceland, Japan, and Australia, the closest and most similar nations were used as the bordering countries. For the majority of nations, however, the nations that bordered the target country were used. For example, for Canada, the United States was used; for Sweden, Norway and Finland were used; and for Panama, Colombia and Costa Rica were used. The idea is that if a country is surrounded by nations that are much poorer or much richer, this should serve as a comparison basis for the citizens of the target nation and therefore influence their SWB. Although we cannot be sure that adjacent nations are always the primary referent countries, because of their propinquity and relatively greater similarity, it seems plausible that comparison

Table 1 Values of mean SWB and specific predictor variables

Nation	SWB	Last nat. survey	Purchas. power	Civil rights	GDP growth	Soc. comp neighbor	Income Gini	Triandis indiv.	Ethnic divers.	Sample N
Iceland	1.11	1.22			1.2	18,610	0.32	7	1	690
Sweden	1.03	1.22	80.5	4.41	1.8	24,595	0.40	8	1	1,038
Australia	1.02	1.30	76.4	4.42	1.7	4,700	0.33	9	1	2,208
Denmark	1.00	1.38	79.4	4.46	2.1	22,730	0.34	8	1	1,000
Canada	0.97	0.97	91.0	4.97	2.4	21,700	0.34	9	3	1,254
Switzerland	0.94	1.30	95.9	4.96	1.7	19,089	0.30	9	4	998
USA	0.91	0.73	100.0	4.58	2.2	11,470	0.34	10	2	1,526
Colombia	0.82		23.8	10.25		1,838		3	3	(91)
Luxembourg	0.82	0.89			3.9	19,217		8	1	300
New Zealand	0.82		67.3	4.42	2.0	17,080	0.38	9	1	(314)
N. Ireland	0.78	0.97				9,550		5		304
Norway	0.77	0.32	80.1	4.88	2.7	20,917	0.31	7	1	1,233
Finland	0.74	1.06	73.1	4.43	3.1	16,600	0.31	8	2	1,003
Britain	0.69	0.32	73.1	4.84	2.5	14,515	0.32	9	2	1,300
Netherlands	0.68	1.06	70.2	4.42	1.4	19,085	0.27	9	1	1,000
Ireland	0.57	0.32	42.4	5.71	1.1	16,070	0.31	5	1	1,000
Brazil	0.57	0.49	26.3	7.18	0.6	1,499	0.60	4	3	1,000
Tanzania	0.51		2.5	10.76	-3.0	353		3	5	(222)
Belgium	0.51	0.49	71.7	4.46	1.2	22,075	0.27	7	3	1,000
Singapore	0.43	0.57	55.7	9.57	5.7	2,340		5	4	1,006
Bahrain	0.36				-3.0	10,613		3		(275)
W. Germany	0.18	0.49	80.7	4.58	4.0	18,014	0.33	8	1	1,000
Austria	0.15	0.57	72.8	5.65	2.0	14,070		8	1	1,584

Table 1 (continued)

Nation	SWB	Last nat. survey	Purchas. power	Civil rights	GDP growth	Soc. comp neighbor	Income Gini	Triandis indiv.	Ethnic divers.	Sample N
Chile	0.13		27.7	11.62	-2.0	1,383	0.45	6	3	(256)
Philippines	0.10	0.00	10.9	4.87	-1.5	1,260	0.49	4	4	9,961
Malaysia	0.08	0.08	26.6	10.94	2.5	990		4	4	502
Cuba	0.00	0.00		10.96		6,518		4	3	992
Israel	-0.18	-0.33	60.5	7.01	1.5	888	0.33	6	2	354
Mexico	-0.28	-1.72	31.6	9.55	-0.9	8,190	0.52	5	3	2,204
Bangladesh	-0.29		5.1	10.26	2.0	280		1		(262)
France	-0.38	-0.33	77.8	4.54	1.7	21,250	0.35	7	1	1,000
Spain	-0.41	-0.17	50.5	5.10	2.7	12,185	0.32	6	3	1,000
Portugal	-0.41	-0.49	36.0	5.01	2.4	10,920	0.41	5	1	1,000
Italy	-0.44	-0.33	71.6	6.03	2.2	18,513	0.36	6	1	1,000
Hungary	-0.48	-0.41	30.4	9.45	1.5	6,016		6	2	1,464
Puerto Rico	-0.51	-0.17				820		7		1,417
Thailand	-0.62	0.08	17.2	9.01	5.6	763	0.42	4	2	500
S. Africa	-0.63	-0.49		11.08	-0.9	765		5	4	5,587
Jordan	-0.77		26.4		1.0	4,819		3	1	(279)
Egypt	-0.78	-0.74	16.4	10.86	2.1	5,630	0.40	5	2	499
Yugoslavia	-0.81	-1.14		9.57	-0.9	7,146		6	4	1,523
Japan	-0.86	-0.41	74.9	5.03	3.5	2,409	0.28	4	1	
Greece	-0.89	-0.90	33.9	4.85	0.8	2,050		7	2	1,000
Poland	-0.90	-0.90	25.8	10.70	1.2	5,913		5	1	1,464
Kenya	-0.92		6.1	9.88	-1.0	206	0.55	3	4	(268)

Table 1 (continued)

Nation	SWB	Last nat. survey	Purchas. power	Civil rights	GDP growth	Soc. comp neighbor	Income Gini	Triandis indiv.	Ethnic divers.	Sample N
Turkey	-1.02		21.1	10.97	3.0	2,767	0.49	4	2	(287)
India	-1.13	-0.17	4.6	8.81	3.2	253	0.40	4	4	1,000
S. Korea	-1.15	-0.17	28.8	9.17	8.9	867	0.37	3	1	1,500
Nigeria	-1.31	-1.31	5.5	10.20	-3.0	480		3	3	1,200
Panama	-1.31	-1.31	25.8	6.31	-2.0	1,575		4	4	642
E. Germany	-1.52	-0.41		10.13		9,190	0.56	6	1	2,000
U.S.S.R.	-1.70		38.7	11.37		4,066		6	4	(116)
China	-1.92		6.5	12.58	9.5	552		2	2	(149)
Cameroon	-2.04		15.9	10.69	6.0	902		2	4	(159)
Dom. Repub.	-3.92	-3.92	15.6	6.08	-0.4	370		4	3	814
Mean	-0.2	6.4	44.7	7.6	1.8	8,484.9		5.6	2.3	1,143.4
SD	1.0	1.2	29.4	2.8	2.6	7,645.2		2.2	1.2	1,478.4

Note: SWB refers to the mean standardized value of four surveys (three national surveys plus student survey). Last Nat. Survey is the SWB from last national probability survey. Purchas. Power refers to the per capita income of each nation expressed as percent of the U.S. figure in terms of purchasing power. Civil Rights, a low number denotes greater rights. GDP growth refers to the percentage growth rate of the national gross domestic product. Soc. Comp. Neighbor refers to the income in adjacent nations or the nearest neighbors. Income Gini (income equality) can vary from 0 (complete equality) to 1.0 (complete inequality). Triandis indiv. refers to the national ratings of individualism provided by Harry Triandis. Ethnic divers, refers to the 1 to 5 ethnic diversity of the nations, where 1 is the most homogeneous. Sample N's refer to last national probability sample, except they refer to college student sample where no national samples were available (shown in parentheses).

with neighboring nations is on average more likely than comparison to distant countries.

Measure 2: The second method of analyzing social comparison effects was based on the skew of income distributions within nations. The positive skews of the income distributions within nations were computed based on data contained in the *World Development Report* (1994). The skew was based on the most widely available distribution information, namely the incomes of the lowest, second, and highest income quintiles. A highly skewed distribution resulted when the lowest and second income quintiles were relatively close to each other but far below the richest quintile. To the extent that the second quintile was relatively equidistant between the lowest and highest quintiles, the distribution was less positively skewed. Nations varied from virtually unskewed (Egypt and Portugal) to highly positively skewed (e.g., Chile and Brazil). The prediction was that nations with highly positively skewed income distributions would have lower mean SWB because most individuals would be far below the top incomes.

Measure 3: The third approach to analyzing social comparison was not a single measure, but rather was the correlation between income spread and SWB spread across countries. Income distribution data were obtained from the *World Development Report* (1994) and from World Bank (1994). We calculated income spread by computing a ratio of the highest income quintile to the lowest income quintile in terms of earnings. So, for example, in Bangladesh and Spain, the highest quintile income group earns approximately four times as much as the low income group, whereas in Brazil and Panama, the highest income quintile earns approximately 30 times as much as the poorest fifth of people. The standard deviations of SWB within nations were computed based on the last national survey reported by Veenhoven (1993). The income spread ratio was correlated with the standard deviation of SWB in the last national survey. If this correlation is high, it would indicate that nations with a greater range of income also tend to have a greater range of SWB.

Equality. We measured equality of income, of longevity, and of educational access. Measure 1: Equality of income was measured by the Gini coefficients for nations (Veenhoven, 1993). Measure 2: Similarly, the dispersion of length of life was also indexed by Gini coefficients for longevity (Veenhoven, 1993). Gini coefficients range from O (*perfect equality*) to 1.0 (*one individual has all of the resource and others have none*). Measure 3: Equality of the sexes was measured by computing the percent of age-eligible girls attending secondary school compared to the percent of age-eligible boys attending (World Development Report, 1994).

Individualism–collectivism. Measure 1: Hofstede (1991) reports I–C scores for 43 of the nations we studied. These I–C ratings are based on questionnaires given to IBM employees throughout the world. Individualism was based on the reporting of work goals related to personal time, freedom, and challenge, whereas collectivism was related to work goals related to training, use of skills, and physical conditions.

Measure 2: A leading expert in the area of individualism and collectivism, Harry Triandis, rated each of the 55 countries on a 1–10 scale on which 1 was the most collectivistic and 10 was the most individualistic (see Table 1). Triandis was unaware of the data being used and unaware of the hypotheses being examined.

Measure 3: The third measure of I–C was the divorce rate in each nation (1992 Demographic Yearbook, United Nations, 1994). This variable was thought to reflect individualism for several reasons. Nations where divorce is high are more likely to emphasize the rights of individuals over the importance of collective relationships. Divorce represents a decline in obligation, duty, obedience, and other collective values. Instead, divorce is a manifestation of people seeking their own individual goals and happiness. Furthermore, divorce is not just a manifestation of individualism, but in turn is a cause of heightened individualism. The children of divorce, as well as other observers, see that relationships are not necessarily lasting and that individuals may ultimately have to rely heavily on themselves.

Cultural heterogeneity. Measure 1: Estes (1986) reported on several variables for a large number of countries. Among these variables was one labeled cultural homogeneity, which was composed of three factors: the largest percent of the population in a nation speaking the same language, the largest percent of the nation who shared the same or similar ethnic and racial background, and the largest percent of a nation who shared the same religion. Based on this composite, Estes rank ordered the countries from *most homogeneous* (1) to *most heterogeneous* (124), and we used this rank order as one homogeneity score.

Measure 2: Sterling (1974) grouped nations based on their degree of ethnic (culturally distinct groups) homogeneity. We used these groups to assign the following values to nations: 1 = nations with nearly homogeneous ethnic composition; 2 = nations with a single dominant ethnic group; 3 = nations with two major ethnic groups; 4 = nations with several major ethnic groups; and 5 = fragmented nations with many small ethnic groups. These ethnic homogeneity ratings are shown in Table 1.

Measure 3: Our third measure of heterogeneity was a rating by Taylor and Jodice (1983) of separatism within nations. They defined separatism as group activity seeking greater autonomy for a group or region, or the structural preconditions for such activity. An example of the latter is where a region populated by an ethnic group was forcibly incorporated into a nation during the twentieth century. Taylor and Jodice rated the intensity of separatist activity as well as the percent of the population in the society that is involved. Our separatist score is the product of the intensity times the percent figures for the latest year for which figures were available.

Results

Descriptive Data

Values for selected major variables for each country are presented in Table 1. The nations are ordered from the highest in mean subjective well-being to the lowest. The SWB that is shown in the left column of numbers is the mean figure derived across the four surveys (three national surveys and one college student survey, see below). Several nations scored unexpectedly high in SWB (Colombia and Tanzania), perhaps because only the student survey was available from those societies. The mean SWB figures can be compared to the level of subjective well-being found in the last national survey (shown in the next right column). Although the last National Survey is based on Veenhoven's (1993) zero to ten value, we report the scores here as in terms of standard scores across the last survey so that the scale values can be more easily compared to the mean of all four surveys.

The value of one predictor variable from each concept is shown in Table 1. In addition, the sample size of the last national survey is listed (or the N of the college survey if no national surveys were available). As can be seen, there was substantial variation on all variables, thus permitting correlations to emerge. Because of missing data for some nations, the following analyses contain somewhat different Ns.

Convergence of SWB Surveys

The convergence between the four SWB surveys is shown in Table 2. As can be seen, there was a high degree of convergence between SWB scores. The national surveys, conducted in different years with different measures, correlated an average of 0.71 with each other, and the measures from the college student survey correlated at a moderately high level with the national surveys (mean $r = 0.55$). When the four surveys of SWB were analyzed using principal-components analyses, one strong component emerged (eigenvalue $= 3.01$) which accounted for 75% of the variance in SWB scores. No other eigenvalue exceeded one and the plot of eigenvalues also indicated a one-factor solution. With only one component, no rotation of factors was possible. The component loadings were: Last National Survey $= 0.76$; Average Happiness $= 0.94$; Average Satisfaction $= 0.92$; College Student Happiness and Satisfaction $= 0.84$. This indicates that the various surveys were assessing the same construct. This component scale had a Cronbach's alpha of 0.88, and correlated highly with the individual scales. In order to create a more stable score with more surveys, and also covering more nations, the mean of the four surveys was computed and is shown in the table as mean SWB.

Table 2 Intercorrelations of SWB measures across nations

Sample and sample size	Mean SWB	Last national survey	Prior happiness	Prior life satisfaction
Number of nations	55	43	32	28
Last national survey	0.91***			
Prior happiness	0.89***	0.65***		
Prior life satisfaction	0.92***	0.67***	0.80***	
College survey ($N = 39$)	0.88***	0.49***	0.46*	0.71***

$^*p < 0.05$; $^{**}p < 0.01$; $^{***}p < 0.001$.

Convergence of Predictor Variables Within Concept

Table 3 shows the intercorrelations of the predictor variables within concept. The numbered variables across the top of the table refer to the corresponding measures within each concept. So, for instance, the intercorrelation of the three individualism measures is shown under Individualism. For example, the Hofstede (measure 1) and the Triandis (number 2) measures correlated with each other 0.83. It should be noted that under equality, girls in high school was scored in the opposite direction from the other two variables, and therefore convergence is indicated by inverse correlations. As can be seen, almost without exception, measures converged well with other measures of the same concept. One clear exception is for social comparison, where the two measures varied inversely.

The correlations between the various survey measures of SWB and the predictor variables are presented in Table 4. In addition to individual measures, the table also shows correlations with a principal-component score for each of the concepts. No component score was created for social comparison because the third index of

Table 3 Convergence of measures within concepts

| | Concept | | |
Measure	1	2	Component loading
Income			
1. GDP per capita			0.95
2. Purchasing power	0.95***		0.98
3. Basic needs	0.76***	0.86***	0.92
Rights			
1. Gross violations			0.94
2. Civil	0.89***		0.98
3. Political	0.83***	0.94***	0.96
Social comparison			
1. Income positive skew			
2. Neighbors' income	−0.38*		
Equality			
1. Income Gini			0.76
2. Longevity Gini	0.66***		0.95
3. Girls sec. school	−0.34	−0.57**	0.70
Individualism			
1. Hofstede measure			0.94
2. Triandis rating	0.83***		0.93
3. Divorce rate	0.78***	0.53***	0.91
Heterogeneity			
1. Ethnic diversity			0.96
2. Cultural heterogeneity	0.86***		0.87
3. Separatism	0.39***	0.48***	0.68

Note. Numbers across the top of the table refer to each of the measures within a concept. Thus, the correlations of variables are shown only within each of the italicized concept groupings.

$*p < 0.05$; $**p < 0.01$; $***p < 0.001$.

Table 4 Correlations of predictor variables with subjective well-being measures

Concept Measure	Mean of 4 surveys	Last national survey	Prior happiness survey	Prior satisfaction survey	College survey
Money					
Component score	0.59***	0.64***	0.51**	0.61**	0.48**
GDP per capita	0.58***	0.66***	0.43*	0.57**	0.47**
Purchasing power	0.61***	0.64***	0.57**	0.64***	0.53***
Basic needs	0.52***	0.55***	0.37*	0.60***	0.38*
Rights					
Component score	−0.48***	−0.40*	−0.53**	−0.65***	−0.62***
Gross violations	−0.46***	−0.36*	−0.50**	−0.66***	−0.57***
Civil	−0.46***	−0.40*	−0.48**	−0.61***	−0.61***
Political	−0.46***	−0.38*	−0.52**	−0.61***	−0.60***
Income growth					
GDP/capita growth	−0.08	0.40*	−0.22	−0.21	−0.44**
Social comparison					
Income positive skew	−0.10	−0.13	−0.03	−0.25	0.04
Neighbors' income	0.58***	0.55***	0.49*	0.61***	0.58***
Equality					
Component score	−0.48*	−0.43	−0.52*	−0.62**	−0.10
Income Gini	−0.43*	−0.49**	−0.10	−0.15	−0.24
Longevity Gini	−0.40*	−0.35	−0.39*	−0.56**	−0.04
Relative % girls in secondary school	0.43**	0.16	0.34	0.59**	0.41*
Individualism					
Component score	0.77***	0.73***	0.60**	0.74***	0.72***
Hofstede measure	0.61***	0.65***	0.51**	0.58**	0.58***
Triandis rating	0.55***	0.59***	0.40*	0.59***	0.61***
Divorce	0.31	0.50**	0.04	0.57**	0.37*
Heterogeneity					
Component score	−0.22	−0.21	0.09	−0.26	−0.21
Ethnic diversity	−0.21	−0.27	0.05	−0.29	−0.09
Cultural heterogeneity	−0.13	−0.12	0.09	−0.21	−0.11
Separatism	−0.25	−0.22	−0.01	−0.27	−0.35*

Note. For rights and equality, a low score indicates more of that quality. GDP = gross domestic product.
*$p < 0.05$; **$p < 0.01$; ***$p < 0.001$.

social comparison was an overall correlation instead of individual nation scores and because the other two variables correlated inversely. The principal-components loadings are shown in the right column in Table 3. As can be seen in Table 3, the component loadings were high. The eigenvalues and percent of variance accounted for by each component were: Income 2.72 (91%); Rights 2.77 (92%); Equality 1.97 (66%); Individualism 2.58 (86%); and Heterogeneity 2.18 (73%). High alphas for the components also provided evidence that the three variables for each concept formed homogeneous scales: Income = 0.95; Individualism = 0.92; Rights = 0.96; Equality = 0.73; and Homogeneity = 0.80.

Predictors of SWB

As can be seen in Table 4, income, individualism, and human rights were consistent and significant predictors of SWB. Virtually without exception these three predictors replicated across the SWB measures as highly significant correlates of SWB. Linear regression analysis indicated the income, rights, individualism, and equality component scores produced a multiple R with mean SWB of 0.85, $F(4, 12) = 8.03$, $p < 0.01$. Not only did the component scores consistently correlate with SWB, but each of the individual measures usually did as well. It is interesting to note that the satisfaction survey produced stronger correlations with the predictor variables than did the happiness survey. This finding suggests that the predictors may more strongly influence cognitive judgments of well-being than they influence positive affective reactions.

For equality all correlations were in the expected direction, but not all were significant. Heterogeneity tended to be inversely correlated with SWB, but virtually none of the correlations were significant. Growth produced two significant correlations that were in the opposite direction of each other, and three non-significant correlations.

For social comparison, neighbor's income produced an effect opposite to that predicted—nations with wealthy neighbors were happier (to be analyzed further below). The positive skewing of income did not correlate with the SWB of nations. Furthermore, the correlation between the spread of income of nations and the spread of SWB was small and nonsignificant, $r(23) = 0.19$. Thus, for the three social comparison measures, only one was significant—and it was in the opposite direction to that predicted by a simple social comparison approach.

Further analyses were conducted on the neighbor income comparison. The correlation between a nation's per capita income and that of its neighbors was $r(53) = 0.80$, $p < 0.001$. This indicates that income is highly regionalized in the world, with some areas being predominantly poor and other regions being predominantly wealthy. The regionalization of wealth means that the income of one's neighbors correlated positively with SWB because a nation with wealthy neighbors was itself likely to be wealthy. Therefore, we also computed a partial correlation in which the effect of neighbors' income was correlated with mean SWB when the income component of nations was controlled. The partial correlation with 43 degrees of freedom was 0.22, ns, indicating that social comparison across neighboring nations did not strongly influence SWB. Indeed, this partial correlation remained in the opposite direction to that predicted by social comparison.

Similar neighboring country analyses were computed for rights (political), individualism (Triandis rating), and equality (income Gini). When a neighboring nation possessed more rights, the target nation had higher SWB: $r(53)=-0.50$, $p < 0.001$, and this correlation remained even after partialing out the target nation's level of rights: $r(46) = -0.31$, $p < 0.05$. The individualism of neighboring nations also correlated significantly with the mean SWB of the target country: $r(53) = 0.51$, $p < 0.001$, but this association became nonsignificant when the target nation's individualism was partialed out: $r(52) = 0.17$. The neighboring nations' equality did not correlate significantly with mean SWB. Thus, across four dependent variables, an analysis of neighboring nations produced no support for a social comparison and SWB link, and in several cases was in the opposite direction.

Basic Needs and Income

An important question is whether income correlates with SWB beyond the influence of basic need fulfillment. In order to control the effects of basic needs, partial correlations between GDP/person and SWB, and Purchasing Power and SWB were calculated with the Basic Need Fulfillment score held constant: GDP/person and Mean SWB $r(50)=0.33$, $p < 0.05$; and Purchasing Power and Mean SWB $r(43)=0.37$, $p < 0.05$. In other words, although the correlations decreased when basic need fulfillment was controlled, the correlations remained significant.

Another way to approach the question of basic needs versus purchasing power in terms of their influence on SWB is to examine the plots of these variables. Figure 1 shows the relation of basic needs to purchasing power. There is a clear curvilinear shape to this relation in that there is a steep rise in basic need fulfillment across the lower income nations, but once nations reach 40% of the purchasing power of the United States there is little further increase in meeting basic needs. This conclusion based on visual inspection of Fig. 1 is supported by a regression analysis that includes the quadratic component of Purchasing Power. Whereas the linear component of Purchasing Power produces an R^2 of 0.73 with basic needs, the R^2 increases to 0.85 when the quadratic component is included (quadratic beta$=-1.52$, $p < 0.001$). In contrast, Fig. 2 shows the relation between Purchasing Power and Mean SWB.

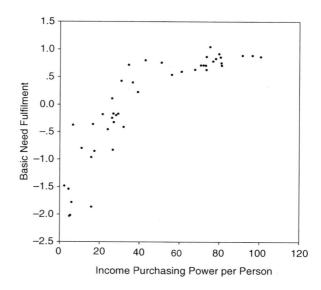

Fig. 1 The relation between basic need fulfillment and purchasing power

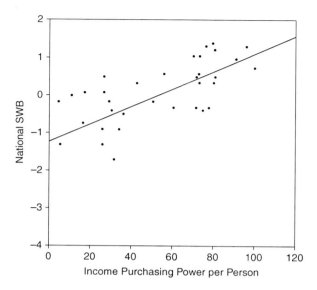

Fig. 2 The relation between subjective well-being and purchasing power

No curvilinear effect can be seen, and there is not a levelling off of mean SWB at a Purchasing Power of 40. The regression analysis supports this conclusion in that the linear R^2 is virtually identical to the R^2 that includes the quadratic component, 0.372 versus 0.375 (quadratic beta = 0.23, NS). For SWB and GDP/capita there also was no curvilinear component.

Interrelation of Predictors

Table 5 presents the intercorrelations of the Predictor Component Scores with each other, as well as with the income growth variable. It is evident that several of the predictors correlated significantly and substantially with each other. Thus, we explored the independent influence on SWB of several of the predictors with the

Table 5 Intercorrelation of predictors

Predictors	Income component	Individualism component	Rights component	Heterogeneity component	Equality component
Individualism component	0.80***				
Rights component	−0.80***	−0.75***			
Heterogeneity component	−0.50***	−0.21**	0.44***		
Equality	−0.84***	−0.32	0.80***	0.59*	
Income growth	0.17	0.14	0.03	−0.44**	−0.37

Note. Low scores on equality and rights indicate more of that quality.
$^* p < 0.05;\ ^{**} p < 0.01;\ ^{***} p < 0.001$.

Table 6 Partial correlations of predictor variables and Mean SWB

Correlation of predictor variable & SWB	Zero order r	Controlling for:			
		Income	Individualism	Rights	Equality
Income	0.59***		−0.08	0.40**	0.40
Individualism	0.77***	0.62***		0.72***	0.75***
Rights	−0.48***	−0.01	0.24		−0.17
Equality	−0.48*	0.04	−0.39	−0.19	

Note. SWB = subjective well-being.
$^* p < 0.05$; $^{**} p < 0.01$; $^{***} p < 0.001$.

effects of other predictors controlled. Income, individualism, equality, and human rights were selected because they were the ones that correlated significantly and consistently with SWB, as well as with each other. Table 6 reveals the correlations of each component score with SWB when each of the other component scores was controlled. As can be seen, individualism remained a very strong predictor when each of the other components was controlled. The strong relation between individualism and SWB is shown in Fig. 3. In contrast, the partial correlations for rights and equality all dropped to nonsignificance when the other variables were controlled. Income dropped to nonsignificance when individualism or equality were controlled. Thus, only individualism showed consistently unique variance in predicting SWB.

We also partialed out the effects of income growth on the correlation between SWB and income. The partial correlation of the income component and the mean SWB score with growth controlled was (41) 0.62, $p < 0.001$. In contrast, when the income component was partialed from the income growth and mean SWB relation, the correlation was inverse and nonsignificant, (41) −0.23.

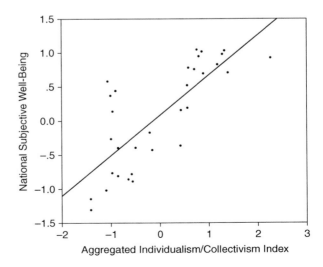

Fig. 3 Individualism and subjective well-being

Rank-Order Correlations

It could be argued that the surveys provide a rank-order estimate of the SWB of nations rather than an interval estimate. Therefore, Spearman rank-order correlations were also computed. The results were slightly stronger than for the Pearson correlations reported in Table 4. For example, the average Spearman correlation between the three national surveys was 0.81. Because the Spearman correlations produced no dramatic differences, only Pearson correlations were reported.

Discussion

The strong covariation among surveys, despite different years, sample populations, wording, and response formats, is encouraging. This indicates that, at least at the level of self-report, various scales for measuring SWB tend to yield similar results across countries. The construct validity of the SWB measures is strengthened by the finding that objective variables can predict them across cultures. The findings also suggest that data based on college students give a moderately accurate estimate of the relative SWB of the populations of nations, but do not converge as highly as national samples do. The high convergence of SWB surveys is desirable, but future research should also explore non-self-report methods of measuring SWB. For example, do measures of smiling, of memories for good events, and of peer reports of SWB also converge well across nations? An interesting lead for future research is whether life satisfaction is more influenced by money and other resources than is affective "happiness" (see also Diener & Fujita, 1995).

Three concepts showed replicable and strong relations with SWB—income, individualism, and human rights. These three concepts produced consistent results across four different surveys and across three different measures of each concept. Although some might object to a particular measure to reflect the concept in question (e.g., basic needs fulfillment as a measure of income), it should be noted that the pattern of correlations replicated across virtually all measures. Also, concepts were intercorrelated and with the exception of individualism, tended not to correlate with SWB when the other concepts were controlled. Thus, there appears to be a general trend of national development including higher income, equality, and human rights, and this general trend correlates with SWB. The covariation of SWB and individualism was so strong, however, that it persisted even when the general economic developmental trend was controlled. Not only is a larger sample needed to completely disentangle the effects of these four variables, but longitudinal and causal modeling procedures are also desirable. What can be stated with some certainty is that people in industrially developed nations (with high levels of income, individualism, equality, and human rights) report greater SWB than do people in less developed societies. Together these four predictors accounted for 73% of the variance between nations in mean SWB.

We explored the relation between income, basic need fulfillment, and SWB in more depth because base need fulfillment is not isomorphic with national income. There is clear evidence that income correlated with SWB even when basic needs were controlled. This indicates that economic development has an impact on well-being that transcends meeting basic biological needs such as food, water, health, and sanitation. Even above income levels of $15,000 per person, it is possible that there are increases in interesting leisure pursuits, in potential health benefits, and in self-development through education. It may be, however, that income continues to correlate with SWB even among wealthier nations because there is a common goal of a high level of affluence that few have attained, but after which many strive.

Individualism was a strong predictor of SWB across all surveys. One potential reason that this might be so is that individualistic societies afford an individual more freedom to choose his or her own life course. Another related reason is that successful people in individualistic societies may be more likely to attribute success to themselves. Although individualists may have a weaker social network in times of distress, in favorable times they have more freedom to pursue their individual goals. The individualist-collectivist correlation with SWB is intriguing, and deserves further research effort.

Income growth did not correlate consistently with SWB, and its effect was not positive when absolute levels of income were controlled. In contrast, income correlated moderately strongly with SWB, and did not decrease when income growth was controlled. These findings indicate that income has a direct influence on SWB that is not mediated by people's past level of income. Thus, there was no evidence for the relative standards approach to SWB that states that it is one's present position relative to one's past position that influences SWB.

The three social comparison approaches did not show any evidence that comparing one's income with that of others influences one's SWB. Indeed, positive correlations existed between the income (and rights) of neighboring nations and a country's SWB, suggesting that having neighbors with positive qualities is beneficial and does not make the citizens of a nation dissatisfied. Even when the rights of the target nations were controlled, there was a significant correlation with the rights in neighboring nations and a nation's SWB. The degree of positive skew of income within nations did not correlate with SWB, and the range of incomes within countries did not correlate with the range of SWB in those societies. These findings cast doubt on social comparison theory explanations of long-term SWB. As such, they are congruent with the findings of Fujita (1993) and E. Diener et al. (1993). Fujita found that the level of one's roommates and friends on important characteristics did not influence one's own satisfaction ratings in those areas, and Diener et al. found that people with a specific income who were living in either a poorer or richer neighborhood did not differ in SWB. Fox and Kahneman (1992) report evidence that suggests that social comparison judgments may follow from well-being rather than cause it, and Wood (1989) reviews evidence that indicates that social comparison can be used in a very flexible way to enhance one's well-being. Thus, other evidence also points to the fact that exposure in natural settings to others who are better off will not automatically influence one's moods in a negative way.

Social comparison might nevertheless influence SWB in ways not explored here. For example, perhaps people in countries look to other nations which are not necessarily on their borders. For example, southern Europeans might look to Northern Europe rather than to their closest neighbors. Or all nations may look to the USA because a wealthy version of its lifestyle is widely portrayed in television and movies in many societies. These alternative manifestations of social comparison await testing in future research. What would be required is an a priori specification of which individuals or nations people compare themselves to in each society. It should be noted, however, that direct tests of social comparison have often failed, whereas support for social comparison as a theory of satisfaction has often come from post-hoc explanations of findings. For example, it has been noted that Greece, France, Italy, and Spain report lower levels of SWB than one might expect based on their GDP per person. Is this because these countries are proximal to very prosperous nations such as Switzerland? The problem with this explanation is that other less prosperous European nations such as Ireland, Britain, and the Netherlands who have wealthy neighbors also have relatively high levels of SWB. Furthermore, an alternative explanation for low SWB in Southern Europe is in terms of cultural norms in these societies. Thus, the explanation for the comparatively low levels of SWB in Southern Europe may not be because of social comparisons across countries. It may be that social comparison is such a flexible cognitive process for achieving heightened SWB that comparisons imposed by one's local environment are not a major cause of differences in long-term SWB.

Cultural homogeneity, a nation of people sharing the same language, level of wealth, culture, and religion, also did not relate to higher SWB. The fact that homogeneity correlates with other factors that correlate with well-being (e.g., income and rights) makes it even more surprising that there is so little relation between this variable and SWB. It may be that cultural homogeneity has costs as well as benefits. For example, culturally homogeneous societies may be less varied and interesting. Alternately, most people's everyday lives may be largely confined to interactions with their own cultural group, and therefore homogeneity may not have an impact. Nations differ greatly in their homogeneity, a factor often overlooked by researchers. It is unknown why this variable does not influence SWB in this set of surveys, but given the apparent importance of this variable, further exploration of it is warranted.

Responses people give in reporting their happiness and life satisfaction relate in systematic ways to some predictor variables and not to others. The current results indicate with some certainty that the SWB of a nation correlates with income, rights, and the degree to which basic needs are fulfilled for the majority of its citizens. This pattern suggests that efficacy in terms of meeting one's needs, and an ability to pursue one's goals may be important cross-cultural factors in achieving SWB. Income allows one to achieve material goals, whereas rights and equality mean that a greater percentage of citizens have freedom and opportunity to pursue a wide variety of goals. Furthermore, individualism continued to be a strong correlate of SWB even when other predictors were controlled. Thus, a feeling of autonomy may be important in achieving SWB. In contrast to the successful predictors of SWB, relative standards approaches—social comparison and change from the past—failed to predict levels of SWB. This suggests either that long-term well-being is based on universal needs and desires, or that it is based on people's ability to select and pursue their goals. The relative standards we assessed did not have a large impact on SWB, and therefore it seems that these particular comparison standards were not critical in determining people's goals. These data indicate that having rights, material prosperity, individual freedom, and equality are more important to long-term SWB in the modern world than is how many resources others have or how many resources one had in the past.

Acknowledgments Our sincere thanks are extended to Alex Michalos and to Ruut Veenhoven. The efforts of these two in compiling cross-nation data is an outstanding service to the scholarly community. Their efforts are greatly appreciated; without them, the present study would not have been possible. Our appreciation is extended to Harry Triandis who provided individualism and collectivism ratings for the nations. Finally, we thank Marilyn George for her efforts in compiling the written paper.

References

Balatsky, G., & Diener, E. (1993). Subjective well-being among Russian students. *Social Indicators Research, 28*, 225–243.
Diener, E. (1984). Subjective well-being. *Psychological Bulletin, 95*, 542–575.
Diener, E. (1994). Assessing subjective well-being: Progress and opportunities. *Social Indicators Research, 31*, 103–157.
Diener, E., & Fujita, F. (1995). Resources, personal strivings, and subjective well-being: A nomothetic and idiographic approach. *Journal of Personality and Social Psychology, 68*, 926–935.
Diener, E., & Larsen, R. J. (1993). The experience of emotional well-being. In M. Lewis & J. M. Haviland (Eds.), *Handbook of emotions* (pp. 405–415). New York: Guilford.
Diener, E., Sandvik, E., Seidlitz, L., & Diener, M. (1993). The relationship between income and subjective well-being: Relative or absolute? *Social Indicators Research, 28*, 195–223.
Easterlin, R. A. (1974). Does economic growth improve the human lot?: Some empirical evidence. In P. A. David & W. R. Levin (Eds.), *Nations and households in economic growth* (pp. 98–125). Palo Alto, CA: Stanford University Press.
Emmons, R. A. (1986). Personal strivings: An approach to personality and subjective well-being. *Journal of Personality and Social Psychology. 51*, 1058–1068.
Estes, R. J. (1986, September). *Trends in global social development*. Paper presented at the Global Development Conference, College Park, MD.
Eurobarometer (1991). *Trends 74–90 BI*. The public opinion in the E. C. Brussels, Belgium: Commission of the European Community.
Fox, C. R., & Kahneman, D. (1992). Correlations, causes and heuristics in surveys of life satisfaction. *Social Indicators Research, 27*, 221–234.
Fujita, F. (1993). *The effects of naturalistic social comparison on life satisfaction*. Unpublished doctoral dissertation, University of Illinois, Urbana-Champaign.
Fujita, F., Diener, E., & Gallagher, D. (1994). *The effects of naturalistic social comparison on subjective well-being*. Unpublished manuscript, University of Illinois, Urbana-Champaign.
Gallup, G. H. (1976). Human needs and satisfactions: A global survey. *Public Opinion Quarterly, 40*, 459–467.

Gupta, D. K., Jongman, A. J., & Schmid, A. P. (1994, July). *Assessing country performance in the field of human rights.* Paper presented at the XIII ISA Congress, Bielefeld, Germany.

Headey, B., & Wearing, A. (1992). *Understanding happiness.* Melbourne, Australia: Longman Chesire.

Hoffman, M. S. (Ed.). (1991). *The world almanac and book of facts: 1992.* New York: Pharos Books.

Hofstede, G. (1980). *Culture's consequences: International differences in work-related values.* Beverly Hills, CA: Sage.

Hofstede, G. (1991). *Cultures and organizations: Software of the mind.* London: McGraw-Hill.

Inglehart, R., & Rabier, J. R. (1986). Aspirations adapt to situations-But why are the Belgians so much happier than the French? A cross-cultural analysis of the subjective quality of life. In F. Andrews (Ed.), *Research on the quality of life* (pp. 1–56). Ann Arbor: University of Michigan.

International Monetary Fund. (1992). *International financial statistics yearbook.* Washington, DC: IMF Statistics Department.

Kish, L. (1965). *Survey sampling.* New York: Wiley.

Markus, H. R., & Kitayama, S. (1991). Culture and the self: Implications for cognition, emotion, and motivation. *Psychological Review, 98.* 224–253.

Maslow, A. H. (1954). *Motivation and personality.* New York: Harper & Row.

Michalos, A. C. (1991). *Global report on student well-being.* New York: Springer-Verlag.

Myers, D., & Diener, E. (1995). Who is happy? *Psychological Science, 6,* 10–19.

Parducci, A. (1984). Value judgments: Toward a relational theory of happiness. In J. R. Eiser (Ed.), *Attitudinal judgments* (pp. 3–21). New York: Springer-Verlag.

Shao, L. (1993). *Multilanguage comparability of life satisfaction and happiness measures in mainland Chinese and American students.* Unpublished master's thesis, University of Illinois, Urbana-Champaign.

Smith, R. H., Diener, E., & Wedell, D. (1989). The range-frequency model of happiness applied to temporal and social comparisons. *Journal of Personality and Social Psychology, 56,* 317–325.

Sterling, R. W. (1974). *Macropolitics: International relations in a global society.* New York: Knopf.

Suh, E., Diener, E., & Fujita, F. (1996). Events and subjective well-being: Only recent events matter. *Journal of Personality and Social Psychology, 70,* 1091–1102.

Taylor, C. L., & Jodice, D. A. (1983). *World handbook of political and social indicators. Third Edition: Cross-national attributes and rates of change* (Vol. 1). New Haven: Yale University Press.

Triandis, H. C. (1989). The self and social behavior in differing cultural contexts. *Psychological Review, 96,* 506–520.

United Nations. (1994). *1992 Demographic yearbook* (Department for Economic and Social Information and Policy Analysis). New York: United Nations.

Veenhoven, R. (1991). Is happiness relative? *Social Indicators Research, 24,* 1–34.

Veenhoven, R. (1993). *Happiness in nations.* Rotterdam, The Netherlands: Risbo.

Wood, J. V. (1989). Theory and research concerning social comparisons of personal attributes. *Psychological Bulletin, 106,* 231–248.

World Bank. (1994). *Social indicators of development 1994.* Baltimore: John Hopkins University Press.

World Development Report 1994: Infrastructure for development (1994). Oxford: Oxford University Press (published for the World Bank).

Wright, J. W. (Ed.). (1992). *The universal almanac: 1993.* Kansas City, MO: Andrews & McMeel.

Cross-Cultural Correlates of Life Satisfaction and Self-Esteem

Ed Diener and Marissa Diener

Abstract College students in 31 nations ($N = 13,118$) completed measures of self-esteem, life satisfaction, and satisfaction with specific domains (friends, family, and finances). The authors assessed whether cross-cultural variations in the strength of associations were related to societal dimensions including income and individualism. At the national level, individualism correlated -0.24 (ns) with heterogeneity and 0.71 ($p < 0.001$) with wealth. At the individual level, self-esteem and life satisfaction were correlated 0.47 for the entire sample. This relation, however, was moderated by the individualism of the society. The associations of financial, friend, and family satisfactions with life satisfaction and with self-esteem also varied across nations. Financial satisfaction was a stronger correlate of life satisfaction in poorer countries. It was found that life satisfaction and self-esteem were clearly discriminable constructs. Satisfaction ratings, except for financial satisfaction, varied between slightly positive and fairly positive.

Subjective well-being (SWB) is now the focus of intense research attention (see Campbell, Converse, & Rodgers, 1976; Diener, 1984; Diener & Larsen, 1993). Subjective well-being is a person's evaluative reactions to his or her life—either in terms of life satisfaction (cognitive evaluations) or affect (ongoing emotional reactions). A number of correlates of SWB have been examined in the search for an understanding of the causes of SWB, for example: (a) personality variables, such as self-esteem (Campbell, 1981), (b) income (Veenhoven, 1991), and (c) social support variables, such as family satisfaction (Campbell, 1981). Little attention has been given, however, to whether the predictors of SWB differ in various cultures. It seems likely that the variables that influence people's evaluations of their lives do vary across cultures. In the present study, we systematically related predictors of life satisfaction to characteristics of the societies: individualism (Hofstede, 1980) versus collectivism, income per person, and cultural homogeneity. We hypothesized that the correlates of SWB would differ across nations with differing characteristics.

E. Diener (✉)
Department of Psychology, University of Illinois, Champaign, IL 61820, USA
e-mail: ediener@uiuc.edu

E. Diener (ed.), *Culture and Well-Being: The Collected Works of Ed Diener*, Social Indicators Research Series 38, DOI 10.1007/978-90-481-2352-0_4,
© Springer Science+Business Media B.V. 2009

Self-Esteem and Subjective Well-Being

Past research in the West has shown that self-esteem is a strong predictor of life satisfaction. For example, Campbell (1981) found that self-esteem was the strongest predictor of life satisfaction in a national sample of adults in the United States: The correlation between the two was 0.55. However, Kitayama and Markus (in press) questioned the universal importance of self-esteem. They pointed out that in Western culture it is "taken for granted that individuals are motivated to feel good about themselves." They noted, however, that in collectivist cultures "the primary task of interdependent selves is to fit in, to engage, to belong or to become part of the relevant social relationships." In Western cultures people are taught to like themselves, and doing so is a sign of mental adjustment. In cultures in which the collective is stressed, however, feeling good about oneself may be a sign of maladjustment.

We predicted that the importance of the self to life satisfaction would vary systematically across cultures, with greater predictive value of self-esteem in individualistic cultures (Hofstede, 1980; Triandis, 1989). In contrast, we also predicted that family and friendship satisfaction would be stronger correlates of life satisfaction in collectivist cultures. In collectivist cultures a person's life satisfaction may be derived much more from his or her ingroup (family, friends, and coworkers) than from self-esteem. Given that the family is usually the most important ingroup (Triandis, 1989), we predicted that family satisfaction would correlate most highly with life satisfaction in collectivist cultures.

Financial Satisfaction and Life Satisfaction

We predicted that the importance of financial satisfaction also would vary across cultures. In this case, we hypothesized that financial satisfaction would vary as a predictor of life satisfaction depending on the economic level of the society. Veenhoven (1991) hypothesized that income has a stronger relation to global well-being in poorer nations. Maslow (1954) posited that physiological needs are prepotent over other needs, such as belonging and self-actualization, which appear only after the lower-order needs are fulfilled. Thus, in an impoverished society in which income is low for many people, the most basic needs may not be met for everyone. In contrast, in a wealthier society most people will have fulfilled their physiological needs, and therefore needs such as belonging, which are less tied to income will be prepotent for many individuals. Thus, Maslow's hierarchy of needs can be used to predict that life satisfaction is most strongly correlated with financial satisfaction in the poorest nations. In support of this hypothesis, E. Diener, Sandvik, Seidlitz, and M. Diener (1993) found only a very weak relation in the United States between income and SWB. Veenhoven found that, across nations, the correlation between SWB and income was strongest in the poorest nations. Our analysis is a conceptual replication of Veenhoven's finding but an extension to financial satisfaction.

Cultural Homogeneity and Life Satisfaction

We used an additional national variable, cultural homogeneity, in analyzing the differences in trends across cultures. *Cultural homogeneity* refers to the degree to which people in a society share the same culture. When a nation is homogeneous, people share the same characteristics, such as language, values, and religion. In a homogeneous society, the family, friends, and self may not stand out as different and therefore may not be as salient of concepts. Therefore, we included a measure of cultural homogeneity to determine whether it moderated the correlation of life satisfaction with friend satisfaction, family satisfaction, and self-satisfaction.

Note that cultural heterogeneity might have been mistaken for the individualism–collectivism dimension in past work. That is, although cultures certainly differ in the degree to which they emphasize the individual versus the group, they also differ in the degree to which people in the culture are similar. It may have been that cultural similarity is separable from individualism but that the two have been conflated in past theoretical work. Thus, an ancillary purpose of the present study was to examine the correlation between individuality and heterogeneity and to determine their joint impact on life satisfaction.

Life Satisfaction Compared with Self-Esteem

Life satisfaction and self-esteem are variables that both represent global evaluations: in the former case an evaluation of a person's entire life and in the latter case a judgment of oneself. Life satisfaction is a construct that is central to the subdiscipline of SWB (e.g., Andrews & Withey, 1976; Diener, 1984), and self-esteem is a cardinal concept in personality research (e.g., Singer, 1984). Although one could argue that these two concepts are distinct because the target of evaluation is different, we asked whether they are empirically distinct: Do participants discriminate these evaluations? We explored the issue in several ways. For example, the constructs ought to show the same pattern of relations with other variables if they are isomorphic. In addition, other variables ought to add little to the prediction of life satisfaction once self-esteem is controlled if the two constructs are virtually identical.

Absolute Levels of Satisfaction

Another purpose of this study was to describe the levels of life satisfaction, self-esteem, and domain satisfactions of college students in various countries. Are most college students satisfied with their lives, with their life domains, and with themselves? The 7-point scale we used to measure satisfaction in this study had a neutral point of 4; above this point were various levels of positive satisfaction, and below this point were varying levels of dissatisfaction. E. Diener and C. Diener (1993) maintained that most people in the United States have a positive level of SWB but also suggested that although most Americans are happy, they rarely report extremely high SWB at the top of the scale. E. Diener and C. Diener hypothesized that there is a set point near the level of "somewhat satisfied" around which SWB fluctuates. Cross-cultural data are needed in part because one potential underpinning for a positive level of well-being in the United States is socialization for positive emotions E. Diener & C. Diener, 1993). If, however, the pattern of somewhat positive well-being persists across nations, this indicates that socialization may not be the reason for widespread reports of moderate SWB.

Sex Differences and Similarities

The last area we examined was the similarity between women and men in their levels of satisfaction. It might be predicted that women have lower levels of life satisfaction and self-esteem because they have traditionally possessed less power and fewer resources than men, whereas in most cultures men possess more freedom and status. Nevertheless, many studies have found only small differences between men and women in SWB (e.g., Herzog, Rodgers, & Woodworth, 1982). Although women often report more negative affect than men, recent studies have shown that, in the United States, their levels of global happiness are close to those of men (Fujita, Diener, & Sandvik, 1991). In the present study we sought to expand past findings in this area in several directions. First, we examined women's and men's life satisfaction in many nations, including non-western societies. Second, we assessed not only global life satisfaction but also satisfaction with the self, family, friends, and finances. Finally, we examined the similarity between the correlates of well-being for women and men. It may be, for instance, that because of socialization practices, satisfaction with self and finances is more predictive of life satisfaction for men, whereas for women the best predictors of life satisfaction are friendship and family satisfaction.

Summary

In the present study we sought to determine whether the correlates of life satisfaction differ across cultures and whether characteristics of the societies could predict these variations. We also hoped to determine whether the predictors of self-esteem varied across cultures. Third, we endeavored to discover whether life satisfaction and self-esteem are discriminable constructs. Another purpose of the study was to explore the generality of the pattern of well-being noted in the United States by E. Diener and C. Diener (1993)—that most people are somewhat satisfied but do not score in the extremely satisfied range. Finally, we examined across cultures the similarity of SWB, self-esteem, and domain satisfaction ratings between women and men.

Method

Participants

The participants were 13,118 college students, 6,519 of whom indicated that they were women and 6,590 of whom indicated that they were men (and 9 who did not indicate their gender). All analyses have somewhat fewer participants than this total, because for a few participants we were missing data for each variable. The participants were from 49 universities in 31 countries on five continents. Colleagues of Alex Michalos of Guelph University collected data in a global study of college students. These colleagues were located at prestigious universities, smaller private colleges, and one junior college. Thus, the respondents represented a broad spectrum of students, although they came primarily from private and elite institutions. The data used here are the same as those described in Michalos (1991), except that several nations and some participants were dropped from this analysis. The data from several countries were unreadable or unavailable in a standard computer format and so were not included. Furthermore, the data of some individual participants were irregular and were deleted before the data analyses. Michalos reported that students came primarily from various introductory classes and therefore more than half of the participants were in their first or second year of college. The major area of study of respondents did not influence the results. Eighty percent of the sample were in the 17- to 25-year-old age range, 90% were single, and 63% were not employed. The vast majority of respondents were native-born citizens in the nation where the data were collected. Michalos (1991) argued that, although the sample cannot be considered representative of the world's college students, it is the most diverse and broad college student sample collected to date.

   The analyses in each nation were computed across all respondents in that country. The nations that were sampled were diverse and came from the following areas: Africa (5), Asia (5), Europe (8), Latin America (3), Middle East (4), North America (3, including Mexico), and the Pacific (3). In some countries only one university participated (e.g., Chile), in several nations two or three colleges were represented (e.g., Philippines), and in other nations there were four or more universities participating (e.g., Canada). To later examine the impact of status of university on the findings, we rated the colleges from 1 (the most prestigious university in the nation) to 4 (a junior college). When several colleges in a nation participated, we computed a mean status value across the universities.

Measures

Respondents completed a demographic sheet that contained questions about age, gender, and other general information. On the following page they rated their satisfaction with 12 life domains (e.g., family, friends, and finances) on a scale from 1 (*terrible*) to 7 (*delightful*), with the option of also responding with *no opinion*. Of the 12 domain satisfaction reports, we used satisfaction with family, friends, self, and finances in this study. Satisfaction with life as a whole was measured on the same 7-point *delighted–terrible* scale at the end of the 12 domains. Family, friendships, and finances were rated toward the beginning, satisfaction with self was rated 10th (followed by transportation and education), and life satisfaction was rated last. The order of ratings was the same in all locations. We counted the no-opinion responses as missing data. The following are the percentages of respondents who expressed no opinion in each domain: Life satisfaction, 3%; Self-esteem, 2%; Family satisfaction, 1%; Financial satisfaction, 2%; and Friendship satisfaction, 1%.

The questionnaire also contained many comparative judgments (e.g., how the participants compare with others) that were not analyzed in this study and came after the ratings we analyzed. The questionnaires were translated from English into the native language in 19 of the nations and were typically administered in large group settings. Investigators collected the data from both classroom volunteers and from participant-pool respondents, depending on the location. On request, Michalos (1991) provided the findings to researchers who had assisted in collecting the data.

External Nation Data

We obtained gross national product (GNP) data from Michalos (1991), except for Puerto Rico, which we obtained from Hoffman (1991). The income figures reflect per capita GNP for 1983 (and for 1985 for Puerto Rico). These years were used because the self-reports were collected in 1984–1986. The mean income per person was $4,676, with a standard deviation of $4,297. Ratings of the 31 countries on a 10-point scale of individualism versus collectivism were obtained from H. C. Triandis (personal communication, August 1, 1992). A 1 denoted the most collectivistic country and 10 denoted the most individualistic. The mean collectivism score on a scale of 1–10 was 5.4, with a standard deviation of 2.3. The rater was unaware of the data set being used and the questions being asked in this study. The individualism ratings correlated substantially with the individualism index of nations reported by Hofstede (1980), $r(19) = 0.72$, $p < 0.001$. A heterogeneity rating of nations was obtained from Estes (except for Bahrain and Puerto Rico). Estes (1986) ranked nations on their cultural homogeneity versus heterogeneity by summing three variables: the percent speaking the most common language, the percent sharing the dominant religion, and the percent of the nation who were in the same ethnic group. He ordered the nations from most homogeneous (a score of 1) to most heterogeneous (a score of 124). The objective ratings of nations can be seen in Table 1. The heterogeneity ratings are identical for some nations because countries received the same score when there were ties.

Table 1 Characteristics of nations

Nation	GDP/person	Ind.–collectivism[a]	Heterogeneity[b]
Austria	9,218	8	11
Bahrain	10,401	3	–
Bangladesh	129	1	17
Brazil	2,032	4	1
Cameroon	845	2	122
Canada	12,284	9	85
Chile	1,920	6	53
Egypt	672	5	28
Finland	10,725	8	11
Germany	11,403	8	17
Greece	3,932	7	1
India	262	4	85
Israel	5,420	6	74
Japan	10,154	4	1
Jordan	1,690	3	11
Kenya	347	3	114
Korea	1,978	3	17
Mexico	2,154	5	62
Netherlands	9,869	9	53
New Zealand	7,709	9	44
Norway	4,007	7	1
Philippines	724	5	108
Puerto Rico	5,477	7	–
Singapore	6,653	5	78
South Africa	2,424	3	96
Spain	4,780	6	61
Tanzania	240	3	124
Thailand	810	4	44
Turkey	1,210	4	28
United States	14,172	10	34
Yugoslavia	2,500	6	89

Note. GDP = gross domestic product; Ind. = individualism. Dashes indicate data not available.
[a] Numbers are ratings on a scale that ranged from 1 (*most collectivistic*) through 10 (*most individualistic*).
[b] Numbers are ratings on a scale that ranged from 1 (*most homogeneous*) to 124 (*most heterogeneous*).

Results

Correlates of Life Satisfaction

Four variables (satisfaction with self, family, friends, and finances) were correlated with life satisfaction across all respondents in all nations. All correlations were moderately strong, and with approximately 12,600 participants, were all highly significant: self-esteem, $r = 0.47$; family satisfaction, $r = 0.36$; satisfaction with finances, $r = 0.37$; and satisfaction with friends, $r = 0.39$. The four types of satisfaction were used to predict life satisfaction in a linear regression equation. Self-esteem was the strongest predictor, although all variables had highly significant standardized βs. The multiple R with 4 and 12,267 df was 0.61 ($p < 0.0001$) and the standardized βs were: self-esteem, 0.32; financial satisfaction, 0.24; friendship satisfaction, 0.21; family satisfaction, 0.15.

The correlations between the predictors and life satisfaction within individual nations can be seen for women in Table 2 and for men in Table 3. The Ns for respondents who reported both life satisfaction and gender data are also shown for each country. The average correlations shown at the bottom of the tables were computed by transforming the rs to zs, averaging the zs, and then transforming the average zs back to rs. As can be seen, the averages of the correlations within nations were very similar to the correlations across all participants. Note that the four variables

Table 2 Correlations between life satisfaction and satisfaction with self, finances, and family for women

Nation	N^a	Self-esteem	Finances	Family	Friends
Austria	194	0.52	0.23	0.28	0.45
Bahrain	221	0.21	0.53	0.41	0.22
Bangladesh	88	0.27	0.52	0.33	−0.05*
Brazil	163	0.40	0.43	0.43	0.43
Cameroon	29	0.07*	0.36*	0.00*	0.12*
Canada	985	0.60	0.26	0.33	0.41
Chile	115	0.57	0.37	0.31	0.33
Egypt	118	0.45	0.41	0.39	0.22
Finland	161	0.65	0.41	0.56	0.45
Germany	257	0.51	0.34	0.33	0.48
Greece	80	0.51	0.34	0.20	0.33
India	83	0.08*	0.39	0.33	0.31
Israel	154	0.22	0.11*	0.29	0.42
Japan	218	0.44	0.45	0.31	0.09*
Jordan	54	0.30	0.51	0.52	0.12*
Kenya	115	0.59	0.52	0.50	0.56
Korea	50	0.61	0.33	0.20	0.36
Mexico	65	0.42	0.48	0.35	0.25
Netherlands	194	0.47	0.24	0.40	0.56
New Zealand	202	0.58	0.42	0.27	0.41
Norway	136	0.47	0.19	0.15*	0.22
Philippines	645	0.42	0.45	0.44	0.37
Puerto Rico	132	0.52	0.36	0.47	0.21
Singapore	213	0.49	0.30	0.38	0.40
South Africa	154	0.39	0.35	0.29	0.24
Spain	138	0.38	0.34	0.17*	0.22
Tanzania	70	0.62	0.67	0.46	0.33
Thailand	307	0.37	0.40	0.31	0.28
Turkey	90	0.35	0.52	0.10*	0.44
United States	819	0.60	0.36	0.41	0.41
Yugoslavia	155	0.47	0.29	0.46	0.32
M	6,405	0.45	0.39	0.34	0.33

^{a} N for life satisfaction.
* ns at $p < 0.05$.

Table 3 Correlations between life satisfaction and satisfaction with self, finances, family, and friends for men

Nation	N[a]	Self-esteem	Finances	Family	Friends
Austria	125	0.55	0.38	0.44	0.47
Bahrain	54	0.44	0.52	0.23*	0.28
Bangladesh	174	0.04*	0.22	0.19	0.17
Brazil	105	0.31	0.44	0.37	0.46
Cameroon	130	0.42	0.40	0.39	0.46
Canada	615	0.59	0.25	0.39	0.49
Chile	141	0.37	0.26	0.43	0.35
Egypt	156	0.24	0.34	0.24	0.27
Finland	109	0.56	0.40	0.35	0.41
Germany	283	0.49	0.24	0.37	0.45
Greece	84	0.35	0.46	0.31	0.36
India	151	0.40	0.35	0.24	0.34
Israel	163	0.42	0.31	0.40	0.53
Japan	982	0.34	0.29	0.29	0.37
Jordan	225	0.37	0.50	0.36	0.24
Kenya	153	0.42	0.48	0.38	0.43
Korea	191	0.57	0.53	0.35	0.36
Mexico	155	0.43	0.36	0.31	0.44
Netherlands	158	0.35	0.21	0.26	0.51
New Zealand	112	0.61	0.09*	0.28	0.44
Norway	86	0.59	0.36	0.29	0.39
Philippines	308	0.41	0.44	0.37	0.28
Puerto Rico	165	0.50	0.34	0.40	0.56
Singapore	43	0.62	0.16*	0.57	0.41
South Africa	121	0.25	0.36	0.29	0.25
Spain	137	0.39	0.41	0.35	0.41
Tanzania	152	0.54	0.69	0.43	0.25
Thailand	264	0.41	0.34	0.35	0.35
Turkey	197	0.38	0.33	0.44	0.39
United States	415	0.56	0.40	0.41	0.48
Yugoslavia	177	0.50	0.45	0.43	0.63
M	6, 331	0.44	0.37	0.36	0.40

[a] *N* for life satisfaction.
* *ns* at $p < 0.05$.

were significant correlates of life satisfaction in most nations for both genders. Only a few of the correlations within nations were not significantly different from 0. For example, of the correlations between self-esteem and life satisfaction, only 3 of 62 correlations were not significant at $p < 0.05$.

The conclusion from the above analyses is that satisfaction in the four life domains are highly significant predictors of life satisfaction across all respondents and also within virtually all nations. Despite the general pattern, we should also inquire whether the correlations were homogeneous across nations. We conducted a meta-analysis of the correlations within each of the four domains within each sex across the 31 countries (Hedges & Olkin, 1985). We asked whether the 31 correlations for each predictor (within the same sex) were drawn from the same population. These meta-analyses revealed a significant amount of heterogeneity in virtually every case. For example, the chi-square value of 157.60 (30, $N = 31$) for women for the correlations between self-esteem and life satisfaction indicates that the 31 correlations form a heterogeneous set that is not drawn from the same underlying distribution. Except for the correlations for men between family and life satisfaction, all the distributions of correlations showed significant heterogeneity at $p < 0.01$ or less.

The next question is whether the size of the correlations can be predicted from characteristics of the societies. For the self, family, and friend satisfaction correlations, the individualism–collectivism of the nations was used to predict the size of the correlations. We transformed the correlations within each sex within each nation to zs and correlated these with the individualism scores across societies. The individualism of the nations correlated significantly for women, $r(29) = 0.53$, $p < 0.01$, with the size of the life satisfaction and self-esteem relation. This was also true for men, $r(29) = 0.53$, $p < 0.01$, indicating that the size of the relation between life satisfaction and satisfaction with the self was higher in individualistic nations and lower in collectivistic countries. We examined whether this relation might be affected by the variability within nations. Collectivism correlated with variability for men for both life satisfaction and self-esteem (rs $= -0.40$ and -0.41, ps < 0.05) but not for women. When variability (as reflected in the within-nation standard deviations) of life satisfaction and self-esteem was controlled in the life satisfaction and self-esteem correlation as it related to individualism, it made virtually no change in the correlations for either men or women. Because the status of colleges ranged from the most elite to a junior college, we also controlled the ranking of colleges in the major finding above. College status ranking across nations did not correlate with the individualism of the countries, nor did controlling it change the impact of individualism on the life satisfaction and self-esteem relation.

We also correlated the level of individualism with the transformed correlations for family and friendship satisfaction. Contrary to expectation, the family correlations did not differ with the individualism of nations; the relations were quite small and nonsignificant. Recall that for men there was not significant heterogeneity in correlations for family satisfaction across countries. For friend satisfaction, there was a strong positive relation between individualism and the size of the correlations between friend satisfaction and life satisfaction for women, $r(29) = 0.53$, $p < 0.01$; and for men, $r(29) = 0.59$, $p < 0.001$. These correlations indicate that the size of the relation between friendship satisfaction and life satisfaction was strongly dependent on the degree of individualism of the country, with the correlation between friendship satisfaction and life satisfaction being stronger in individualistic nations. In contrast, the homogeneity of the society did not significantly moderate the relation between life satisfaction and any of the predictor variables. Furthermore, we found that homogeneity did not, when used as a control variable, change the impact of individualism on the life satisfaction and self-esteem correlation. It is noteworthy that the individualism of a society correlated only -0.24, ns, with its heterogeneity.

In the domain of financial satisfaction, we correlated the transformed correlations with life satisfaction across countries with the income per person of the society. The size of the relation between financial satisfaction and life satisfaction (r to z transformed) across countries varied inversely with income for women, $r(29) = -0.36$, $p < 0.05$, and was of borderline significance for men, $r(29) = -0.32$, $p < 0.10$. Thus, financial satisfaction tended to be a stronger predictor of life satisfaction in poor than in wealthy nations.

Correlates of Self-Esteem

Self-esteem covaried significantly with each of the three other satisfaction domains across the entire sample: friend satisfaction, $r(12, 848) = 0.31$, $p < 0.001$; family satisfaction, $r(12, 816) = 0.28$, $p < 0.001$; and financial satisfaction, $r(12, 782) = 0.19$, $p < 0.001$. A regression equation predicting self-esteem revealed that friendship satisfaction was the strongest predictor (standardized $\beta = 0.24$, $p < 0.0001$), followed by family satisfaction (standardized $\beta = 0.19$, $p < 0.0001$). Although financial satisfaction was a weaker predictor (standardized $\beta = 0.11$), it was also highly significant given the large sample size. The covariation between self-esteem and the predictors is presented for both sexes in Table 4. As can be seen, the average correlation with self-esteem was strongest for satisfaction with friends and weakest for satisfaction with finances. Self-esteem covaried significantly with friend and family satisfaction in most societies for both sexes. In contrast, financial satisfaction was not a significant correlate of self-esteem in about one half of the nations.

We computed meta-analyses for each predictor variable separately for each sex. All distributions of correlations were significantly heterogeneous, with the female friend correlations reaching $p < 0.05$ and the other distributions being significant at $p < 0.01$. For example, the chi-square $(30, N = 31)$ for the female family correlations was 77.63 ($p < 0.01$), indicating that the correlations within nations were drawn from different distributions.

However, unlike the case for life satisfaction, the self-esteem correlations were not related to the individualism of the nations, or to their income levels. We found that the correlation between self-esteem and family satisfaction in countries depended significantly on the heterogeneity of the nation: female $r(27) = 0.45$, $p < 0.05$; male $r(27) = 0.42$, $p < 0.05$. In more homogeneous nations there was a smaller relation between self-esteem and satisfaction with one's family.

Life Satisfaction Compared with Self-Esteem

We conducted a number of analyses to explore the discriminant validity of self-esteem and life satisfaction. First we made a comparison of the extent to which the two covary with the predictor variables. Across all respondents, life satisfaction correlated more strongly with the predictors than did self-esteem: family satisfaction ($r = 0.36$ vs. 0.28, $p < 0.001$), friend satisfaction ($r = 0.39$ vs. 0.31, $p < 0.001$),

Table 4 Predictors of self-esteem

	Women			Men		
Nation	Friends	Family	Finances	Friends	Family	Finances
Austria	0.32	0.24	0.11*	0.40	0.26	0.22
Bahrain	0.17	0.31	0.20	0.35	0.36	0.24*
Bangladesh	0.19*	0.17*	0.18*	0.32	0.10*	0.06*
Brazil	0.31	0.21	0.10*	0.09*	0.24	0.14*
Cameroon	0.31*	0.46	−0.04*	0.29	0.22	0.04*
Canada	0.29	0.25	0.21	0.39	0.24	0.17
Chile	0.40	0.11*	0.10*	0.19	0.20	0.17
Egypt	0.27	0.21	0.16*	0.18	0.29	0.03*
Finland	0.33	0.44	0.22	0.38	0.14*	0.26
Germany	0.35	0.22	0.08*	0.30	0.13	0.06*
Greece	0.28	0.17*	0.25	−0.01*	−0.15*	0.19*
India	0.32	0.25	0.30	0.21	0.13*	0.23
Israel	0.26	0.22	0.12*	0.36	0.39	0.12*
Japan	0.32	0.34	0.30	0.30	0.26	0.15
Jordan	−0.12*	0.24*	0.49	0.28	0.32	0.27
Kenya	0.57	0.56	0.53	0.39	0.37	0.03*
Korea	0.41	−0.04*	0.02*	0.30	0.17	0.17
Mexico	0.42	0.43	0.20*	0.36	0.28	−0.01*
Netherlands	0.30	0.25	0.13*	0.30	0.21	0.13*
New Zealand	0.27	0.20	0.30	0.34	0.20	−0.06*
Norway	0.23	0.26	0.00*	0.44	0.23	0.22
Philippines	0.27	0.38	0.22	0.35	0.37	0.31
Puerto Rico	0.34	0.33	0.19	0.46	0.24	0.19
Singapore	0.34	0.16	0.15	0.29*	0.21*	0.28*
South Africa	0.19	0.30	0.11*	0.20	0.29	0.08*
Spain	0.24	−0.06*	0.16*	0.12*	0.08*	0.10*
Tanzania	0.43	0.48	0.42	0.46	0.32	0.44
Thailand	0.34	0.20	0.16	0.30	0.24	0.02*
Turkey	0.16*	0.15*	0.17*	0.28	0.25	0.16
United States	0.33	0.30	0.28	0.38	0.38	0.27
Yugoslavia	0.26	0.23	0.21	0.50	0.40	0.07*
M	0.30	0.26	0.20	0.31	0.24	0.15

* ns at $p < 0.05$.

and financial satisfaction ($r = 0.37$ vs. 0.19, $p < 0.001$). This same pattern can be seen in the average correlations across nations, with the life satisfaction relations being stronger.

Perhaps the strongest case for discriminant validity can be seen in correlations of variables across the two sexes. When mean levels of life satisfaction and self-esteem for nations were correlated across gender, there was strong convergence of the same variables: female and male average life satisfaction correlated $r(29) = 0.92$, $p < 0.001$, and female and male average self-esteem covaried at $r(29) = 0.84$, $p < 0.001$. In contrast, female life satisfaction varied with male self-esteem $r(29) = 0.52$, $p < 0.01$, and male life satisfaction covaried with female self-esteem only $r(29) = 0.25$, ns. The convergent correlations are both significantly larger (McNemar, 1969) than the two multitrait correlations (all $ps < 0.01$). Thus, although self-esteem and life satisfaction appear to be related, men and women from the same nations strongly converge only when the same variable is in question.

Finally, the divergence of life satisfaction and self-esteem can be explored through an analysis of variance (ANOVA) across nations in which life satisfaction and self-esteem were treated as repeated measures (within-subjects) variables. There was not only a significant difference between the two variables, $F(1, 12, 550) = 741.51$, $p < 0.001$, but there also was a significant interaction between variables and nation, $F(30, 12, 550) = 41.45$, $p < 0.001$, indicating that life satisfaction and self-esteem differed in their relative positions when considered across nations.

Satisfaction Levels

Tables 5 and 6 display the mean satisfaction scores for each variable for all nations for women and men, respectively. It can be seen that most means for all five types of satisfaction were positive. Other than financial satisfaction, 247 of 248 means (variables × gender × nations) were above the neutral point of 4.0. This was significantly different than the number of means above neutral that one would expect by chance ($p < 0.0001$). Only Korean women's satisfaction with self fell slightly below the neutral point. The average score across all participants for life satisfaction was 4.82, and for self-esteem it was 5.06. For financial satisfaction, only 38 of 62 means were above neutral, a number not significantly different than what one would expect by chance. The mean across all participants for financial satisfaction was 4.14.

Table 7 shows the percent of women and men in each nation who responded *above* the neutral point for the two key variables of life satisfaction and self-esteem. These figures support the conclusion that the majority of respondents in most nations were above neutral for life satisfaction and self-esteem. As can be seen, a majority of individuals were satisfied with the self (except respondents in Korea and Japan, and women in Spain). Life satisfaction was low not only in the two nations with low self-esteem but also in several very poor countries (e.g., Bangladesh and Cameroon). Across all nations, 70% of women reported a positive level of life satisfaction, and 73% of women reported a positive level of self-esteem. For men, 63% reported positive life satisfaction, and 70% reported a positive level of self-esteem. In contrast, only 8% of women and 14% of men reported life satisfaction below neutral, and 8% of women and 12% of men reported self-esteem below the neutral point of the scale. For financial satisfaction, only 48% of women and 41% of men were above neutral. Thus, with the exception of financial satisfaction, it appears that the majority of respondents reported positive levels of satisfaction in all domains. The highest levels of satisfaction were expressed with friends and family (the percent of positive responses varied from 76 to 81).

Most participants, however, did not report life satisfaction at the top of the scale. Only 4% of the total sample reported a 7 for life satisfaction, a response indicating that their life is "delightful." In the most satisfied nation, only 12% scored at the top of the life satisfaction scale. This small percentage is consistent with E. Diener and C. Diener's (1993) conclusion that, although most respondents are positive,

Table 5 Means and standard deviations for satisfaction with self, finances, family, friends, and life for women

Nation	Self		Finances		Family		Friends		Life	
	M	SD	M	SD	M	SD	M	SD	M	SD
Austria	4.8	1.2	4.3	1.2	5.1	1.3	5.2	1.1	5.0	0.9
Bahrain	5.6	1.3	5.1	1.3	5.8	1.4	5.7	1.2	4.9	1.2
Bangladesh	5.1	1.2	4.4	1.0	5.7	1.2	5.5	1.2	4.5	1.3
Brazil	5.8	1.0	3.9	1.3	5.6	1.3	5.3	1.2	5.0	1.0
Cameroon	5.6	1.0	3.6	1.2	5.1	1.0	5.0	1.0	4.4	0.6
Canada	5.1	1.1	4.0	1.4	5.4	1.2	5.5	1.1	5.1	0.9
Chile	5.0	1.1	4.3	1.1	5.3	1.1	5.3	1.0	4.9	0.8
Egypt	5.1	1.5	4.9	1.0	5.3	1.5	5.5	1.3	4.5	1.1
Finland	5.2	1.1	4.8	1.3	5.9	1.1	5.5	1.2	5.5	1.1
Germany	4.7	1.1	4.1	1.2	5.1	1.3	5.1	1.2	4.7	0.9
Greece	5.0	1.0	4.6	0.8	5.4	1.0	5.2	1.1	4.8	1.0
India	5.1	1.0	4.6	1.1	5.5	1.2	5.2	1.2	4.8	1.0
Israel	5.5	0.9	3.6	1.3	5.7	1.1	5.3	1.1	4.9	0.9
Japan	4.3	1.3	4.0	1.1	5.2	1.3	5.2	1.1	4.3	1.1
Jordan	5.7	1.4	4.7	1.2	5.8	1.3	5.3	1.5	4.5	1.0
Kenya	4.9	1.4	3.7	1.2	5.0	1.4	4.8	1.3	4.4	1.0
Korea	3.9	1.5	4.0	1.4	4.6	1.4	4.6	1.3	4.0	1.4
Mexico	5.4	0.9	4.6	0.9	5.4	1.2	5.2	1.0	5.1	0.8
Netherlands	4.8	1.2	4.7	1.2	5.3	1.4	5.5	1.2	5.2	1.0
New Zealand	4.9	1.0	4.0	1.2	5.2	1.3	5.6	0.9	5.1	1.0
Norway	4.9	1.2	3.9	1.3	5.2	1.1	5.4	1.1	5.1	0.9
Philippines	5.3	0.9	4.6	1.0	5.3	1.2	5.7	1.0	5.0	0.9
Puerto Rico	5.2	1.1	4.7	1.1	5.4	1.1	5.4	1.0	5.0	1.0
Singapore	4.8	0.9	4.3	1.2	4.9	1.0	5.3	1.0	4.8	0.9
South Africa	5.4	1.1	3.3	1.4	5.5	1.0	5.3	1.1	4.6	1.2
Spain	4.3	1.1	4.0	1.1	5.0	1.0	5.2	0.9	4.6	0.9
Tanzania	5.4	1.2	3.8	1.4	5.3	0.8	5.2	0.8	5.0	1.1
Thailand	5.3	1.1	4.2	1.1	5.6	1.3	5.1	1.1	4.6	0.9
Turkey	5.1	1.1	4.2	1.0	5.1	1.3	4.7	1.2	4.2	1.0
United States	5.1	1.2	4.2	1.4	5.5	1.3	5.6	1.1	5.3	1.0
Yugoslavia	4.9	1.3	4.2	1.1	5.3	1.3	5.1	1.2	4.7	1.1

they are not so positive that they report that their life is perfect. In contrast to the life satisfaction findings, 11% of respondents scored at the top of the scale for self-esteem. This percentage is significantly higher than that for life satisfaction, χ^2 (1, $N = 12,934$) $= 389.51$, $p < 0.0001$. In the most positive nation, 33% scored at the top of the self-esteem scale.

Sex Comparisons

Although there were scattered differences between the responses of women and men, the similarities between the two are striking. As mentioned previously, the means across nations for women and men strongly covaried for life satisfaction

Table 6 Means and standard deviations for satisfaction with self, finances, family, friends, and life for men

Nation	Self M	Self SD	Finances M	Finances SD	Family M	Family SD	Friends M	Friends SD	Life M	Life SD
Austria	5.1	1.2	4.3	1.2	4.9	1.4	5.0	1.2	4.9	1.1
Bahrain	6.0	1.1	4.8	1.3	6.0	1.3	5.7	1.4	5.1	1.1
Bangladesh	5.0	1.2	3.9	1.2	5.5	1.4	5.2	1.3	4.2	1.0
Brazil	5.8	1.0	3.6	1.4	5.5	1.4	5.4	1.3	4.9	1.0
Cameroon	5.0	1.3	3.0	1.2	4.6	1.1	4.7	1.1	4.1	1.0
Canada	5.2	1.1	4.1	1.4	5.4	1.2	5.4	1.2	5.1	1.0
Chile	5.3	1.0	4.1	1.1	5.3	1.2	5.1	1.2	5.0	0.9
Egypt	5.3	1.3	4.3	1.3	5.4	1.3	5.5	1.2	4.6	1.1
Finland	5.2	1.2	4.8	1.3	5.4	1.0	5.0	1.1	5.4	0.9
Germany	5.0	1.1	4.2	1.3	4.9	1.1	5.0	1.2	4.7	0.9
Greece	5.1	1.0	4.6	1.2	5.6	1.0	5.3	1.2	5.0	0.9
India	5.2	1.3	4.5	1.3	5.4	1.3	5.1	1.5	4.7	1.1
Israel	5.5	0.9	3.5	1.5	5.6	1.2	5.0	1.0	5.0	0.9
Japan	4.0	1.3	3.8	1.2	5.0	1.3	5.0	1.2	4.1	1.0
Jordan	5.5	1.3	4.3	1.4	5.7	1.3	5.5	1.2	4.5	1.2
Kenya	5.2	1.2	3.5	1.3	5.3	1.1	5.1	1.3	4.5	1.0
Korea	4.2	1.5	4.0	1.5	5.3	1.4	5.2	1.2	4.3	1.5
Mexico	5.3	0.9	4.3	1.0	5.3	1.0	5.1	0.9	5.1	0.8
Netherlands	5.3	1.0	4.5	1.4	5.4	1.1	5.6	1.1	5.1	1.0
New Zealand	5.0	1.0	4.3	1.3	5.2	1.3	5.2	1.1	5.1	0.9
Norway	5.0	1.0	4.4	1.3	5.3	1.0	5.1	1.1	5.2	0.9
Philippines	5.3	1.0	4.8	1.0	5.5	1.2	5.7	1.1	5.2	1.0
Puerto Rico	5.6	1.1	4.6	1.0	5.6	1.0	5.5	1.0	5.3	0.9
Singapore	5.2	0.9	4.6	1.0	4.4	1.5	5.1	1.0	4.7	0.9
South Africa	5.3	1.1	2.8	1.4	5.4	1.2	5.3	1.1	4.4	1.1
Spain	4.7	1.1	3.8	1.3	4.7	1.1	5.2	0.9	4.5	0.9
Tanzania	5.6	1.2	3.7	1.4	5.4	1.0	5.2	1.0	5.0	1.3
Thailand	5.5	1.2	3.8	1.2	5.3	1.3	5.1	1.1	4.6	1.0
Turkey	5.2	1.1	4.0	0.9	5.2	1.3	4.9	1.2	4.2	1.0
United States	5.3	1.1	4.2	1.4	5.3	1.3	5.5	1.2	5.3	1.0
Yugoslavia	5.0	1.3	4.2	1.3	5.3	1.3	5.1	1.3	4.7	1.2

and self-esteem. They also covaried for family satisfaction, $r(29) = 0.65$, $p < 0.001$; friend satisfaction, $r(29) = 0.65$, $p < 0.001$; and financial satisfaction, $r(29) = 0.79$, $p < 0.001$. There was also strong convergence for the percentages of people above neutral. For example, the percentage of women and percentage of men in countries who scored above neutral on life satisfaction correlated 0.95 across nations.

At the individual level, the correlational patterns between life satisfaction and the predictors were similar for men and women, and this also was true in the case of self-esteem. The covariation across individual participants between self-esteem and life satisfaction was 0.47 for women and 0.48 for men (ns difference). None of the correlations between self-esteem and the predictors were significantly different for women and men: family satisfaction ($rs = 0.29$ and 0.28), friendship satisfaction ($rs = 0.30$ and 0.33), and financial satisfaction ($rs = 0.20$ and 0.17). For life

Table 7 Percentage of respondents above neutral on well-being

Nation	Men		Women	
	Life satisfaction	Self-esteem	Life satisfaction	Self-esteem
Austria	71	72	70	64
Bahrain	72	87	72	83
Bangladesh	27	67	33	77
Brazil	70	90	70	90
Cameroon	35	69	45	89
Canada	78	77	79	75
Chile	76	79	73	73
Egypt	63	78	52	76
Finland	87	74	84	79
Germany	66	68	65	59
Greece	68	85	66	69
India	62	75	67	78
Israel	75	88	76	88
Japan	36	34	37	46
Jordan	60	85	54	87
Kenya	53	75	56	71
Korea	49	45	44	38
Mexico	83	86	80	83
Netherlands	80	82	78	60
New Zealand	79	75	73	68
Norway	83	75	83	73
Philippines	81	84	76	82
Puerto Rico	87	81	76	75
Singapore	58	83	69	68
South Africa	59	80	59	86
Spain	54	60	61	42
Tanzania	69	81	71	77
Thailand	56	81	52	78
Turkey	39	78	47	78
United States	83	78	82	72
Yugoslavia	66	73	61	63
Across nations	63	70	70	73

satisfaction, family satisfaction was not a differential predictor for the two sexes ($rs = 0.36$ and 0.35). Because of the large sample, small differences in correlations were significant in the case of life satisfaction and friendship satisfaction, $rs = 0.37$ and 0.40, $t(12, 658) = 2.36$, $p < 0.05$ and financial satisfaction, $rs = 0.34$ and 0.38, $t(12, 590) = 2.70$, $p < 0.01$. Striking similarities in the average correlations across sexes can be seen in Tables 2, 3, and 4.

In the case of means, ANOVAs revealed significant sex differences for most variables, however, the discrepancies were quite small in absolute terms. Across all respondents, women and men did not differ significantly on life satisfaction ($Ms = 4.78$ and 4.79). On the other four variables, there were small but significant differences (female means listed first): self-esteem, $Ms = 5.07$ versus 5.18, $F(1, 12, 924) = 18.28$, $p < 0.001$; family satisfaction, $Ms = 5.34$ versus 5.28, $F(1, 12, 980) = 5.29$, $p < 0.05$; friend satisfaction, $Ms = 5.27$ versus 5.21,

$F(1, 13,014) = 6.24$, $p < 0.05$; and financial satisfaction, $Ms = 4.23$ versus 4.09, $F(1, 12,948) = 24.25$, $p < 0.001$. The picture is one of striking similarities rather than dramatic differences.

Discussion

Life satisfaction was significantly correlated with satisfaction with the self, both across the entire sample and also in most nations. The correlations were found, however, to significantly differ in size across societies. When the individualism of the countries was related to the correlations, we found that the covariation between self-esteem and life satisfaction was lower in collectivistic nations. Similarly, satisfaction with friends and with family covaried with life satisfaction, and these correlations also varied significantly and systematically across nations. The individualism of a society correlated positively with the friendship satisfaction and life satisfaction relation, indicating that satisfaction with friends was a weaker correlate of life satisfaction in collectivistic societies. Contrary to expectations, the relation between family satisfaction and life satisfaction was not stronger in collectivistic societies. Finally, the strength of the financial satisfaction and life satisfaction relation was dependent on the income of a country; there was a stronger covariation of financial satisfaction with life satisfaction in poorer societies.

Our results on financial satisfaction support Veenhoven's (1991) hypothesis that the economic condition of a nation moderates the relation between financial satisfaction and life satisfaction. There was a greater correlation between financial satisfaction and life satisfaction in less wealthy countries, supporting the idea of a need hierarchy in which finances become less important to people once they have met their basic physical needs. Similarly, E. Diener et al. (1993) found a curvilinear relation in the United States between income and SWB, showing that income had little influence at the upper levels of wealth. These findings point to a decreasing marginal utility for money as one climbs the income ladder. Once most people obtain an adequate level of a resource such as money to meet the goals prescribed by societal norms, that resource may correlate less with SWB. In poor societies, however, many people probably still lack the goods and services that are seen as important to happiness in that culture, and therefore the amount of money the person has is a stronger causal factor in her or his happiness. The importance of the present finding is in showing that finances can vary in importance to SWB, depending on objective characteristics of the society. People certainly vary in financial satisfaction in wealthier nations, but this has little impact on their life satisfaction, because other goals have come to the fore.

Our findings do not support the contention that wealthier nations are more materialistic, valuing material good to the exclusion of all else. For example, family satisfaction was high and correlated with life satisfaction in wealthier nations. This set of findings supports the idea of a postindustrial society in which attention turns from the acquisition of material goods to self-development and other pursuits.

The correlates of self-esteem also differed across nations. Financial satisfaction, family satisfaction, and friendship satisfaction, all showed significantly varying correlations with self-esteem across countries. In this case, however, heterogeneity of the society in some cases moderated the relations. The covariation between self-esteem and family satisfaction was lower in homogeneous nations for both men and women. Several explanations of this relation are possible. It might be, for example, that a person's feelings about him- or herself are more dependent on the family in a heterogeneous culture because it is primarily within the family that values are shared. Or it may be that in a heterogeneous culture one's self and family stand out together as separate from the society. The relation between self-esteem and family satisfaction deserves further research attention.

The results of the present study have clear implications for the importance of cross-cultural replication of psychological findings. Self-esteem and life satisfaction have been found to be closely related in studies within the United States. If we stopped with this finding alone, however, we would be unaware that the relation between self-esteem and life satisfaction differs across cultures. Indeed, even if we replicated the finding in a nonwestern culture, we might find that self-esteem and life satisfaction were correlated significantly greater than 0, and thus not recognize the influence of culture. Thus, our findings point to the necessity of replicating studies across diverse cultures before they can be accepted as universal. Furthermore, our results point to the need for examining whether effect sizes systematically vary across cultures.

The fact that the influence of self-esteem on life satisfaction differs by cultures follows theoretically from the idea that individualists are socialized to attend to their own internal attributes. Thus, a person's unique attitudes, emotions, and cognitions are highly salient characteristics when making judgments about life in individualistic cultures. Therefore, it is not surprising that how a person feels about him- or herself is more strongly correlated with life satisfaction when the individual is the focus of attention. In contrast, collectivists are socialized to view their place in the social order as of utmost importance. Collectivists are socialized to fit into the community and to do their duty. Thus, how a collectivist feels about him- or herself is less relevant to his life satisfaction than is his or her view of whether he or she behaves properly in the organized social order. Thus, life satisfaction for the collectivist may be more externally based. In fact, life satisfaction itself is less likely to be a salient concept for the collectivist and therefore may correlate at lower levels with predictor variables because it is a less well-formed judgment and therefore more likely to be influenced by momentary or normative factors (Diener, Suh, Smith, & Shao, 1995).

An additional explanation for the differential importance of self-esteem in collectivist and individualistic nations is in terms of the socialization of affect. Diener et al. (1995) found that students in the United States believe positive affect to be more normative, whereas students in Korea and China were more accepting of the experience of negative affect. On the basis of this finding, one can hypothesize that life satisfaction may be based more on positive feelings in individualistic nations, for example feelings, about the self. Conversely, in collectivist nations life satisfaction might be influenced by a more prevalent negative focus and therefore be more dependent on how many problems and social conflicts the person faces.

There has been a search in the SWB literature for *the* causes of well-being. This study clearly reveals that those causes may differ across cultures. Veenhoven (1991) showed that the influence of income on SWB differs across nations. Diener and Fujita (1995) found that the predictors of individual SWB differed in an analogous manner. Based on a person's goals, different resources predicted her or his happiness. Taken together, these results clearly indicate that there are different predictors of happiness for different people and in different societies.

One issue we addressed in the present article is whether self-esteem and life satisfaction are truly discriminable constructs, and our data indicate that they are. The level of life satisfaction of men correlated very strongly across nations with the level of life satisfaction of women in that country, but at a much lower level with self-esteem. Similarly, the levels of self-esteem of men and women correlated quite strongly across nations, but at a weaker level with life satisfaction. More important, variables such as financial and family satisfaction are related to life satisfaction beyond the influence of self-esteem. Finally, life satisfaction and self-esteem change their relative positions in comparison with each other across nations. Thus, although self-esteem is likely to influence life satisfaction (or vice versa), the two variables are clearly discriminable.

The present study demonstrates that college students from around the world are predominantly satisfied with their lives, with themselves, and with the social domains of family and friends. This conclusion, however, must be circumscribed in several ways. First, it is based on college students rather than on nationally representative samples. The second point that must be made in delimiting the present findings is that the majority of university students were satisfied with their finances in only slightly more than half of the countries. Across societies, only 44% of college students showed slight to strong satisfaction with their finances. If positive levels of satisfaction are the rule, why might college students be dissatisfied with their finances? They may have very high aspirations but be unable to meet them, or they may feel that their current finances are marginal but that their situation will improve dramatically when they graduate. College students may not adapt their aspirations to their financial level in order to be more satisfied because they expect their financial status to improve dramatically.

The results also support the arguments of E. Diener and C. Diener (1993) in that most respondents, although positive, were not extremely positive: Most did not respond at the top of the scale. The picture drawn by Diener and Diener is that most people in the United States are somewhat happy and satisfied but have room for improvement. The international college student data present the same picture.

It is notable that cultural homogeneity and collectivism were not significantly correlated. In fact, the correlation was in the direction that more heterogeneous societies were more collectivistic. This finding suggests that there may be two important dimensions that influence how people view their social worlds. One dimension influences whether others are viewed as similar or dissimilar, and the second dimension affects whether one makes sharp distinctions between ingroup and outgroup members. Conceptualizing societies with these two dimensions suggests a fourfold typology in which strangers may be seen as similar but either as outgroup members or as simply other individuals who are not differentiated according to the outgroup categorization. Similarly, one's close associates may be either relatively similar to oneself or relatively different from oneself in homogeneous versus heterogeneous cultures, respectively. The differential impact of these national characteristics on the factors that influence life satisfaction suggests that they are theoretically separable. Viewing people as similar or dissimilar from oneself appears to be distinct from viewing people in terms of their group identity or as individuals.

The last set of findings that is noteworthy is the striking similarity between the data for men and women. The strong convergence between the satisfaction responses of the sexes was consonant with most past research, although this research has primarily been conducted in western nations. Most past studies, however, have focused on the similarity of mean levels between men and women, whereas the present research extends the similarity findings to predictors of life satisfaction and self-esteem. Men and women were similar in satisfaction across domains, suggesting that aspiration levels shift to some degree to match one's life. The marked resemblance between the SWB of women and men in this study may, however, be due to the use of college students as respondents. It may be that college women and men are more similar than others who are following more traditional roles.

The present study possesses several notable strengths: the inclusion of diverse and less westernized nations, a very large sample size and the inclusion of many nations, and a number of important predictor variables. The participants were, however, all college students. This fact may have reduced the differences between the sexes and created higher levels of satisfaction. It should be noted, however, that the homogeneity of the sample is a strength in some respects. For example, the differences between the correlates of life satisfaction and self-esteem across nations are all the more impressive because the participants were all students. Because students are likely to share many attributes and life circumstances across even very different nations, the differences in correlations between various nations is more likely to be due to differences in culture.

There were several unexpected findings in the present research that present interesting directions for additional study. The relation between family satisfaction and life satisfaction was not moderated by collectivism. Further conceptual and empirical examination of the issue seems warranted. The stronger relation between friendship satisfaction and life satisfaction in individualistic cultures was the opposite of our prediction. Post hoc explanations for this finding are certainly possible. For example, it is possible that friends are more important in individualistic cultures because they are chosen rather than imposed. Another possible explanation is that people define "friends" more narrowly in individualistic cultures, so these individuals are quite important to one's life satisfaction.

Acknowledgments Our appreciation is extended to Harry C. Triandis for his assistance in providing individualism–collectivism ratings of the nations and for his comments on drafts of this article. Our warm thanks are also given to Alex Michalos for organizing the raw data on which this article is based. We appreciate the assistance of Marilyn George in preparing the manuscript. Finally, we express our gratitude to Carol Diener for her comments on the article. In a cross-cultural study related to this report, E. Diener, M. Diener, and C. Diener (1995) explored how objective characteristics of nations predict subjective well-being levels in those societies.

References

Andrews, F. M., & Withey, S. B. (1976). *Social indicators of well-being: America's perception of life quality*. New York: Plenum Press.

Campbell, A. (1981). *The sense of well-being in America: Recent patterns and trends*. New York: McGraw-Hill.

Campbell, A., Converse, P. E., & Rodgers, W. L. (1976). *The quality of American life*. New York: Russell Sage Foundation.

Diener, E. (1984). Subjective well-being. *Psychological Bulletin, 95*, 542–575.

Diener, E., & Diener, C. (1993). *Most people in the United States are happy and satisfied*. Unpublished manuscript.

Diener, E., Diener, M., & Diener, C. (1995). Factors predicting the subjective well-being of nations. *Journel of Personality and Social Psychology, 69*, 851–864.

Diener, E., & Fujita, F. (1995). Resources, personal strivings, and subjective well-being: A nomothetic and idiographic approach. *Journal of Personality and Social Psychology, 68*, 926–935.

Diener, E., & Larsen, R. J. (1993). The experience of emotional well-being. In M. Lewis & J. M. Haviland (Eds.), *Handbook of emotions* (pp. 405–415). New York: Guilford Press.

Diener, E., Sandvik, E., Seidlitz, L., & Diener, M. (1993). The relationship between income and subjective well-being: Relative or absolute? *Social Indicators Research, 28*, 195–223.

Diener, E., Suh, E., Smith, H., & Shao, L. (1995). National differences in reported subjective well-being: Why do they occur? *Social Indicators Research, 34*, 7–32.

Estes, R. J. (1986, September). *Trends in global social development, 1970–1986*. Paper presented at the Global Development Conference, College Park, MD.

Fujita, F., Diener, E., & Sandvik, E. (1991). Gender differences in negative affect and well-being: The case for emotional intensity. *Journal of Personality and Social Psychology, 61*, 427–434.

Hedges, L. V., & Olkin, I. (1985). *Statistical methods for meta-analysis*. San Diego, CA: Academic Press.

Herzog, A. R., Rodgers, W. L., & Woodworth, J. (1982). *Subjective well-being among different age groups*. Ann Arbor: University of Michigan Institute for Social Research.

Hoffman, M. S. (1991). *The world almanac and book of facts: 1992*. New York: Pharos Books.

Hofstede, G. (1980). *Culture's consequences*. Beverly Hills, CA: Sage.

Kitayama, S., & Markus, H. R. (in press). Construal of the self as cultural frame: Implications for internationalizing psychology. In H. K. Jacobsen (Ed.), *Internationalization and higher education*.

Maslow, A. H. (1954). *Motivation and personality*. New York: Harper & Row.

McNemar, Q. (1969). *Psychological statistics*. New York: Wiley.

Michalos, A. C. (1991). *Global report on student well-being*. New York: Springer-Verlag.

Singer, J. L. (1984). *The human personality*. San Diego: Harcourt Brace Jovanovich.

Triandis, H. C. (1989). The self and social behavior in differing cultural contexts. *Psychological Review, 96*, 506–520.

Veenhoven, R. (1991). Is happiness relative? *Social Indicators Research, 24*, 1–34.

Goals, Culture, and Subjective Well-Being

Shigehiro Oishi and Ed Diener

Abstract The present studies examined the role of independent and interdependent goal pursuits in the subjective well-being (SWB) of Asian and European American college students. In Study 1, the authors found that independent goal pursuit (i.e., goal pursuit for fun and enjoyment) increased the benefit of goal attainment on SWB among European Americans but not among Asian Americans. In Study 2, the authors found that interdependent goal pursuit (i.e., goal pursuit to please parents and friends) increased the benefit of goal attainment on the SWB of Asian Americans, whereas it did not increase the benefit of goal attainment on the SWB of European Americans. In Study 3, the authors found that whereas interdependent goal pursuit increased the benefit of goal attainment, independent goal pursuit did not increase the benefit of goal attainment among Japanese college students. Altogether, the present findings suggest that independent and interdependent goal pursuits result in divergent affective consequences across cultures.

From daily experiences, all of us must recognize the pervasive role of goals in our lives, because achieving a goal or failing to do so makes our everyday lives enjoyable or miserable. For example, breaking one's personal record in a 5K race, receiving a rejection letter from a journal editor, hosting a successful cocktail party, and giving a horrible lecture are all likely to, at least temporally, influence a person's sense of well-being. Indeed, there is ample evidence that goal attainment is associated with positive emotional experience (Brunstein, 1993) and life satisfaction (Emmons, 1986; see Cantor & Blanton, 1996; Emmons, 1996, for review). But is goal attainment equally good for anyone? Recently, researchers found that the effect of goal attainment on well-being varies depending on individuals' motives (e.g., Brunstein, Schultheiss, & Graessman, 1998; Emmons, 1991; Oishi, Diener, Suh, & Lucas, 1999; Sagiv & Schwarz, 2000; Sheldon & Kasser, 1998). For instance, Sheldon and Kasser (1998) found that goal attainment had a very positive effect for those who pursued their goals for intrinsic reasons (i.e., for the fun and enjoyment they provide)

S. Oishi (✉)
Department of Psychology, University of Virginia, Charlottesville, VA 22904, USA
e-mail: soishi@virginia.edu

E. Diener (ed.), *Culture and Well-Being: The Collected Works of Ed Diener*, Social Indicators Research Series 38, DOI 10.1007/978-90-481-2352-0_5,
© Springer Science+Business Media B.V. 2009

but did not have any positive effect for those who pursued their goals for extrinsic reasons. The question regarding the effect of goal attainment on well-being takes on additional importance in light of cultural variation in goal motivation (e.g., Heine, Lehman, Markus, & Kitayama, 1999; Heine, Takata, & Lehman, 2000; Iyengar & Lepper, 1999; Kitayama, Markus, Matsumoto, & Norasakkunkit, 1997; Markus & Kitayama, 1991, 1994; Triandis, 1995). That is, is the type of person who benefits most from goal attainment the same or different across cultures? The present article tackles this question from the cultural psychological perspective (e.g., Heine et al., 1999; Markus & Kitayama, 1994; Miller, 1999) and examines the role of culture in the link between goal attainment and well-being.

Goals and Culture

Goals have been central constructs in cross-cultural and cultural psychology (e.g., Schwartz, 1992; Triandis, 1995). Most notably, Triandis (1995) distinguished individualist cultures from collectivist cultures by the type of goals that people pursue. He argued that people in individualist cultures tend to pursue personal goals that reflect personal desires, wishes, and needs, whereas people in collectivist cultures tend to pursue communal goals that reflect the desires, wishes, and needs of ingroup members (see also Schwartz, Sagiv, & Boehnke, 2000, for the link between values and daily concerns). In their seminal *Psychological Review* article, Markus and Kitayama (1991) also emphasized the interconnected nature of goals in the interdependent culture and noted that "the goals of others may become so focal in consciousness that the goals of others may be experienced as personal goals" (p. 229). Consistent with this thesis, Iyengar and Lepper (1999) have recently discovered that Asian American schoolchildren enjoyed and performed anagram and math problems better in an imposed condition (i.e., when they were told that the task was chosen by their mother or classmates) than in a free-choice condition. In contrast, European American schoolchildren enjoyed and performed the same problems better in a free-choice condition than in a chosen condition.

Based on the cultural variation in the type of salient goals, Markus and Kitayama (1994) proposed the culture-specific genesis of emotional well-being. These researchers posited that the attainment of culturally prescribed goals, or engagement in culturally appropriate behavior, should feel "good." To the extent that culturally prescribed goals in an independent culture are to stand out, feelings of separation and pride should lead to good feelings in an independent culture. On the other hand, to the extent that culturally prescribed goals in an interdependent culture are to fit in and have harmonious relationships, feelings of connection should lead to good feelings in an interdependent culture. Consistent with these hypotheses, Kitayama, Markus, and Kurokawa (2000) found that the frequency of good feelings was most closely associated with the frequency of friendly feelings in Japan, whereas it was most highly correlated with the frequency of pride in the United States. Also, consistent with the basic idea of Markus and Kitayama (1994), self-esteem (E. Diener & M. Diener, 1995) and freedom (Oishi, Diener, Lucas, & Suh,

1999) were significantly stronger predictors of life satisfaction in individualist cultures than in collectivist cultures. Similarly, relationship harmony had a predictive power of life satisfaction above and beyond self-esteem among Hong Kong students but not among American students (Kwan, Bond, & Singelis, 1997). In addition, the perception of a person's life by important others played a prominent role in predicting Asians' life satisfaction but played only a minor role in predicting European Americans' life satisfaction (Radhakrishnan & Chan, 1997; Suh, 1999). These findings suggest that the well-being of Asians may depend not only on how they view themselves but also on how they are viewed by important others (Heine et al., 1999; Triandis, 1995). Furthermore, the salience of the external perspective among Asians (Suh, 1999) suggests that the type of goal progress conducive to Asians' well-being might be different in an important way from European Americans'.

The Present Studies

Although the previous cross-cultural studies (E. Diener & M. Diener, 1995; Heine & Lehman, 1999; Kwan et al., 1997; Oishi et al., 1999; Suh, 1999; Suh, Diener, Oishi, & Triandis, 1997) found important cultural variations in correlates of well-being, they were limited in two ways. First, because the previous studies relied entirely on global self-reports at one point in time, knowledge of specific processes and causal chains involving subjective well-being (SWB) was notably missing. What predicts changes in well-being? And how do these predictors differ across cultures? Second, despite the fact that goals have been an integral part of the cultural theory of the self (Markus & Kitayama, 1991) and individualism–collectivism (Triandis, 1995), they have not been directly measured and tested in the context of SWB in the previous research. Therefore, the role of goal attainment in SWB has never been examined in the cross-cultural context.

We conducted three studies to address these limitations from the previous research. In these studies, we tested the role of goal attainment and motivation in temporal changes in the well-being of Asians and European Americans. In all studies, participants first evaluated their recent life satisfaction at Time 1. Next, the participants listed the five most important goals for the next month (Study 1) or week (Studies 2 and 3) and rated the degree to which they pursued these goals for independent (Studies 1 and 3) or interdependent (Studies 2 and 3) reasons. Following Sheldon and Kasser (1998), we defined independent goal pursuit as pursuing a goal for the enjoyment and fun that it provides to them. We defined interdependent goal pursuit as pursuing a goal to make parents and friends happy. At Time 2 (i.e., 1 month later in Study 1 and 1 week later in Studies 2 and 3), the participants rated their well-being and their degree of goal attainment. Based on cultural variation in the function of motivation (Heine et al., 1999; Iyengar & Lepper, 1999; Markus & Kitayama, 1991), we hypothesized that progress toward goals pursued for interdependent reasons would lead to positive changes in well-being among Asians, whereas progress toward goals pursued for independent reasons would lead to positive changes in well-being among European Americans. The present studies extend the previous research by (a) providing more direct information on process and causal chains of SWB and (b) examining culture-specific functions of goals and motivation in SWB.

Study 1

Method

Participants

Participants were 87 European Americans (28 men, 57 women, 2 unknown) and 19 Asian Americans (7 men, 12 women) in a semester-long course on personality and well-being at the University of Illinois. The median age for European Americans was 20 years (range from 18 to 25 and older), whereas the median age for Asian Americans was 21 years (range from 18 to 23 years old). Eight of the 19 Asian American participants were born in the United States, and all but 3 participants have lived in the United States for at least 6 years.

Measures and Procedure

Monthly life satisfaction was measured by a 5-item scale based on the Satisfaction With Life Scale (SWLS) (Diener, Emmons, Larsen, & Griffin, 1985). Sample items include, "In most ways my life during the past month was close to ideal," "The conditions of my life during the past month were excellent," and "During the past month, I was satisfied with my life." Participants indicated their agreement on a 7-point scale ($1 = strongly\ disagree$, $2 = disagree$, $3 = slightly\ disagree$, $4 = neither\ agree\ nor\ disagree$, $5 = slightly\ agree$, $6 = agree$, $7 = strongly\ agree$). The mean Time 1 monthly satisfaction was 24.24 ($SD = 5.81$) for European Americans and 21.42 ($SD = 6.69$) for Asian Americans, $t = 1.86$, $p = 0.06$. Cronbach's alpha for the Time 1 monthly satisfaction scale was 0.89 for European Americans and 0.90 for Asian Americans. At Time 1, after completing the monthly life satisfaction scale, the participants listed their five most important goals in the coming month on a separate sheet of the paper. We assessed independent goal pursuit by using the scale developed by Sheldon and Kasser (1998); that is, for each goal, participants indicated their agreement on the statement, "I pursue this goal because of the fun and enjoyment that it provides me" using the 7-point scale ($1 = not\ at\ all\ true$, $7 = absolutely\ true$). The index of independent goal pursuit was computed by taking the average of the ratings for this statement across the five goals. The mean independent goal pursuit was 3.93 ($SD = 1.22$) for European Americans and 3.67 ($SD = 1.56$) for Asian Americans, $t = 0.82$, ns. At Time 2 (exactly 1 month after the first assessment), the participants first rated their monthly satisfaction using the scale described above. The mean Time 2 monthly life satisfaction was 24.88 ($SD = 5.23$) for European Americans and 22.79 ($SD = 6.17$) for Asian Americans, $t = 1.52$, $p = 0.13$. Cronbach's alpha for the Time 2 monthly satisfaction scale was 0.86 for European Americans and 0.91 for Asian Americans.

Then, the goal list was given back individually and the participants rated the degree of goal progress on each goal (i.e., How much did you achieve this goal?) on the 7-point scale ($1 = 0\%$, $4 = $ about 50%, $7 = 100\%$). The index of goal progress was computed by averaging the ratings for the five goals. The mean goal progress was 4.80 ($SD = 1.02$) for European Americans and 4.51 ($SD = 1.32$) for Asian Americans, $t = 0.98$, ns. We did not find any gender difference regarding weekly satisfaction. Also, the key interaction between goal progress and goal motives did not differ across gender in all three studies. Thus, we did not include gender in our analyses below.

Results and Discussion

Time 2 monthly life satisfaction was predicted from Time 1 monthly life satisfaction, independent goal pursuit, goal progress, and the interaction between independent goal pursuit and goal progress for each cultural group using a regression analysis with the centering procedure outlined by Aiken and West (1991). This analysis allowed us to examine the degree to which changes in monthly life satisfaction were predicted from independent goal pursuit, goal progress, and the interaction between independent goal pursuit and goal progress (see Cohen & Cohen, 1983, for details). Replicating the findings of Sheldon and Kasser (1998), we found a significant two-way interaction between goal progress and independent goal pursuit among European Americans ($B = 1.27$, $\beta = 0.22$, $p < 0.05$). As shown by the dotted lines in Fig. 1, the degree of goal progress was, on average, positively associated with an increase in monthly life satisfaction. Furthermore, for European Americans, this tendency was significantly stronger for those who pursued the goals for independent reasons; that is, goal attainment was particularly beneficial to those who pursued their goals for independent reasons among European Americans. On the other hand, the interaction between independent goal pursuit and goal progress was not only nonsignificant but also negative among Asian Americans ($B = -0.24$, $\beta = -0.07$, ns). In other words, the benefit of goal progress was not greater for those Asian Americans who pursued their goals for independent reasons. In fact, the benefit of goal progress for those who pursued their goals for independent reasons was slightly smaller than those who pursued their goals for interdependent reasons (see solid lines in Fig. 1). Thus, Study 1 indicates that whereas independent goal pursuit increases the positive effect of goal attainment on the well-being of European Americans, the positive function of independent goal pursuit does not seem to operate among Asian Americans.

Study 2

We conducted Study 2 to extend Study 1 in several ways. First, because of the small sample size of Asians, the estimates in Study 1 might not be as reliable as desired.

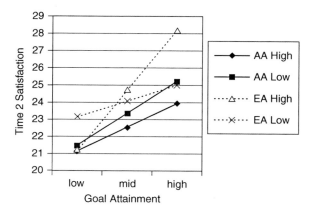

Fig. 1 Adjusted Time 2 monthly satisfaction as a function of goal attainment for Asian Americans with high independent goal pursuit (AA High), Asian Americans with low independent goal pursuit (AA Low), European Americans with high independent goal pursuit (EA High), and European Americans with low independent goal pursuit (EA Low).

Note. The estimated regression equations for European Americans and Asian Americans are as follows: EA : LS2 = 20.04 + 0.18 LS1 + 2.20 GA + 0.30IGP + 1.27GA∗IGP; AA : LS2 = 13.73 + 0.43 LS1 + 1.63 GA − 0.41IGP − 0.24GA∗IGP, where LS2 = Time 2 monthly satisfaction, LS1 = Time 1 monthly satisfaction, GA = standardized goal attainment, and IGP = standardized independent goal pursuit. Following Aiken and West (1991), goal attainment and independent goal pursuit were standardized around the mean before forming the interaction term. The regression *lines* described above were computed using the mean Time 1 monthly satisfaction and 1 *SD* above (*high*) or below (*low*) the mean independent goal pursuit

Thus, we obtained more Asian participants in Study 2. Second, Study 1 did not provide any information as to factors that could contribute to positive changes in the well-being of Asians. Finally, retrospective judgment of life satisfaction and goal attainment over 1 month might have led participants to use their general levels of life satisfaction and goal attainment. To reduce such a memory bias in assessment of goal progress and life satisfaction, we shortened the interval from 1 month to 1 week. This time frame should allow for more reality-based judgment of life satisfaction and goal progress in Study 2 than Study 1. Based on Iyengar and Lepper's (1999) findings on Asian Americans, we predicted that interdependent goal pursuit, or goal pursuit to make parents and friends happy, would enhance the positive effect of goal attainment on the well-being of Asian Americans.

Method

Participants

Participants were 67 European Americans (34 men, 27 women, 6 unknown) and 64 Asian Americans (29 men, 30 women, 5 unknown) enrolled in an introductory psychology course at the University of Illinois.

Measures and Procedure

Weekly satisfaction was assessed by a three-item scale based on the SWLS. The items include, "I am satisfied with the past 1 week of my life" and "The conditions of my life during the last week were excellent." Participants indicated their agreement on a 7-point scale (1 = *strongly disagree*, 4 = *neither agree nor disagree*, 7 = *strongly agree*). The index of weekly satisfaction was computed by taking the average of the ratings for three statements. The mean weekly satisfaction was 4.14 ($SD = 1.22$) for European Americans and 4.12 ($SD = 1.38$) for Asian Americans, $t = 0.09$, *ns*. Cronbach's alpha of the Week 1 satisfaction scale was 0.88 for European Americans and 0.87 for Asian Americans. At Time 1, participants listed the five most important goals for the next 7 days. Then, for each goal, they indicated their agreement with the statement, "I pursue this goal because I want to make my parents and friends happy" on a 7-point scale (1 = *not at all true*, 4 = *somewhat true*, 7 = *absolutely true*). The mean interdependent goal pursuit was 3.70 ($SD = 1.57$) for European Americans and 3.71 ($SD = 1.34$) for Asian Americans, $t = 0.01$, *ns*. At Time 2 (1 week later), the participants returned to the same experimental laboratory and completed the weekly satisfaction scale. The mean Week 2 satisfaction was 4.38 ($SD = 1.35$) for European Americans and 4.57 ($SD = 1.36$) for Asian Americans, $t = -0.70$, *ns*. Cronbach's alpha for the Week 2 satisfaction scale was 0.92 for European Americans and 0.91 for Asian Americans. Next, participants were provided with their own goal lists from Time 1 and rated their progress on each goal ("How much did you achieve this goal?") on the 7-point scale (1 = 0%, 4 = about 50%, 7 = 100%). The index of goal progress was computed by taking the average of the ratings for these five items. The mean goal progress was 4.83 ($SD = 1.16$) for European Americans and 4.75 ($SD = 0.95$) for Asian Americans, $t = -0.40$, *ns*.

Results and Discussion

As in Study 1, Week 2 satisfaction was predicted from Week 1 satisfaction, interdependent goal pursuit, goal progress, and the interaction between interdependent goal pursuit and goal progress for each group. Consistent with Sheldon and Kasser's (1998) findings, there was a significantly negative interaction between interdependent goal pursuit and goal progress among European Americans ($B = -0.32$, $\beta = -0.26$, $t = 2.29$, $p < 0.05$). Among European Americans, the degree to which goal attainment was associated with positive changes in weekly satisfaction was significantly less for those who pursued their goals to make parents and friends happy than for those who did not pursue the goals for interdependent reasons (see dotted lines in Fig. 2). On the other hand, the interaction between interdependent goal pursuit and goal progress was positive and nearly significant among Asian Americans ($B = 0.35$, $\beta = 0.20$, $t = 1.46$, $p = 0.15$) (see solid lines in Fig. 2). The 95% confidence interval for the unstandardized regression coefficient for the interaction term obtained in the Asian sample ranged from -0.13 to 0.82, which excludes the unstandardized regression coefficient for the interaction term

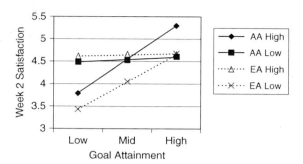

Fig. 2 Adjusted Week 2 satisfaction as a function of goal attainment for Asian Americans with high interdependent goal pursuit (AA High), Asian Americans with low interdependent goal pursuit (AA Low), European Americans with high interdependent goal pursuit (EA High), and European Americans with low interdependent goal pursuit (EA Low).
Note. The estimated regression equations for European Americans and Asian Americans are as follows: EA : LS2 = 2.36+0.48 LS1+0.29GA+0.29DGP−0.32GA∗DGP; AA : LS2 = 3.63+ 0.22LS1+0.40GA+0.00DGP+0.35GA∗DGP, where LS2 = Week 2 satisfaction, LS1 = Week 1 satisfaction, GA = goal attainment, and DGP = interdependent goal pursuit. The regression *lines* described above were obtained using the same procedure as in Study 1

obtained in the European American sample ($B = -0.32$). Furthermore, a regression analysis including both Asian and European Americans (i.e., predicting Week 2 satisfaction from Week 1 satisfaction, culture, goal progress, interdependent goal pursuit, and all the interaction terms) revealed a significant three-way interaction among culture (European vs. Asian Americans), interdependent goal pursuit, and goal progress ($B = -0.33$, $\beta = -0.23$, $t = 2.50$, $p = 0.01$). The three-way interaction indicates the contrasting role of interdependent goal pursuit on the effect of goal attainment on the well-being of Asian and European Americans. As seen in Fig. 2, among Asians, goal progress was more conducive to weekly satisfaction for those who pursued their goals for interdependent reasons, whereas among European Americans, goal progress was less conducive to weekly satisfaction for those who pursued their goals for interdependent reasons. In short, although it replicated the previous research (Sheldon & Kasser, 1998) among European Americans, Study 2 revealed that interdependent goal pursuit, which was considered to be detrimental to well-being, could have a beneficial role in the well-being of Asian Americans.

Study 3

We conducted Study 3 to address three remaining issues from the first two studies. First, although the first two studies provided support for our hypothesis, we did not examine independent and interdependent goal pursuits in the same study. Second, although we followed the previous studies (e.g., Sheldon & Kasser, 1998) in measuring intrinsic goal pursuit ("because of fun and enjoyment that it provides me"), the item we used in Study 1 might not convey the concept of independent goal pursuit well. Also, the item we used for measuring interdependent goal pursuit in

Study 2 ("because I want to make my friends and family happy") might not entirely represent the traditional definition of extrinsic motivation. Third, although we found the expected three-way interaction in Study 2, the two-way interaction between goal attainment and interdependent goal pursuit was not statistically significant among Asian Americans. This could be due to the fact that Asians in Study 2 lived in the United States. Indeed, previous research shows that Asians living in North America tend to show patterns of self-esteem and self-descriptions more individualistic than Asians living in Asia (e.g., Heine et al., 1999; Rhee, Uleman, Lee, & Roman, 1995). To address these issues, in Study 3, we examined both independent and interdependent goal pursuits, included two more items capturing the independent and interdependent nature of goal pursuit, and collected data from Japanese college students living in Japan.

Method

Participants

Participants were 70 Japanese students (20 men, 50 women) at Meisei University in Tokyo, Japan, who were enrolled in a research method course in psychology.

Measures and Procedure

All the materials were prepared in Japanese by the first author and administered in Japanese. Weekly satisfaction was measured by the same three-item scale used in Study 2. The mean weekly satisfaction was 4.44 ($SD = 1.64$) at Time 1. Cronbach's alpha for this scale was .89 at Time 1. As in Study 2, participants listed the five most important goals for the next 7 days at Time 1. Then, for each goal, they indicated their agreement with the following two statements used in Studies 1 and 2 (i.e., "I pursue this goal because of the fun and enjoyment that it provides me," "I pursue this goal because I want to make my parents and friends happy") on a 7-point scale ($1 = $ not at all true, $4 = $ somewhat true, $7 = $ absolutely true). In addition, for each goal, they indicated their agreement with two additional statements: "I pursue this goal for myself, not for others" and "I pursue this goal to meet expectations of others," again on a 7-point scale ($1 = $ not at all true, $4 = $ somewhat true, $7 = $ absolutely true). The descriptive statistics and correlations among four types of goal pursuit (i.e., the mean goal pursuit score across five goals) are shown in Table 1.

At Time 2 (1 week later), the participants returned to the same experimental laboratory and completed the weekly satisfaction scale. The mean Week 2 satisfaction was 4.28 ($SD = 1.57$) at Time 2. Cronbach's alpha for the Week 2 satisfaction scale was 0.93. Next, participants were provided with their own goal lists from Time 1 and rated their attainment on each goal ("How much did you achieve this goal?") on the 100-point scale, ranging from 0 to 100%. To make the rating easier, we changed the goal attainment scale from the artificially devised 7-point scale used in Study 2 to the more natural, 100% scale in this study. The index of goal attainment was computed by taking the average of the ratings for the five goals. The mean goal attainment

Table 1 Descriptive statistics and correlations among four goal motives among Japanese participants in Study 3

Goal motives	1	2	3	4
1. For fun and enjoyment	—	−0.16	0.29*	0.24*
2. For self		—	−0.36**	−0.11
3. For family and friends			—	0.67**
4. For expectations of others				—
M (SD)	3.38 (1.41)	6.49 (0.65)	2.86 (1.27)	2.85 (1.39)

Note. $N = 70$. Goal motives are reasons why they pursued their goals.
*$p < 0.05$; **$p < 0.01$.

was 54.93% ($SD = 20.96$). As recommended by Judd and McClelland (1989, p. 526), we transformed the percentage ratings provided by the participants using a logit transformation to normalize the distribution and the psychological meaning of intervals in percentages. The logit-transformed goal attainment score was used in the following analyses.

Results and Discussion

Goal motives. As seen in Table 1, Japanese participants pursued their goals for themselves to a greater extent than to make friends and family happy, $t(69) = 18.76$, $p < 0.01$, to meet the expectations of others, $t(69) = 19.05$, $p < 0.01$, or for fun and enjoyment, $t(69) = 15.86$, $p < 0.01$. As expected, goal pursuit for self was negatively correlated with goal pursuit to make friends and family happy. Also, as expected, goal pursuit to make friends and family happy was highly correlated with goal pursuit to meet the expectations of others. Interestingly, intrinsic goal pursuit (i.e., for fun and enjoyment) was positively correlated with goal pursuit to make friends and family happy and to meet the expectations of others. Thus, the descriptive statistics and patterns of correlations among goal motives reveal an interesting picture of the Japanese participants. On one hand, these Japanese showed that they pursued their goals for independent reasons. On the other hand, the goals they pursued to make friends and family happy and to meet the expectations of others were the goals that were fun and enjoyable. Here, one can see that so-called extrinsic goal motives (e.g., Sheldon & Kasser, 1998) are highly internalized among the Japanese participants.

Hypothesis testing. As in Studies 1 and 2, Week 2 satisfaction was predicted from Week 1 satisfaction, goal pursuit, goal progress, and the interaction between goal pursuit and goal progress. We repeated this multiple regression analysis for each goal pursuit separately. Consistent with Study 1, the interaction between goal progress and intrinsic goal pursuit (i.e., goal pursuit for fun and enjoyment) was nonsignificant among Japanese college students ($B = 0.02$, $\beta = 0.01$, $t = 0.11$, *ns*); that is, goal progress was no more beneficial for the Japanese who pursued their goals for fun and enjoyment than for those who did not. Similarly, the interaction between goal progress and independent goal pursuit (i.e., goal pursuit for self, not for others) was also nonsignificant ($B = 0.06$, $\beta = 0.06$, $t = 0.41$). Therefore, goal progress was no more beneficial for the Japanese who pursued their goals for themselves than for those who did not. In other words, the previous findings on the positive benefit of intrinsic goal pursuit (e.g., Sheldon & Kasser, 1998) were not replicated with the Japanese.

On the other hand, consistent with Study 2, the interaction between goal progress and goal pursuit to make friends and family happy was marginally positive ($B = 0.37$, $\beta = 0.19$, $t = 1.73$, $p = 0.09$). A simple slope analysis (Aiken and West, 1991) revealed that for the Japanese who pursued their goals to make friends and family happy (1 SD above the mean), goal attainment was associated with a positive change in well-being (e.g., 1 SD increase in goal progress corresponded to 0.52 increase in Week 2 satisfaction). On the other hand, for the Japanese who did not pursue their goals to make their friends and family happy, 1 SD increase in goal attainment corresponded to 0.21 decrease in Week 2 satisfaction. Indeed, the obtained regression equation indicates that when goal attainment was average, those low in this goal pursuit reported slightly higher Week 2 satisfaction than those high in this goal pursuit (4.44 vs. 4.10). Nevertheless, when goal attainment was high, those high in family/friends' goal pursuit reported substantially higher Week 2 satisfaction than those low in parental goal pursuit (4.62 vs. 4.23). Consistent with Study 2, therefore, goal progress translated into a positive change in weekly satisfaction for the Japanese who pursued their goals to make their friends and family happy, whereas it did not bring more satisfaction for the Japanese who did not pursue their goals to this end.

Finally, consistent with our hypothesis, the interaction between goal progress and goal pursuit to meet others' expectations was significantly positive ($B = 0.46$, $\beta = 0.27$, $t = 2.31$, $p = 0.02$). A simple slope analysis revealed that, as can be seen in Fig. 3, 1 SD increase in goal attainment corresponded to 0.70 increase in Week 2 satisfaction for the Japanese high in this goal pursuit. On the other hand, 1 SD increase in goal attainment corresponded to 0.22 decrease in Week 2 satisfaction for the Japanese low in the goal pursuit for others' expectations. More specifically, when goal attainment was high (1 SD above the mean), the Japanese high in this goal pursuit reported much higher satisfaction than those low in this goal pursuit (4.75 vs. 4.25), although when goal attainment was average, the Japanese high in the extrinsic goal pursuit were not as satisfied as those low in the extrinsic goal pursuit (4.08 vs. 4.47). Therefore, goal progress had a more positive benefit for the Japanese who pursue their goals to meet the expectations of others than for those who do not.

General Discussion

In three studies, we examined the role of independent and interdependent goal pursuit on the well-being of Asians and European Americans. Based on recent cross-cultural findings on motivation (Iyengar & Lepper, 1999) and self-construals (Heine et al., 1999; Markus & Kitayama, 1991), we predicted that the function of

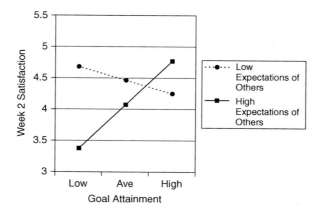

Fig. 3 Adjusted Week 2 satisfaction as a function of goal attainment for Japanese high in goal pursuit to meet expectations of others and low in goal pursuit to meet expectations of others in Study 3.

Note. The estimated regression equation was as follows: $LS2 = 2.34 + 0.436LS1 + 0.244GA - 0.20GPE + 0.46GA^*GPE$, where $LS2$ = Week 2 satisfaction, $LS1$ = Week 1 satisfaction, GA = standardized goal attainment, and GPE = standardized goal pursuit to meet others' expectations. With the mean Week 1 satisfaction = 4.44 in the equation, simple slopes for high and low in goal pursuit to meet the expectations of others (1 SD above or below mean) are as follows: High: $LS2 = 4.08 + 0.70$ GA; Low: $LS2 = 4.48 - 0.216GA$

independent and interdependent goal pursuit on well-being would differ between Asians and European Americans. Consistent with our predictions, Study 1 showed that independent goal pursuit did not enhance the positive effect of goal attainment on the well-being of Asians while amplifying the benefit of goal attainment on the well-being of European Americans. Furthermore, Study 2 demonstrated that interdependent goal pursuit tended to increase the benefit of goal progress among Asians while diminishing the effect of goal progress among European Americans. Finally, Study 3 showed that goal progress was particularly beneficial for the well-being of the Japanese who pursued their goals to make their friends and family happy and to meet the expectations of others. Altogether, the present findings provide evidence that processes through which Asians and European Americans attain their well-being are different. European Americans appear to gain and maintain their well-being by achieving goals that they pursue for their own enjoyment and fun. On the other hand, Asian Americans seem to attain and maintain their well-being by achieving goals that they pursue to make important others happy and meet the expectations of others.

In American psychology, personal choice independent of others has been the sine qua non of spontaneous behavior (Lepper, Greene, & Nisbett, 1973) and mental health (Maslow, 1947; Rogers, 1961). To the extent that individuals pursue and achieve self-chosen goals, and to the extent that individuals feel that they are the driving forces of their lives, they feel good (Sheldon & Kasser, 1998). This theory perfectly captures American icons such as Michael Jordan and Bill Gates.

As evidenced by the idealization of the self-made billionaire, the founder of the Softbank Masayoshi Son in Japan, self-determination has recently become a popular ideology in Asia as well. Indeed, Study 3 showed that on average, Japanese college students pursued their goals for themselves (6.49) much more frequently than to make family and friends happy (2.86) or to meet the expectations of others (2.85). Also, on average, the degree to which Asian participants in Studies 1 and 2 pursued their goals for intrinsic reasons or to make friends and family happy was very similar to European American counterparts. In other words, Japanese participants in Study 3 as well as Asian participants in Studies 1 and 2 are not as "collectivist" or "interdependent" as cultural theorists (e.g., Markus & Kitayama, 1991, 1994; Triandis, 1995) might assume in terms of goal motives. What is interesting, however, is that despite the similar levels of independent and interdependent goal motives across cultures, the very function of goal motives differed considerably across cultures. That is, although both Japanese and European Americans pursue their goals for themselves, such independent goal pursuit does not generate as positive an outcome for Japanese as for European Americans.

Why does independent goal pursuit not work for Asians? One possibility is that because of the traditional value of conformity and deference to authority figures among Asians (e.g., Bond, 1988; Schwartz, 1994), Asians who subscribe to independent goal pursuit are more prone to psychological conflict than European Americans. This conflict, in turn, results in the lack of positive consequence of independent goal pursuit among Asian Americans. Although this explains the cultural difference in the function of independent goal pursuit, this does not fully explain the positive function of interdependent goal pursuit among Asians. Given the ubiquity of the idealization of independence in American culture (Wolfe, 2000), Asians who hold traditional Confucian values may be prone to psychological conflict between conformity and self-determination as much as Asians who prefer the mainstream American values. Thus, the value conflict hypothesis does not seem to fully account for the positive function of interdependent motivation among Asians. Alternatively, a more viable explanation for the current findings can be offered from the cultural theory of the self (Markus & Kitayama, 1991, 1994). According to this theory, Asians' self-concepts are so intertwined with expectations and perceptions by important others that expectations from important others could become their own goals among Asians' interdependent selves. To the extent that their goals overlap with expectations from important others, making their parents and friends happy becomes a key to their own sense of satisfaction. The flip side of this reasoning is that even if Asians achieved the goal they set for themselves, they would not feel satisfied if their parents or friends were not happy about their goals.

Different processes governing the well-being of Asians and European Americans also have an implication for cultural differences in mean levels of SWB. For years, researchers found that people in East Asia were less satisfied with their lives than European and North Americans (e.g., E. Diener, M. Diener, & C. Diener, 1995; Veenhoven, 1993). Whereas the necessary and sufficient condition for happiness for European Americans appears to be to make themselves happy by achieving their self-chosen goals, there seem to be more conditions for Asians. That is, for Asians to be happy they must not only satisfy themselves but also satisfy their parents and friends. To the extent that meeting one condition is easier than multiple ones, European Americans on the average can feel good about their lives more readily than Asians. Although this possibility must be examined more fully in the future, it seems evident that the processes through which people with different self-construals attain their well-being have an immense implication for the mean level of well-being.

Future Directions

In the past, intrinsic motivation was viewed as fundamental and as innate as biological needs such as thirst and hunger (Maslow, 1947; Rogers, 1961). While evidence for the paramount importance of intrinsic motivation among European Americans continues to accumulate, the current findings suggest that intrinsic motivation may not be as biological or fundamental as once thought. Instead, the present findings suggest that the function of motivation is tailored in an important way by culture. Independent goal pursuit appears to be instilled early in life and positively reinforced by the mainstream American culture, whereas consideration for important others seems to be desirable and sometimes demanded in Asian American communities. As a result, expectations from important others seem to be deeply internalized and become integral parts of the self among Asians, which in turn provide standards for evaluating their own life experiences.

It should be noted, however, that the present explanation from the cultural theory of the self (Markus & Kitayama, 1991) remains incomplete in two respects. First, we did not measure self-concepts of Asians and European Americans. Thus, the above explanation is based on the assumption that the interdependent aspect of the self was salient for Asian Americans, whereas the independent aspect of the self was salient for European Americans in the present studies. Second, it is difficult to pinpoint a crucial factor responsible for cultural differences obtained in the present studies. Is it the salience of "I" versus "We"? Is it the value of conformity versus hedonism? Or is it the familiarity of personal choice and independent decision making? These questions still remain. It is critical, therefore, that future research identify the parsimonious conditions for these cultural differences by examining specific factors, such as accessibility of key concepts (e.g., Gardner, Gabriel, & Lee, 1999; Oishi, Wyer, & Colcombe, 2000) and thinking styles (Peng & Nisbett, 1999) in the context of goal progress, motivation, and SWB.

Acknowledgments We thank Professor Hideki Okabayashi for collecting data used in Study 3. We also thank Christie Napa Scollon and Sumie Okazaki for their helpful comments on earlier versions of this article.

References

Aiken, L. S., & West, S. G. (1991). *Multiple regression: Testing and interpreting interactions.* Newbury Park, CA: Sage.
Bond, M. H. (1988). Finding universal dimensions of individual variation in multicultural studies of values: The Rokeach and Chinese value surveys. *Journal of Personality and Social Psychology, 55,* 1009–1015.

Brunstein, J. (1993). Personal goals and subjective well-being: A longitudinal study. *Journal of Personality and Social Psychology, 65,* 1061–1070.

Brunstein, J. C., Schultheiss, O. C., & Graessman, R. (1998). Personal goals and emotional well-being: The moderating role of motive dispositions. *Journal of Personality and Social Psychology, 75,* 494–508.

Cantor, N., & Blanton, H. (1996). Effortful pursuit of personal goals in daily life. In P. M. Gollwitzer & J. A. Bargh (Eds.), *The psychology of action: Linking cognition and motivation to behavior* (pp. 338–364). New York: Guilford.

Cohen, J., & Cohen, P. (1983). *Applied multiple regression/correlational analysis for the behavioral sciences* (2nd ed.). Hillsdale, NJ: Lawrence Erlbaum.

Diener, E., & Diener, M. (1995). Cross-cultural correlates of life satisfaction and self-esteem. *Journal of Personality and Social Psychology, 68,* 653–663.

Diener, E., Diener, M., & Diener, C. (1995). Factors predicting the subjective well-being of nations. *Journal of Personality and Social Psychology, 69,* 851–864.

Diener, E., Emmons, R. A., Larsen, R. J., & Griffin, S. (1985). The Satisfaction With Life Scale. *Journal of Personality Assessment, 49,* 71–75.

Emmons, R. A. (1986). Personal strivings: An approach to personality and subjective well-being. *Journal of Personality and Social Psychology, 51,* 1058–1068.

Emmons, R. A. (1991). Personal strivings, daily life events, and psychological and physical well-being. *Journal of Personality, 59,* 453–472.

Emmons, R. A. (1996). Striving and feelings: Personal goals and subjective well-being. In P. M. Gollwitzer & J. A. Bargh (Eds.), *The psychology of action: Linking cognition and motivation to behavior* (pp. 313–337). New York: Guilford.

Gardner, W. L., Gabriel, S., & Lee, A. Y. (1999). "I" value freedom, but "we" value relationships: Self-construal priming mirrors cultural differences in judgment. *Psychological Science, 10,* 321–326.

Heine, S. J., & Lehman, D. R. (1999). Culture, self-discrepancies, and self-satisfaction. *Personality and Social Psychology Bulletin, 25,* 915–925.

Heine, S. J., Lehman, D. R., Markus, H. R., & Kitayama, S. (1999). Is there a universal need for positive self-regard? *Psychological Review, 106,* 766–794.

Heine, S. J., Takata, T., & Lehman, D. R. (2000). Beyond self-presentation: Evidence for self-criticism among Japanese. *Personality and Social Psychology Bulletin, 26,* 71–78.

Iyengar, S. S., & Lepper, M. R. (1999). Rethinking the value of choice: A cultural perspective on intrinsic motivation. *Journal of Personality and Social Psychology, 76,* 349–366.

Judd, C. M., & McClelland, G. H. (1989). *Data analysis: A model-comparison approach.* Orlando, FL: Harcourt Brace Jovanovich.

Kitayama, S., Markus, H. R., & Kurokawa, M. (2000). Culture, emotion, and well-being: Good feelings in Japan and the United States. *Cognition and Emotion, 14,* 93–124.

Kitayama, S., Markus, H. R., Matsumoto, H., & Norasakkunkit, V. (1997). Individual and collective processes in the construction of the self: Self-enhancement in the United States and self-criticism in Japan. *Journal of Personality and Social Psychology, 72,* 1245–1267.

Kwan, V. S. Y., Bond, M. H., & Singelis, T. M. (1997). Pancultural explanations for life satisfaction: Adding relationship harmony to self-esteem. *Journal of Personality and Social Psychology, 73,* 1038–1051.

Lepper, M. R., Greene, D., & Nisbett, R. E. (1973). Undermining children's intrinsic interest with extrinsic rewards: A test of the "overjustification" hypothesis. *Journal of Personality and Social Psychology, 28,* 129–137.

Markus, H. R., & Kitayama, S. (1991). Culture and the self: Implications for cognition, emotion, and motivation. *Psychological Review, 98,* 224–253.

Markus, H. R., & Kitayama, S. (1994). The cultural construction of self and emotion: Implications for social behavior. In S. Kitayama & H. R. Markus (Eds.), *Emotion and culture* (pp. 89–130). Washington, DC: American Psychological Association.

Maslow, A. (1947). *Motivation and personality.* New York: Harper & Row.

Miller, J. (1999). Cultural psychology: Implications for basic psychological theories. *Psychological Science, 10,* 85–91.

Oishi, S., Diener, E., Lucas, R. E., & Suh, E. M. (1999). Cultural variation in predictors of life satisfaction: A perspective from needs and values. *Personality and Social Psychology Bulletin, 25*, 980–990.

Oishi, S., Diener, E., Suh, E. M., & Lucas, R. E. (1999). Value as a moderator in subjective well-being. *Journal of Personality, 67*, 157–184.

Oishi, S., Wyer, R. S., Jr., & Colcombe, S. (2000). Cultural variation in the use of current life satisfaction to predict the future. *Journal of Personality and Social Psychology, 78*, 434–445.

Peng, K., & Nisbett, R. E. (1999). Culture, dialectics, and reasoning about contradictions. *American Psychologist, 54*, 741–754.

Radhakrishnan, P., & Chan, D.K.-S. (1997). Cultural differences in the relation between self-discrepancy and life satisfaction. *International Journal of Psychology, 32*, 387–398.

Rhee, E., Uleman, J. S., Lee, H. K., & Roman, R. J. (1995). Spontaneous self-descriptions and ethnic identities in individualistic and collectivistic cultures. *Journal of Personality and Social Psychology, 69*, 142–152.

Rogers, C. (1961). *On becoming a person.* Boston: Houghton-Mifflin.

Sagiv, L., & Schwarz, S. H. (2000). Value priorities and subjective well-being: Direct relations and congruity effects. *European Journal of Social Psychology, 30*, 177–198.

Schwartz, S. H. (1992). Universals in the content and structure of values: Theoretical advances and empirical tests in 20 countries. In M. Zanna (Ed.), *Advances in experimental social psychology* (Vol. 25, pp. 1–65). Orlando, FL: Academic Press.

Schwartz, S. H. (1994). Beyond individualism-collectivism: New cultural dimensions of values. In U. Kim, H. C. Triandis, C. Kagtcibasi, S.-C. Choi, & G. Yoon (Eds.), *Individualism and collectivism: Theory, method, and applications* (pp. 85–122). Thousand Oaks, CA: Sage.

Schwartz, S. H., Sagiv, L., & Boehnke, K. (2000). Worries and values. *Journal of Personality, 68*, 309–346.

Sheldon, K. M., & Kasser, T. (1998). Pursuing personal goals: Skills enable progress, but not all goal progress is beneficial. *Personality and Social Psychology Bulletin, 24*, 1319–1331.

Suh, E. M. (1999). *Self and the use of emotion information: Joining culture, personality, and situational influences.* Unpublished manuscript, University of California, Irvine.

Suh, E., Diener, E., Oishi, S., & Triandis, H. C. (1997). The shifting basis of life satisfaction judgments across cultures: Emotions versus norms. *Journal of Personality and Social Psychology, 74*, 482–493.

Triandis, H. C. (1995). *Individualism and collectivism.* Boulder, CO: Westview.

Wolfe, A. (2000, May 7). The pursuit of autonomy. *New York Times Magazine*, 53–56.

Veenhoven, R. (1993). *Happiness in nations: Subjective appreciation of life in 56 nations 1946–1992.* Rotterdam, the Netherlands: Erasmus University Rotterdam.

Cross-Cultural Variations in Predictors of Life Satisfaction: Perspectives from Needs and Values

Shigehiro Oishi, Ed Diener, Richard E. Lucas and Eunkook M. Suh

Abstract The authors tested for cross-cultural difference in predictors of life satis-faction. In Study 1 (39 nations, $N = 54,446$), they found that financial satisfaction was more strongly associated with life satisfaction in poorer nations, whereas home life satisfaction was more strongly related to life satisfaction in wealthy nations. In Study 2 (39 nations, $N = 6,782$), the authors found that satisfaction with esteem needs (e.g., the self and freedom) predicted global life satisfaction more strongly among people in individualist nations than people in collectivist nations. The present investigation provides support for the needs and values-as-moderators model of subjective well-being at the cultural level. The need for theories that account for culture-specific as well as universal predictors of life satisfaction will be discussed.

What predicts people's life satisfaction? To answer this question, subjective well-being (SWB) researchers have investigated various demographic and personality variables, ranging from income, education, and marital status to self-esteem, op-timism, extraversion, and neuroticism (see Myers & Diener, 1995, for a review). Prior research has shown that personality variables such as self-esteem, optimism, and frequent positive emotional experiences predict one's level of life satisfaction (e.g., Diener, 1996; Diener, Suh, Lucas, & Smith, 1999; Lucas, Diener, & Suh, 1996). The initial evidence for the importance of personal domains, however, mostly came from studies in the United States and other Western nations. It is possible that the centrality of internal attributes found in previous studies is unique to individu-alist cultures. Recent cross-cultural research has provided preliminary evidence for such culture-specific correlates of SWB. For example, Kwan, Bond, and Singelis (1997) found that relationship harmony was a more important predictor of life sat-isfaction in Hong Kong than in the United States. Similarly, Suh, Diener, Oishi, and Triandis (1998) found that norms for life satisfaction (e.g., How satisfied should the ideal person be with his or her life?) were more strongly associated with the level of life satisfaction in collectivist nations than in individualist nations. It appears, there-fore, that standards for life satisfaction judgments vary across cultures and that such

S. Oishi (✉)
Department of Psychology, University of Illinois, Champaign, IL 61820, USA
e-mail: soishi@virginia.edu

E. Diener (ed.), *Culture and Well-Being: The Collected Works of Ed Diener*, Social Indicators Research Series 38, DOI 10.1007/978-90-481-2352-0_6,
© Springer Science+Business Media B.V. 2009

cross-cultural variations are systematically related to salient cultural values. The purpose of the present study is to identify sources of systematic cross-cultural differences in correlates of SWB from the perspectives of the need-gratification (Maslow, 1970; Veenhoven, 1991) and the value-as-a-moderator models (Oishi, Diener, Suh, & Lucas, 1999).

The Need-Gratification Models of SWB

Maslow (1970) proposed a need-gratification theory of well-being, stating that the "degree of basic need gratification is positively correlated with degree of psychological health" (p. 67). In his hierarchical organization of basic needs, physiological needs (e.g., food, thirst) are most basic, followed by safety needs (e.g., security, protection), love needs (e.g., affection, belongingness), esteem needs (e.g., self-respect, freedom), and idiosyncratic self-actualization needs at the top of the hierarchy. Maslow postulates that higher needs become salient as lower needs are gratified. Higher need gratification is also assumed to produce more profound happiness than is lower need gratification (Maslow, 1970, p. 99).

Although this theory is usually tested at the individual level, Maslow (1970) suggests that higher needs depend on outside conditions such as "familial, economic, political, education, etc." (p. 99) to make them possible. Because people in poorer nations often suffer from a lack of financial security and adequate housing, physiological and safety needs are more salient in these nations than in wealthy nations. Similarly, because people's physiological and safety needs are more often met in wealthy nations, love and esteem needs are more likely to be salient concerns for people in wealthy nations than in poor nations. Taken together, Maslow's need-gratification theory predicts that (a) people in wealthier nations tend to be more satisfied with their lives and (b) people in wealthier nations tend to base their life satisfaction judgments on the level of gratification of higher needs. People in poorer nations should tend to base their life satisfaction judgments on the level of gratification of more basic needs.

Veenhoven (1991) tested these hypotheses based on Maslow's (1970) theory with data gathered in 22 nations between 1975 and 1985 (e.g., the World Value Survey I and the biannual Eurobarometer surveys; see Veenhoven, 1992, for details). Consistent with the first hypothesis, Veenhoven (1991) found that the mean life satisfaction of the nation was significantly positively correlated with the gross national product (GNP) per capita of the nation ($r = 0.84$). In addition, Veenhoven tested the second hypothesis, examining the correlation between individuals' income and life satisfaction within nations. He found that the correlation between individual's income and life satisfaction was higher in poorer nations than in rich nations ($r = -0.35$). Presumably, income is related to safety needs. Thus, Veenhoven's finding is consistent with the second hypothesis based on Maslow's theory: When making life satisfaction judgments, people in poorer nations weigh their income more heavily than do people in wealthier nations.

E. Diener and M. Diener (1995) also examined the second hypothesis based on Maslow's (1970) theory among college students from 31 nations. Consistent with

Veenhoven (1991), E. Diener and M. Diener (1995) found that the size of within-nation correlation between financial satisfaction and life satisfaction was negatively correlated with the income per person of the nation ($rs = -0.36$ for women, -0.32 for men). That is, people in poorer nations based their life satisfaction judgments more heavily on financial satisfaction than did people in wealthier nations.

In sum, Maslow's (1970) need-gratification theory accounts for variation in predictors of life satisfaction across nations that differ in affluence. This theory does not, however, provide any variation in predictors of life satisfaction among equally wealthy nations. According to Maslow's theory, esteem needs are equally salient in nations A and B so long as these nations provide living conditions that satisfy physiological and safety needs to the same extent.

The Value-as-a-Moderator Model of SWB

In the present investigation, we seek to extend Maslow's (1970) need-gratification theory by applying the value-as-a-moderator model of SWB (Oishi et al., 1999) to the cultural level. The fundamental postulate of this model is that when making life satisfaction judgments, individuals weigh value-congruent domain satisfactions more heavily than value-incongruent domain satisfactions. Oishi et al. (1999) tested this model through intra-individual (i.e., a daily diary study) and inter-individual level analyses of life satisfaction judgments. For example, satisfaction with grades was a strong predictor of life satisfaction among individuals who valued achievement, whereas satisfaction with friends was a major predictor among individuals who valued benevolence. This study suggests that even among individuals whose physiological and safety needs are approximately equally gratified, there are considerable individual differences in the salience of esteem and love needs.

In addition, recent research suggests notable cross-cultural differences in the importance of esteem needs, even among nations that are equally wealthy (Schwartz, 1994; Triandis, 1995). The value-as-a-moderator model of SWB postulates that predictors of life satisfaction vary across cultures, depending on salient cultural values. There is some evidence in support of this model at the cultural level. For instance, E. Diener and M. Diener (1995) found that the strength of association between satisfaction with the self and life satisfaction was significantly stronger in individualist nations than in collectivist nations ($r = 0.53$). In brief, the value-as-a-moderator model adds a culture-specific dimension to Maslow's universalistic need model of well-being.

Overview

We conducted two studies to investigate cross-cultural differences in correlates of SWB. In Study 1, we assessed job satisfaction, financial satisfaction, and home satisfaction in 39 nations. Job satisfaction and financial satisfaction represent safety needs, whereas home life satisfaction represents love needs. Based on Maslow's (1970) theory, we predict that financial and job satisfaction will be stronger predictors of life satisfaction in poorer nations than in wealthier nations. Conversely, we predict that home life satisfaction will be a stronger predictor of life satisfaction in wealthier nations than in poorer nations. In Study 2, we extend the list of satisfaction domains to the self and freedom. This will allow us to examine the value-as-a-moderator model as well as Maslow's need-gratification model of SWB. Based on the value-as-a-moderator model, we predict that the gratification of esteem needs, such as self-respect and freedom, will be more strongly associated with the level of life satisfaction in individualist cultures, in which self-esteem and autonomy are valued, than in collectivist cultures, in which self-criticism and interdependency are valued (see Kitayama, Markus, Matsumoto, & Norasakkunkit, 1997; Markus & Kitayama, 1991; Schwartz, 1994; Triandis, 1989, 1996, for cross-cultural differences in values, goals, and self-concept).

Our studies extend earlier research (e.g., E. Diener & M. Diener, 1995; Kwan et al., 1997; Suh et al., 1998; Veenhoven, 1991) in several important ways. First, prior studies used a simple correlational analysis of within-nation correlation coefficients. Researchers computed correlation coefficients within each nation and then computed correlations between the size of the correlation and national characteristics (e.g., the GNP or the level of individualism). This procedure neglects differential reliability of within-nation correlation coefficients. For instance, in E. Diener and M. Diener (1995), the number of participants in each nation ranged from 29 to 985. The correlation coefficient computed in Cameroon (29 subjects) will be necessarily less reliable than the correlation coefficient computed in Canada (985 participants). Yet, these coefficients were treated as if they were equally reliable. Thus, the obtained correlation at the culture level was likely to be biased in prior research.

To address the issue of differential reliability, we use hierarchical linear modeling (HLM) (Bryk & Raudenbush, 1992) to test multilevel interactions. The HLM analysis yields a better estimate of multilevel interactions, such as the interaction between the GNP of the nation and financial satisfaction in predicting life satisfaction (see Results for details). Thus, differential reliability across nations should not be a problem in the present studies.

Second, our studies also improve on previous research by including two large samples (one adult and one college student sample) from many nations. Finally, previous cross-cultural findings (e.g., E. Diener & M. Diener, 1995; Suh et al., 1998; Veenhoven, 1991) were explained either in terms of affluence or the level of individualism–collectivism. Yet, no study tested the unique contribution of each of these highly correlated factors. In the present article, we test the effect of individualism–collectivism on cross-national variations in predictors of life satisfaction, controlling for the effect of wealth (and vice versa).

Study 1

Study 1 is based on data collected by the World Values Study Group (1994). The data consist of responses from 54,446 participants from 39 nations, varying considerably in standard of living. The diversity in wealth and the level of individualism of

the nations provide us with a rare opportunity to test the role of wealth and individualism in the strength of the relation between satisfaction with safety (i.e., finances
and job) and love needs (i.e., home life) and global life satisfaction.

Method

Participants. The World Value Survey (WVS) II data were collected between 1990
and 1993 in 43 societies representing almost 70% of the world's population. This
study covered a large range of economic, political, geographical, and cultural variation. The sampling universe consisted of all adult citizens age 18 or older. In most
nations, selection was made by quota sampling; quotas were assigned based on sex,
age, occupation, and region, using the census data as a guide to the distribution
of each group in the population. This sampling method ensured that the obtained
samples included all socioeconomic groups and properly represented the compos-
ites of the population in respective nations with minimum error margins. In Eastern
Europe, surveys were carried out by the respective national academies of sciences
or university-based institutes. Surveys in other countries were carried out by professional survey organizations, most of whom were members of the Gallup chain
(see World Values Study Group, 1994, for details). The analyses in Study 1 were
based on the responses from 54,446 participants from 39 nations (see Table 1). The
data from Lithuania ($N = 1,000$) and South Korea ($N = 1,250$) were excluded
because the participants were not presented the financial satisfaction item. The data
from Austria ($N = 1,460$) were excluded prior to the analysis because of irregu-
larity in coding of certain responses. The data from Moscow ($N = 1,012$), which
were included in addition to the data from Russia in the original data set, were not
used in the following analyses because Moscow is a city, not a nation. The median
sample size was 1,027 per nation. The mean age of the respondents was 41.9, with
a standard deviation of 16.5.

Measures and Ratings

Global life satisfaction was measured by a single item: "All things considered, how
satisfied are you with your life as a whole these days?" The respondents answered
the question using a 10-point scale ranging from 1 (*dissatisfied*) to 10 (*satisfied*).
Financial satisfaction was measured by asking "How satisfied are you with the
financial situation of your household?" The respondents answered it by using the
same 10-point scale used in the global life satisfaction item. Using the same format, satisfaction with job and satisfaction with home life also were asked. GNP per
capita for each nation was taken from the *World Atlas* (World Bank, 1992). To be
consistent with the period of data collection, we used the GNP per capita in 1991.
We obtained the individualism–collectivism ratings for each nation, when possible,
by averaging the ratings of two leading experts in the field: Geert Hofstede (1980)
and Harry Triandis (personal communication, February 1996). Triandis rated the
degree of individualism–collectivism of the 39 nations on a scale ranging from 1

Table 1 World values survey II: gross national product, mean financial satisfaction, job satisfaction, home life satisfaction, and life satisfaction

Nation	N	GNP	IC	FS	JS	HS	LS
Nigeria	1, 001	290	3.00	5.51 (2.75)	7.48 (2.33)	7.50 (2.38)	6.59 (2.62)
India	2, 500	330	4.40	6.36 (2.42)	7.03 (2.34)	7.24 (2.17)	6.70 (2.28)
China	1, 000	370	2.00	6.12 (2.54)	7.01 (2.42)	7.80 (2.04)	7.29 (2.10)
Romania	1, 103	1,340	5.00	5.05 (2.40)	6.56 (2.29)	6.83 (2.23)	5.88 (2.33)
Turkey	1, 030	1,820	3.85	5.09 (2.10)	5.72 (2.48)	6.70 (2.30)	6.41 (2.45)
Poland	938	1,830	5.00	5.07 (2.49)	8.25 (2.21)	8.56 (2.01)	6.64 (2.35)
Bulgaria	1, 034	1,840	5.00	4.28 (2.25)	6.20 (2.33)	6.22 (2.29)	5.03 (2.29)
Chile	1, 500	2,160	4.15	5.91 (2.49)	7.63 (2.29)	8.32 (2.09)	7.55 (2.21)
Czech-Slovak	1, 396	2,450	7.00	5.02 (2.54)	6.78 (2.27)	7.31 (2.30)	6.30 (2.15)
S. Africa	2, 736	2,530	5.75	5.46 (3.02)	7.45 (2.48)	7.42 (2.71)	6.72 (2.71)
Hungary	999	2,710	4.00	5.19 (2.56)	7.22 (2.36)	7.74 (2.42)	6.03 (2.45)
Argentina	1, 002	2,780	4.80	5.31 (2.48)	7.63 (2.17)	7.91 (2.12)	7.25 (2.03)
Mexico	1, 531	2,870	4.00	6.15 (2.47)	7.66 (2.11)	7.58 (2.14)	7.41 (2.16)
Brazil	1, 780	2,920	3.90	5.51 (2.76)	7.52 (2.40)	8.25 (2.14)	7.37 (2.40)
Belarus	1, 015	3,110	4.00	5.02 (2.42)	6.10 (2.37)	6.48 (2.66)	5.52 (2.24)
Russia	1, 961	3,220	6.00	4.98 (2.56)	6.28 (2.49)	6.71 (2.64)	5.37 (2.40)
Latvia	903	3,410	4.00	4.21 (2.60)	6.45 (2.49)	5.89 (2.48)	5.70 (2.44)
Estonia	1, 008	3,830	4.00	5.01 (2.57)	6.66 (2.36)	6.13 (2.22)	6.00 (2.13)
Portugal	1, 185	5,620	3.85	5.94 (2.49)	7.42 (2.26)	8.07 (2.04)	7.07 (2.10)
Ireland	1, 000	10,780	6.00	6.75 (2.37)	7.81 (2.00)	8.54 (1.72)	7.88 (1.92)
Spain	4, 147	12,460	5.55	6.23 (2.01)	6.99 (2.10)	7.63 (1.83)	7.15 (1.90)
Britain	1, 484	16,750	8.95	6.45 (2.59)	7.42 (2.06)	8.22 (1.86)	7.49 (1.93)
Netherlands	1, 017	18,560	8.50	7.50 (2.00)	7.48 (1.67)	8.17 (1.47)	7.77 (1.58)
Italy	2, 010	18,580	6.80	7.00 (2.17)	7.29 (2.08)	7.83 (1.97)	7.30 (2.06)
Belgium	2, 792	19,300	7.25	7.21 (2.12)	7.79 (1.82)	8.07 (1.81)	7.60 (1.89)
France	1, 002	20,600	7.05	5.94 (2.16)	6.78 (1.97)	7.44 (2.01)	6.78 (1.98)
Canada	1, 730	21,260	8.50	7.13 (2.28)	7.88 (1.77)	8.41 (1.70)	7.89 (1.73)
United States	1, 839	22,560	9.55	6.86 (2.41)	7.85 (1.88)	8.41 (1.81)	7.73 (1.83)
Iceland	702	22,580	7.00	6.29 (2.43)	7.86 (1.74)	8.26 (1.63)	8.02 (1.60)
West Germany	2, 101	23,650	7.35	6.74 (2.20)	7.14 (1.78)	7.45 (1.93)	7.22 (1.92)
Denmark	1, 030	23,660	7.70	7.22 (2.48)	8.24 (1.66)	8.69 (1.64)	8.16 (1.89)
Norway	1, 239	24,160	6.95	6.67 (2.35)	7.88 (1.76)	7.97 (1.71)	7.68 (1.77)
Finland	588	24,400	7.15	6.60 (2.29)	7.56 (2.03)	8.00 (1.98)	7.68 (1.88)
Sweden	1, 047	25,490	7.55	6.98 (2.39)	8.08 (1.79)	8.46 (1.68)	7.96 (1.74)
Japan	1, 001	26,920	4.30	6.03 (2.09)	7.66 (2.31)	6.94 (1.80)	6.53 (1.75)
Switzerland	1, 400	33,510	7.90	8.21 (2.05)	8.40 (1.88)	8.60 (1.78)	8.36 (1.75)
East Germany	1, 336	—	6.00	5.94 (2.28)	6.75 (2.11)	7.43 (1.96)	6.72 (1.97)
North Ireland	340	—	5.00	6.67 (2.38)	7.85 (1.89)	8.71 (1.50)	7.88 (1.81)
Slovenia	1, 035	—	5.00	4.67 (2.42)	7.21 (2.15)	7.37 (2.15)	6.29 (2.21)

Note. The numbers in parentheses represent standard deviation. Gross national product (GNP) per capita was based on data in 1991 in U.S. dollars, IC = individualism–collectivism, FS = mean financial satisfaction (10-point scale), JS = mean job satisfaction (10-point-scale), HS = mean home life satisfaction (10-point-scale), and LS = 10-point global life satisfaction item.

(*most collectivist*) to 10 (*most individualist*). Hofstede's individualism–collectivism scores were converted to a 10-point scale compatible with Triandis's ratings. The correlation between the GNP per capita and the individualism–collectivism rating was 0.75 in this sample.

Results and Discussion

We tested our hypotheses using the HLM/2L program (Bryk, Raudenbush, & Congdon, 1994). The two-level analysis of the HLM is conceptually equivalent to multiple regression analyses at two levels. In the present study, at Level 1, life satisfaction was predicted from domain satisfaction for each nation. At Level 2, the within-nation regression slopes that indicate the degree of association between domain satisfaction and life satisfaction were predicted from cultural level variables such as the GNP and the level of individualism. The aggregated correlation approach used in prior studies (E. Diener & M. Diener, 1995; Suh et al., 1998; Veenhoven, 1991) neglects the Level 1 error in estimating Level 2 coefficients, which leads to aggregation bias and measurement error. HLM analysis takes into account errors at both levels and thereby provides more precise estimates of the multilevel interactions.

First, reliability estimates of the Level 1 regression coefficients were computed for each nation and then averaged over all nations. The reliability of the Level 1 regression coefficient is in principle the proportion of sample variance to the total variance (i.e., sample variance + error variance). The precision of estimation of regression coefficients depends both on the sample size and on the variability of the predictor variables (see Bryk & Raudenbush, 1992, for details). The reliability estimates in the present study were 0.98 for the intercept (here, life satisfaction), 0.88 for the Level 1 regression coefficient of financial satisfaction, 0.84 for job satisfaction, and 0.84 for home life satisfaction.

Hypothesis testing. Table 2 shows the intercepts and slopes for the Level 2 analyses. Intercepts that are significantly greater than zero indicate that the relation between domain satisfaction and life satisfaction was, on average, positive. Fixed effects of the GNP and individualism–collectivism indicate the degree to which cross-cultural differences in the size of Level 1 slopes were accounted for by the GNP and the level of individualism. The intercept for financial satisfaction shows that, on average, financial satisfaction was positively associated with life satisfaction. Consistent with our hypothesis, the slope of financial satisfaction was significantly larger in poorer nations, as indicated by significantly negative Level 2 regression coefficients. The slope of financial satisfaction was not, however, related to the level of individualism. The second panel of Table 2 shows that job satisfaction was, on average, positively associated with life satisfaction across nations. The slope of job satisfaction was not, however, related to the GNP or the level of individualism. That is, inconsistent with our hypothesis, job satisfaction was not significantly more strongly associated with life satisfaction in poorer nations. Finally, the bottom panel of Table 2 indicates that home life satisfaction was, on average, positively associated with life satisfaction across nations. Consistent with Maslow's hypothesis, the slope

Table 2 Hierarchical linear modeling analysis in Study 1

Fixed effects	Coefficients	SE	T ratio
Slope for financial satisfaction			
Intercept	0.35	0.01	25.47***
Gross national product (GNP)	−0.00	0.00	−2.51*
Individualism	0.00	0.00	0.28
Slope for job satisfaction			
Intercept	0.35	0.01	27.61***
GNP	−0.00	0.00	−1.08
Individualism	−0.00	0.00	−0.88
Slope for home life satisfaction			
Intercept	0.50	0.01	37.29***
GNP	0.00	0.00	2.32*
Individualism	−0.00	0.00	−1.43

$^*p < 0.05$; $^{***}p < 0.001$.

of home life satisfaction in predicting life satisfaction was significantly stronger in wealthier nations. The level of individualism was not related to the size of slope of home life satisfaction.

In sum, the present analyses supported two of the three hypotheses based on Maslow's (1970) need-gratification model of well-being. In poor nations, financial satisfaction plays an important role in determining overall life satisfaction, presumably because safety needs such as security and stability are not as well satisfied as in wealthy nations. On the other hand, in wealthy nations, home life satisfaction appears to play a more central role in overall life satisfaction. This could be because in these societies physiological and safety needs are mostly met and love and belongingness needs are more salient concerns. Finally, job satisfaction could serve different meanings across cultures. In poor nations, aspects of job related to safety needs such as pay and benefit may be more important criteria for job satisfaction. In wealthy nations, on the other hand, aspects of job related to self-actualization (e.g., how much one can express one's ability and talent through the job) could be more important criteria for job satisfaction. It appears that job serves different needs across cultures. That is, job satisfaction was an equally strong predictor of life satisfaction across cultures, perhaps due to the multiple functions of jobs.

Limitations of Study 1. Study 1 extended previous studies (e.g., E. Diener & M. Diener, 1995; Kwan et al., 1997; Veenhoven, 1991) in terms of data analytic strategy. Samples in this study also were nationally representative and included various age, occupational, and socioeconomic groups. Furthermore, we included a much larger and more diverse set of countries than in previous research. These factors make the present findings more generalizable than previous studies. Because of the primary focus of the WVS II on values and attitudes, however, the number of domains compatible with our research purpose was limited to financial satisfaction, job satisfaction, and home life satisfaction. Accordingly, we could not examine the relation between satisfaction with esteem needs and global life satisfaction across nations in Study 1.

Study 2

We conducted Study 2 to address the limitations of Study 1. Instead of using the single item scales used in Study 1, we used the 5-item Satisfaction With Life Scale (SWLS). In addition, we extended Study 1 by including satisfaction items relevant to esteem needs such as the "self" and "freedom" as well as satisfaction items relevant to physiological and safety needs such as "finances," "food," and "housing." Maslow (1970) defined esteem needs as needs or desires for self-esteem, independence, and freedom (see p. 45 for full descriptions of the esteem needs). Recent cross-cultural studies (e.g., Kitayama et al., 1997) indicate that the independent aspect of the self is salient in individualist cultures, whereas the inter-dependent aspect of the self is salient in collectivist cultures. Therefore, questions about the self might prime different aspects of the self across cultures. When asked how satisfied they are with the self, however, the question is similar to one of the Rosenberg (1965) Self-Esteem Scale items that assesses the independent aspect of the self: "On the whole, I am satisfied with myself." That is, in this context, the question seems to focus on the independent aspect of the self. Given the salience of the independent self in individualist nations, the value-as-a-moderator model of SWB predicts that satisfaction with esteem needs will be more strongly associated with global life satisfaction in individualist nations than in collectivist nations.

Method

Participants. The participants were 6,782 college students from 39 countries (2,625 males, 4,118 females, and 39 unspecified). Although college students are not representative of each nation's population, by using college students, we were able to obtain many samples from diverse cultures. One advantage of using college students is that age and socioeconomic status (SES) are somewhat controlled because most participants are approximately the same age and are from similar socioeconomic backgrounds. The 39 nations and their respective sample sizes are shown in Table 3. These nations represent a diverse selection: 2 nations from North America, 4 from South America, 14 from Asia, 13 from Europe, and 5 from Africa. Of the participants, 84% were between the ages of 18 and 25, and 10% of the participants were between 26 and 35 years old. Due to missing items, the number of participants differed slightly across analyses.

Measures and Ratings

Global life satisfaction. Global life satisfaction, or cognitive assessment of life as a whole, was measured by the SWLS (Diener, Emmons, Larsen, & Griffin, 1985). The SWLS consists of five statements, to which respondents are asked to indicate their degree of agreement using a 7-point scale ranging from 1 (*strongly disagree*) to 7 (*strongly agree*). The total SWLS score ranges from 7 to 35. The SWLS has

Table 3 Predicting the SWLS from Satisfaction With Finances, Foods, housing, the self, and freedom in Study 2: unstandardized simple regression coefficients within-nation

Nation	N	Income	IC	Simple regression coefficients within-nation				
				FS	Housing	Foods	Self	Freedom
Low income								
Lithuania	101	2.99	4.00	1.62	1.72	0.90	1.38	1.62
China	558	3.65	2.00	1.01	0.73	0.85	0.81	0.60
Estonia	119	3.85	4.00	0.97	1.59	0.74*	1.58	0.77*
Ghana	118	4.20	3.00	1.68	1.61	1.21	0.99**	1.68
Indonesia	90	4.22	2.20	1.81	1.46	0.98*	1.99	0.82**
Nepal	99	4.30	3.00	0.83	0.67*	0.47**	1.05	0.76
Nigeria	244	4.33	3.00	1.81	1.26	1.67	2.17	0.94
Turkey	100	4.60	3.85	1.03	0.80	0.90	1.33	0.20**
India	93	4.76	4.00	1.44	1.29	1.63	1.42	1.55
Egypt	120	4.78	4.40	2.95	2.89	3.45	3.19	2.94
Tanzania	96	4.95	3.00	1.44	0.94*	−0.03**	−0.87**	−0.54**
Zimbabwe	109	5.12	3.00	2.19	1.44	0.95*	0.95**	0.79*
Hungary	74	5.30	6.00	1.66	1.14	0.78**	2.38	1.14
Medium income								
Singapore	131	5.42	3.50	2.15	1.45	1.50	2.44	0.81*
Brazil	112	5.66	3.90	1.40	1.00	0.01**	1.51	1.06
Bahrain	124	5.85	3.00	1.37	1.15	0.62**	0.87	1.06
Pakistan	155	5.86	2.20	0.87	1.25	1.15	1.70	1.07
Denmark	91	6.12	7.70	0.79	1.10*	0.81**	1.99	1.78
Peru	129	6.15	2.80	1.65	1.32	0.95	2.29	0.65*
Hong Kong	142	6.30	4.75	1.82	0.75*	1.82	2.39	1.60
Guam	186	6.33	5.00	1.87	1.70	0.93	1.63	1.20
South Africa	373	6.41	5.75	1.91	1.23	1.68	2.34	1.49
Slovenia	50	6.90	5.00	2.26	1.45	1.89	2.90	2.63
Colombia	100	6.95	2.15	1.17	1.60	1.48	2.81	1.06
Germany	108	7.22	7.35	1.38	0.62**	0.46**	2.64	1.38
Austria	164	7.26	6.75	1.50	1.20	1.14	1.89	0.96*
High income								
Spain	327	7.33	5.55	1.24	1.03	1.25	2.20	1.04
Portugal	139	7.37	3.85	1.45	1.65	1.66	1.98	1.90
Greece	129	7.44	5.25	0.58**	1.35	0.41**	2.04	0.76**
Korea	277	7.66	2.40	2.13	1.63	0.72	2.39	1.35
Taiwan	533	7.66	3.85	1.27	2.13	2.28	2.47	1.03
Argentina	90	7.76	4.80	0.05**	0.76*	0.35**	1.28	−0.27**
Puerto Rico	87	7.92	7.00	2.53	2.21	1.21	3.08	2.52
Italy	289	8.04	6.80	1.23	1.31	0.61*	2.58	1.23
Finland	91	8.33	7.15	1.74	1.68	1.55	2.72	3.30
Australia	292	8.52	9.00	1.86	2.08	1.71	2.81	2.14
Japan	200	8.62	4.30	1.86	1.40	0.43**	2.63	1.80
United States	443	9.15	9.55	1.47	1.32	0.69	3.02	1.31
Norway	99	9.18	6.95	2.01	0.99*	2.45	3.09	3.15

Note. SWLS = Satisfaction With Life Scale, IC = individualism–collectivism, FS = mean financial satisfaction (10-point scale), and IC rating denotes the individualism–collectivism ratings given by Triandis (personal communication, February 1996) and Hofstede (1980).
*Denotes nonsignificance at $\alpha = 0.01$; **denotes nonsignificance at $\alpha = 0.05$.

adequate psychometric properties (see Pavot & Diener, 1993) and has demonstrated validity among Korean (Suh, 1994), mainland Chinese (Shao, 1993), and Russian samples (Balatsky & Diener, 1993).

Domain satisfactions. We chose three domains representing safety needs (food, housing, and finances) and two domains representing esteem needs (the self and your freedom). The participants answered how satisfied they were with each of the five domains of their lives using a 7-point scale ranging from 1 (*extremely dissatisfied*) to 4 (*neutral*) to 7 (*extremely satisfied*).

Income. The participants were asked to indicate their family's annual income in U.S. dollars using a 10-point scale: 1 (0–400), 2 (401–1,000), 3 (1,001–2,000), 4 (2,001–4,000), 5 (4,001–6,000), 6 (6,001–8,000), 7 (8,000–10,000), 8 (10,001–25,000), 9 (25,001–50,000), and 10 (50,001 and greater).

Individualism–collectivism ratings. We assessed the level of individualism in the same manner as Study 1.

Procedure. The original questionnaire was constructed by Ed Diener in English. This questionnaire was then translated into Spanish, Japanese, Korean, and Chinese by bilingual individuals. Bilingual individuals other than those who engaged in the initial translation next translated the non-English versions of the questionnaire back to English. Ratings made of the back translations indicated that they showed an excellent fit to the original English version (Shao, 1997). In other nations, local collaborators translated the English version to the local language. The data were collected in university classrooms by local collaborators.

Results and Discussion

Satisfaction with the physiological and safety needs. Table 3 indicates the number of participants, the mean family income, individualism–collectivism ratings, and unstandardized simple regression coefficients predicting the SWLS from each domain satisfaction.

We first examined Maslow's hypothesis. We tested whether the strength of the relation between satisfaction with safety needs and life satisfaction would be stronger in poorer nations. As in Study 1, we performed a two-level analysis of HLM using the HLM/2L program (Bryk et al., 1994). At Level 1 (i.e., within-nation level), this procedure is equivalent to predicting the SWLS from satisfaction with finances, foods, and housing. At Level 2 (i.e., national level), HLM tests whether there were significant differences in regression slopes across nations. If differences exist, HLM detects whether levels of the mean family income or individualism–collectivism can account for the cross-national differences. The correlation between the individualism–collectivism ratings and the mean family income in the 39 nations was 0.64 ($p < 0.01$).

First, the reliability estimates in Study 2 were 0.94 for the intercept (here, the SWLS), 0.69 for the regression coefficient of satisfaction with foods, 0.58 for the regression coefficient of satisfaction with finances, and 0.53 for the regression coefficient of satisfaction with housing.

We summarize the results of the HLM analysis in Table 4. Unlike in Study 1, the slope of financial satisfaction did not vary across nations, either in terms of the mean family income or the levels of individualism. Similarly, the slope of satisfaction with food did not vary across nations. Likewise, the slope of satisfaction with housing did not differ across nations, either in terms of the mean family income or the level of individualism. In brief, Maslow's hypothesis was not supported in Study 2. In other words, satisfaction with safety needs was a significant predictor of life satisfaction even in very wealthy nations (also see regression coefficients in Table 3). Samples in Study 2, however, consist solely of college students. Even in

Table 4 Hierarchical linear model analysis: predicting variations in the slopes from individualism–collectivism ratings and the mean family income

Fixed effects	Coefficients	SE	T ratio
Model for finance: SWLS slopes			
Separate entry			
Individualism	0.03	0.04	0.81
Mean family income	0.05	0.05	0.13
Simultaneous entry			
Individualism	0.04	0.06	0.74
Mean family income	−0.01	0.07	−0.21
Model for housing: SWLS slopes			
Separate entry			
Individualism	0.03	0.04	0.79
Mean family income	0.05	0.04	1.21
Simultaneous entry			
Individualism	−0.01	0.05	−0.17
Mean family income	0.07	0.06	1.19
Model for food: SWLS slopes			
Separate entry			
Individualism	0.03	0.06	0.49
Mean family income	−0.03	0.06	−0.50
Simultaneous entry			
Individualism	0.02	0.08	0.27
Mean family income	0.01	0.09	0.16
Model for self: SWLS slopes			
Separate entry			
Individualism	0.16	0.05	2.92**
Mean family income	0.29	0.06	4.84**
Simultaneous entry			
Individualism	0.11	0.07	1.65*
Mean family income	0.20	0.08	2.67**
Model for freedom: SWLS slopes			
Separate entry			
Individualism	0.09	0.05	1.76*
Mean family income	0.13	0.06	2.24**
Simultaneous entry			
Individualism	0.11	0.07	1.54
Mean family income	0.06	0.08	0.74

Note. SWLS = Satisfaction With Life Scale.
$^*p < 0.05; ^{**}p < 0.01$. A one-tailed test was used because the direction was predicted.

poor nations, college students are likely to have enough food and adequate housing. Therefore, it is plausible that cross-cultural differences in the gratification of safety needs in college samples were not as vast as in Study 1, which in turn suppressed cross-cultural differences in the importance of satisfaction with safety needs.

Satisfaction with esteem needs. Next, we tested cross-national variability in the link between satisfaction with esteem needs and life satisfaction, again using the HLM/2L program (Bryk et al., 1994). The reliability estimates were 0.74 for satisfaction with the self and 0.64 for satisfaction with freedom. Replicating E. Diener and M. Diener (1995), the strength of association between satisfaction with the self and life satisfaction was significantly stronger in individualist nations. However, the size of this association also was significantly related to the mean family income. That is, the association between satisfaction with the self and life satisfaction was significantly stronger in wealthier nations. It should be further noted that levels of individualism significantly predicted the strength of the association, controlling for the mean family income of the nation (see the simultaneous entry in Table 4). Similarly, the mean family income significantly predicted the scale of the association between satisfaction with the self and life satisfaction, controlling for the levels of individualism. Thus, extending E. Diener and M. Diener (1995), the size of the association between satisfaction with the self and life satisfaction varies across nations, depending on both individualism–collectivism and affluence. The more individualist the nation is, the stronger the association. Also, the wealthier the nation, the stronger the association between satisfaction with the self and life satisfaction.

With regard to satisfaction with freedom, the strength of association between satisfaction with freedom and life satisfaction was significantly stronger in individualist nations than in collectivist nations (see the separate entry in Table 4). Likewise, the association was stronger in wealthier nations than in less wealthy nations. Controlling for the levels of individualism, however, the mean family income did not predict the cross-national variation in the strength of the association between satisfaction with freedom and life satisfaction (see the simultaneous entry in Table 4). On the other hand, controlling for the mean family income, individualism marginally significantly predicted variations in the slope of satisfaction with freedom.

In sum, consistent with Maslow's (1970) hypothesis, satisfaction with esteem needs was a stronger predictor of life satisfaction in wealthy nations than in poor nations. Furthermore, controlling for the level of the mean family income, the size of the association between satisfaction with individualistic domains and life satisfaction was consistently larger in individualist nations than in collectivist nations. Although esteem needs are more salient concerns in wealthier nations, self-esteem and satisfaction with one's freedom play a more central role in determining the level of life satisfaction in individualist societies than in collectivist societies.

General Discussion

In the present research, we examined sources of systematic cross-cultural differences in correlates of SWB. Based on Maslow's (1970) need-gratification theory and the value-as-a-moderator model of SWB (Oishi et al., 1999), we tested the roles of culture and economy in predictors of life satisfaction. Consistent with Maslow's theory, satisfaction with safety needs tended to be more strongly associated with global life satisfaction in poorer nations, whereas satisfaction with higher needs, such as love and esteem needs, tended to be stronger predictors of life satisfaction in wealthy nations. Furthermore, consistent with the value-as-a-moderator model, when making life satisfaction judgments, people in individualist nations tended to weigh satisfaction with esteem needs more heavily than did people in collectivist nations. Together, the present findings indicate that predictors of life satisfaction differ across cultures, depending on salient needs and values.

Toward a Comprehensive Theory of SWB

Maslow's (1970) need-gratification theory of well-being suggests that predictors of life satisfaction shift from lower needs to higher needs as lower needs are gratified. Maslow's theory was formulated to explain ontological shifts in an individual's life. We applied his theory to phenomena at the cultural level. The present findings suggest that there is a universal process such that when individuals' lower needs are not met, satisfaction with these domains is a primary predictor of life satisfaction. When individuals' lower needs are met, on the other hand, their life satisfaction is better predicted from satisfaction with higher needs such as love and esteem needs. It is important to note, however, that we found that the importance of esteem needs was stronger in individualist cultures than in collectivist cultures. Thus, although there seem to be universal shifts in predictors of life satisfaction as needs are gratified, once lower needs are met, there is more cross-cultural variation in the degree to which the higher needs relate to overall life satisfaction. Maslow's need-gratification theory does not account for cross-cultural differences in correlates of SWB among equally wealthy nations.

This has an important implication for existing theories of SWB in general. For example, Deci and Ryan's (1985; Ryan, Sheldon, Kasser, & Deci, 1996) self-determination theory of SWB is based on Maslow's (1970) universal need-gratification theory. These researchers assume that progress toward so-called intrinsic goals such as self-acceptance, competence, and community involvement is the only path to happiness. Recent studies in the United States provide support for the self-determination theory of SWB (e.g., Sheldon & Kasser, 1998; Sheldon, Ryan, & Reis, 1996). Cross-cultural variation in the importance of satisfaction with the self and freedom found in this study, however, raises a question as to the universality of such a claim. Does attainment of these intrinsic goals also lead to a sense of happiness in collectivist cultures as much as in individualist cultures? Cross-cultural researchers have long recognized that the types of goals that people pursue differ across cultures (e.g., Markus & Kitayama, 1991; Schwartz, 1994; Triandis, 1995, 1996). In interdependent cultures, the goals that individuals pursue are often shared by in-group members. In these cultures, achieving one's goals also means meeting parental and familial expectations (e.g., Radhakrishnan & Chan, 1997). According to the self-determination theory, however, this form of motivation is considered extrinsic. Thus, the progress toward this type of goals should not lead to a sense of well-being.

Whereas the self-determination theory of SWB (Deci & Ryan, 1985; Ryan et al., 1996) posits universally desirable goals, other goal researchers recognize the importance of individual differences in the types of goals that individuals pursue. In a series of longitudinal studies, Brunstein (1993; Brunstein, Schultheiss, & Grassmann, 1998) found that the degree of progress in domains that are consistent with individuals' goals and needs predicted changes in emotional well-being over time. For individuals with high need for power, for instance, the degree of progress toward power-related goals was indicative of changes in emotional well-being, whereas for individuals with high need for affiliation, the degree of progress toward affiliation-related goals was associated with changes in well-being. Likewise, Diener and Fujita (1995) found that the degree of association between resources and life satisfaction was moderated by individuals' goals. That is, resources (e.g., intelligence, athletic ability) were related to the level of life satisfaction only when they were relevant to goals. Similarly, Oishi et al. (1999) found that satisfaction with value-congruent domains was more strongly associated with global life satisfaction than was satisfaction with value-incongruent domains. In sum, these studies highlight individual differences in desired needs and values and suggest that the way in which individuals gain a sense of satisfaction differs across individuals as a function of salient needs and values. Although the value-as-a-moderator model of SWB (Oishi et al., 1999) was not tested at the cultural level before, the present findings indicate that the process involving SWB is captured better with the theories that take into account both individual and cross-cultural differences in desired goals, needs, and values.

Previous cross-cultural studies found important cross-cultural differences in self-concept (e.g., Campbell et al., 1996), self-enhancement (e.g., Heine & Lehman, 1995, 1997; Kitayama et al., 1997), and SWB (E. Diener & M. Diener, 1995; Suh et al., 1998). However, sources of systematic differences were not rigorously examined in prior research. The present findings suggest that Maslow's (1970) need-gratification theory provides systematic predictions and explanations for cross-national differences in correlates of SWB in terms of living conditions and material wealth. Furthermore, the value-as-a-moderator model extends Maslow's theory and provides predictions and explanations for cross-cultural differences in terms of goals and values.

Limitations, Alternative Explanations, and Future Directions

Before closing, some limitations of the present studies should be mentioned. First, we used only self-report questionnaires. The differential levels of association between financial satisfaction and global life satisfaction could be due to cross-cultural differences in social desirability. That is, it is possible that in poorer nations, placing more importance on financial satisfaction is more accepted than in wealthy nations and that the difference in social desirability may have generated the cross-cultural differences in the degree of association between financial satisfaction and life satisfaction. To address this issue, it is necessary to employ a multimethod approach that includes peer reports.

Second, one might argue that the cross-cultural difference obtained in the present studies could be due to different variability in domain satisfaction across cultures. For instance, if financial satisfaction is more homogeneous in wealthier nations (i.e., restricted range), the association between financial satisfaction and life satisfaction should be smaller in wealthier nations than in poorer nations. As shown in Table 1, however, standard deviations were similar across cultures. Furthermore, given that we employed the HLM analysis, which takes into account differential reliability estimates of Level 1 regression coefficients, this explanation is unlikely to account for the obtained cross-cultural differences. Similarly, one may argue that cross-cultural variations in correlates of life satisfaction may be due to ceiling or floor effects. As shown in Table 1, however, the mean domain satisfactions ranged mostly from 5 to 8 in 10-point scales. Coupled with the small standard deviations (which mostly ranged from 1.50 to 2.00), at least 68% of the observations ($-1\ SD$ to $+1\ SD$) in each sample fell well within this range of the scale. Thus, the restriction-of-range effects due to the floor or ceiling effects are unlikely to have caused serious artifacts in our analyses.

Finally, the present studies as well as most previous cross-cultural studies of SWB are cross-sectional rather than longitudinal. To detect the influence of the economy and levels of individualism–collectivism in predictors of life satisfaction, it also will be important to document within-nation changes over time. Many countries have recently experienced rapid economic growth and Westernization. Researchers should investigate the possible effects of societal changes in the predictors of life satisfaction in the future.

Conclusion

The present studies indicate that people are satisfied with their lives to the extent that their needs and values are satisfied. As predicted by Maslow (1970), there is a shift in predictors of life satisfaction from satisfaction with safety needs to satisfaction with love and esteem needs as the lower needs are gratified. More important, however, we found that the degree to which satisfaction with esteem needs predicts global life satisfaction varies across cultures, depending on salient cultural values. The present findings suggest that universalist theories of SWB (Maslow, 1970; Ryan et al., 1996) need to be supplemented with the theories that account for cross-cultural differences in values. In conclusion, the fundamental question in SWB research (i.e., "What predicts people's life satisfaction?") can be answered by combining the perspectives of need-gratification theory (Maslow, 1970) and the value-as-a-moderator model of SWB (Oishi et al., 1999).

Acknowledgments Richard E. Lucas was supported by a National Science Foundation Graduate Research Fellowship during the preparation of this article. We thank Alexander Grob and Ulrich Schimmack for their insightful comments on an earlier version of this article. We also thank Ronald Inglehart and his colleagues for compiling and allowing public access to the World Values Survey Data and the following international colleagues for providing invaluable data for the present study: Adriana Cudnik de Amato, Argentina; John Brebner, Joe Forgas, Emiko and Yoshi Kashima, Australia; Gerold Mikula, Wofgang Schultz, Austria; Nahid Osseiran, Bahrain; Dela Coleta, Brazil; Ling Shao, China; Fernando Berrera, Colombia; Eggert Peterson, Denmark; Aziz H. Daoud, Egypt; Tomas Niit, Estonia; Katarina Salmela-Aro, Finland; Klaus Fielder, Ulrich Schimmack, Germany; Charity Akotia, Ghana; Loukas Ananikas, Andreas Demetriou, Greece; John Christopher, Guam; Harry Hui, Chung Leung Luk, Hong Kong; Robert Urban, Hungary; Naveen Kaplas, India; Ratna Wulan, Indonesia; Anne Maass, Donatella Martella, Italy; Miyuki Yukura, Japan; Jungsik Kim, Myunghan Zoh, Korea; Danguole Beresneviciene, Lithuania; Murari Prasad Regmi, Nepal; Ruut Veenhoven, the Netherlands; Akinsola Olowu, Nigeria; Joar Vitterso, Norway; Afzal Imama, Pakistan; Reynaldo Alarcon, Peru; Felix Neto, Portugal; Ineana P. Rodriguez-Maldoudado, Puerto Rico; Anthony Kennedy, Singapore; Maja Zupancic, Slovenia; Arvin Bhana, Valerie Moller, South Africa; Maria D. Avia, Rosario Jurado, Jose F. Valencia, Salustiano del Campo Urbano, M. L. Sanchez-Bernardos, Spain; Min-Chieih Tseng, Taiway; K. Okoso Amaa, Tanzania; Saovakon Sudsawasd, Thailand; Sami Guven, Turkey; Sara Staats, United States; Elias Mpofu, Zimbabwe. Data were also collected by Mostafa A. Torki in Kuwait, but they were received after this project was completed. We also wish to thank Dawn Owens-Nicholson for helping us access the World Values Survey Data. Based on the same database, an article titled "The Shifting Basis of Life Satisfaction Judgments Across Cultures: Emotions Versus Norms" authored by Eunkook Suh, Ed Diener, Shigehiro Oishi, and Harry C. Triandis was published in February 1998 in the *Journal of Personality and Social Psychology* (Vol. 74, pp. 482–493). It should be noted, however, that this article examined the role of emotions and norms in life satisfaction judgments and did not overlap with the contents of the present article. Based on the data used in Study 2, an article titled "Culture, Parental Conflict, Parental Marital Status, and the Subjective Well-Being of Young Adults" authored by Carol L. Gohm, Shigehiro Oishi, Janet Darlington, and Ed Diener was also published in May 1998 in the *Journal of Marriage and the Family*. This article explored the relation between marital status and life satisfaction across cultures. Thus, this article also does not overlap with the contents of the current article.

References

Balatsky, G., & Diener, E. (1993). Subjective well-being among Russian students. *Social Indicators Research, 28*, 225–243.

Brunstein, J. C. (1993). Personal goals and subjective well-being: A longitudinal study. *Journal of Personality and Social Psychology, 65*, 1061–1070.

Brunstein, J. C., Schultheiss, O. C., & Grassmann, R. (1998). Personal goals and emotional well-being: The moderating role of motive dispositions. *Journal of Personality and Social Psychology, 75*, 494–508.

Bryk, A. S., & Raudenbush, S. W. (1992). *Hierarchical linear models: Applications and data analysis methods*. Newbury Park, CA: Sage.

Bryk, A. S., Raudenbush, S. W., & Congdon, R. T., Jr. (1994). *Hierarchical linear modeling with the HLM/2L and HLM/3L programs*. Chicago: Scientific Software International.

Campbell, J. D., Trapness, P. D., Heine, S. J., Katz, I. M., Lavallee, L. F., & Lehman, D. R. (1996). Self-concept clarity: Measurement, personality correlates, and cultural boundaries. *Journal of Personality and Social Psychology, 70*, 141–156.

Deci, E. J., & Ryan, R. M. (1985). *Intrinsic motivation and self-determination in human behavior*. Hillsdale, NJ: Lawrence Erlbaum.

Diener, E. (1996). Traits are powerful, but are not enough: Lessons from subjective well-being. *Journal of Research in Personality, 30*, 389–399.

Diener, E., & Diener, M. (1995). Cross-cultural correlates of life satisfaction and self-esteem. *Journal of Personality and Social Psychology, 68*, 653–663.

128000126   S. Oishi et al.

Diener, E., Emmons, R. A., Larsen, R. J., & Griffin, S. (1985). The Satisfaction With Life Scale. *Journal of Personality Assessment, 49*, 71–75.

Diener, E., & Fujita, F. (1995). Resources, personal strivings, and subjective well-being: A nomothetic and idiographic approach. *Journal of Personality and Social Psychology, 68*, 926–935.

Diener, E., Suh, E. M., Lucas, R. E., & Smith, H. L. (1999). Subjective well-being: Three decades of progress: 1967 to 1997. *Psychological Bulletin, 125*, 276–302.

Heine, S. J., & Lehman, D. R. (1995). Cultural variation in unrealistic optimism: Does the West feel more invulnerable than the East? *Journal of Personality and Social Psychology, 68*, 595–607.

Heine, S. J., & Lehman, D. R. (1997). The cultural construction of self-enhancement: An examination of group-serving biases. *Journal of Personality and Social Psychology, 72*, 1268–1283.

Hofstede, G. (1980). *Culture's consequences: International differences in work-related values.* Beverly Hills, CA: Sage.

Kitayama, S., Markus, H. R., Matsumoto, H., & Norasakkunkit, V. (1997). Individual and collective processes in the construction of the self: Self-enhancement in the United States and self-criticism in Japan. *Journal of Personality and Social Psychology, 72*, 1245–1267.

Kwan, V. S. Y., Bond, M. H., & Singelis, T. M. (1997). Pancultural explanations for life satisfaction: Adding relationship harmony to self-esteem. *Journal of Personality and Social Psychology, 73*, 1038–1051.

Lucas, R. E., Diener, E., & Suh, E. (1996). Discriminant validity of well–being measures. *Journal of Personality and Social Psychology, 71*, 616–628.

Markus, H., & Kitayama, S. (1991). Culture and the self: Implications for cognition, emotion, and motivation. *Psychological Review, 98*, 224–253.

Maslow, A. H. (1970). *Motivation and personality.* New York: Harper & Row.

Myers, D. G., & Diener, E. (1995). Who is happy? *Psychological Sciences, 6*, 10–19.

Oishi, S., Diener, E., Suh, E., & Lucas, R. E. (1999). Value as a moderator in subjective well-being. *Journal of Personality, 24*, 1319–1331.

Pavot, W., & Diener, E. (1993). Review of the Satisfaction With Life Scale. *Psychological Assessment, 5*, 164–172.

Radhakrishnan, P., & Chan, D. K. -S. (1997). Cultural differences in the relation between self-discrepancy and life satisfaction. *International Journal of Psychology, 32*, 387–398.

Rosenberg, M. (1965). *Society and the adolescent self-image.* Princeton, NJ: Princeton University Press.

Ryan, R. M., Sheldon, K. M., Kasser, T., & Deci, E. (1996). All goals were not created equal: An organismic perspective on the nature of goals and their regulation. In P. M. Gollwitzer, & J. A. Bargh (Eds.), *The psychology of action: Linking motivation and cognition to behavior.* New York: Guilford.

Schwartz, S. H. (1994). Beyond individualism and collectivism: New cultural dimensions of values. In U. Kim, H. C. Triandis, C. Kagitcibasi, S.-C. Choi, & G. Yoon (Eds.), *Individualism-collectivism: Theory, method, and applications* (pp. 88–122). Newbury Park, CA: Sage.

Shao, L. (1993). *Multilanguage comparability of life satisfaction and happiness measures in mainland Chinese and American students.* Unpublished master's thesis, University of Illinois, Urbana-Champaign.

Shao, L. (1997). *Extraversion and positive affect.* Unpublished doctoral dissertation, University of Illinois, Urbana-Champaign.

Sheldon, K. M., & Kasser, T. (1998). Pursuing personal goals: Skills enable progress, but not all progress is beneficial. *Personality and Social Psychology Bulletin, 24*, 1319–1331.

Sheldon, K. M., Ryan, R. M., & Reis, H. (1996). What makes for a good day? Competence and autonomy in the day, and in the person. *Personality and Social Psychology Bulletin, 22*, 1270–1279.

Suh, E. (1994). *Emotion norms, values, familiarity, and subjective well-being: A cross-cultural examination.* Unpublished master's thesis, University of Illinois, Urbana-Champaign.

Suh, E., Diener, E., Oishi, S., & Triandis, H. C. (1998). The shifting basis of life satisfaction judgments across cultures: Emotions versus norms. *Journal of Personality and Social Psychology, 74*, 482–493.

Triandis, H. C. (1989). The self and social behavior in differing cultural contexts. *Psychological Review, 96*, 506–520.

Triandis, H. C. (1995). *Individualism and collectivism.* Boulder, CO: Westview.

Triandis, H. C. (1996). The psychological measurement of cultural syndromes. *American Psychologist, 51*, 407–415.

Veenhoven, R. (1991). Is happiness relative? *Social Indicators Research, 24*, 1–34.

Veenhoven, R. (1992). *Happiness in nations: Subjective appreciation of life in 56 nations, 1946–1991.* Rotterdam, the Netherlands: Erasmus University Rotterdam.

World Bank. (1992). *World atlas.* Washington, DC: Author.

World Values Study Group. (1994). *World values survey, 1981–1984 and 1990–1993* (computer file, ICPSR version). Ann Arbor, MI: Institute for Social Research.

From Culture to Priming Conditions: Self-Construal Influences on Life Satisfaction Judgments

Eunkook M. Suh, Ed Diener and John A. Updegraff

Abstract Existing cross-cultural research often assumes that the independent versus interdependent self-construal process leads to different cultural behaviors, although few studies directly test this link. Extending from prior cross-cultural findings, two studies were conducted to explicitly test whether self-construal is linked with the differential use of emotions versus social information in judgments of life satisfaction. Study 1 confirmed the prediction that even among Americans, those who view themselves in interdependent terms (allocentrics) evaluate their life satisfaction in a more collectivistic manner (strong reliance on social appraisal) than those who view themselves in independent terms (idiocentrics). Study 2 replicated these findings in two cultural settings (United States and Korea) by using experimental primes of independent versus relational self-construal. Results strongly suggest that differences in self-construal processes underlie cross-cultural differences in life satisfaction judgments.

Psychological research during the past two decades has revealed cultural differences across a wide range of domains. Due to this research effort, most psychologists are now keenly aware that the way people in different cultures think, feel, and act are, in varying degrees, different. Nevertheless, there are still very few research fields, if any, that can point out with precision the exact cause of the cultural difference observed in their research. This difficulty has to do with the fact that many of the existing studies have not clearly identified the precise cultural mechanism producing the outcomes, or when theoretically conceived, failed to directly measure the cultural variable in question (Matsumoto, 1999; Matsumoto & Yoo, 2006; Oyserman, Coon, & Kemmelmeier, 2002).

In this article, we examine in more depth an interesting cross-cultural phenomenon that falls under such a category—cross-cultural differences in the bases of life satisfaction (Schimmack, Radhakrishnan, Oishi, Dzokoto, & Ahadi, 2002; Suh, Diener, Oishi, & Triandis, 1998)—and provide tests of an empirically supported explanation for the differences. When people construct judgments about their

E.M. Suh (✉)
Department of Psychology, Yonsei University, Shinchon-dong, Seoul 120–749, Korea
e-mail: esuh@yonsei.ac.kr

E. Diener (ed.), *Culture and Well-Being: The Collected Works of Ed Diener*, Social
Indicators Research Series 38, DOI 10.1007/978-90-481-2352-0_7,
© Springer Science+Business Media B.V. 2009

overall life satisfaction, different cultural members place relative emphasis on different types of information. Whereas inner emotional experience (relative frequency of positive versus negative affect) is strongly predictive of overall life satisfaction in highly individualistic cultures (e.g., United States, Sweden), life satisfaction is better predicted by social norms (i.e., whether being personally satisfied is perceived as socially acceptable) in collectivistic societies, such as China or India. Such cultural difference emerged from two large sets of international data involving, in total, more than 60,000 respondents from 61 nations (Suh et al., 1998). Schimmack et al. (2002) drew an essentially identical conclusion from another set of international data.

Taking the findings from these three large independent data sets together, the conclusion that life satisfaction judgments are based more heavily on inner emotional experience in individualistic rather than in collectivistic culture is quite robust. However, the precise explanation for this cultural difference has not been documented. Although it was theorized that several defining characteristics of individualism and collectivism (e.g., emphasis on private experience versus relational concerns) played key roles in eliciting the cultural difference, the specific cultural variables were not explicitly measured in these studies.

In terms of Matsumoto and Yoo's (2006) recent distinction of types of cross-cultural research, the Suh et al. (1998) and Schimmack et al. (2002) studies exemplify the Phase III–level research wherein a potential mediator of cultural difference is conceptually identified but not directly measured. The next advancement, suggested by Matsumoto and Yoo, is to conduct a linkage study that attempts to empirically link the observed cultural phenomenon with a specific cultural element that is believed to produce the cultural difference. More specifically, two possible empirical approaches have been suggested. One route is to "unpackage" the influence of culture by replacing culture as an unspecified variable by a more specific individual-level context variable (cf. Matsumoto & Kupperbusch, 2001) and examine whether this measure (e.g., social axioms; Leung et al., 2002) relates with the cultural phenomenon in the predicted direction. Another powerful strategy for demonstrating the linkage between variable X and cultural phenomenon Y is to conduct a priming study, wherein the mind-sets of cultural members are experimentally manipulated in accord with the researcher's theory (e.g., Gardner, Gabriel, & Lee, 1999; Trafimow, Triandis, & Goto, 1991). In line with these suggestions, in this study, we reexamine the life satisfaction judgment pattern observed between cultures at two different levels—at the individual difference level (Study 1) and also through an experimental manipulation (Study 2).

Among the various elements of culture (e.g., beliefs, values, cultural practices), we believe that the way the person defines himself or herself (self-construal) plays a crucial role in influencing the relative use of inner emotional versus more socially nuanced information in judgments of life satisfaction. The most heavily discussed self-construal dimension in reference to culture is the independent versus interdependent self (Markus & Kitayama, 1991). Although important insights have accrued from this framework, the present research is built on the assumption that multiple modes of self-construal exist among all individuals in all cultures (e.g., Brewer & Chen, 2007). Regardless of one's cultural background, all individuals are aware of the unique, personal, and highly independent aspects of self-identity as well as the self-aspects that acquire meaning in relation to others. Although cultures may "sample" (Triandis, 1989) the different aspects of the self to a different degree, all individuals think of themselves in individual, relational, and collective terms. Furthermore, salient contextual cues can temporarily modify self-construal styles, illustrating that the self-system is inherently multiple, flexible, and dynamic rather than singular, fixed, or static (e.g., Gardner et al., 1999; Hong, Benet-Martinez, Chiu, & Morris, 2003; Hong, Morris, Chiu, & Benet-Martinez, 2000).

In the present research, we seek direct empirical evidence for the claim that variation in self-construal is the proximal reason for why life satisfaction judgments are framed differently between cultures (Suh et al., 1998). Although all individuals construe themselves in multiple ways, we are particularly interested in the case when either the individual or the relational self-aspect is relatively more salient than the other. We expect that when the fundamental separateness of the self from others is more accessible than the relational dimension, the person's attention will be directed to the private experiences that affirm his or her uniqueness and individuality (such as emotions). Hence, the "individualistic" life satisfaction judgment pattern—strong reliance on emotions—is expected to emerge in such a self-construal condition. On the other hand, when the relational aspects of the self are at the forefront of attention, we expected that people would go beyond their inner emotions and give considerable weight to social cues in evaluating their overall lives.

In sum, it is believed that the relative salience of the relational versus independent self is a major driving force behind the divergent life satisfaction judgment styles found cross-culturally by Suh et al. (1998) and Schimmack et al. (2002). If this is a valid idea, a parallel style of judgment pattern is expected to occur within a culture, at a chronic individual difference level (Study 1) and also at an experimental level, when either the independent or the relational self-aspects are primed (Study 2). The current predictions, if obtained, will lend strong empirical support for the claim that the self-construal process is strongly linked with the relative weight assigned to affect versus social information in life satisfaction judgments.

Study 1: Idiocentric Versus Allocentric Individuals

Within a culture, individuals vary in the degree to which they define themselves as being separate from or connected with others (Kashima & Hardie, 2000; Matsumoto, Weissman, Preston, Brown, & Kupperbusch, 1997; Sato & McCann, 1998; Singelis, 1994). Triandis, Leung, Villareal, and Clack (1985) proposed the terms *idiocentrism* and *allocentrism* to refer to this individual difference dimension that roughly corresponds with the individualism/collectivism dimension at the cultural level. Triandis, Chan, Bhawuk, Iwao, and Sinha (1995) found that attributes such as dependence on others and sociability characterize allocentrics, whereas separation from groups, independence, and personal competence reflect the core tendencies of idiocentrics. Hence, research suggests that the relational aspects of self-view are salient to allocentric individuals, whereas the unique, independent dimensions of the self are salient to idiocentric individuals.

In this study, we measured how frequently the participants experienced various emotions (affect) as well as their beliefs about how much significant others might approve of their current life (social appraisal). We predicted that idiocentrics would base their life satisfaction prominently on their emotional feelings. Allocentrics, on the other hand, were expected to take a more divergent perspective, consider not only their emotions but also whether significant others approve of their lives.

Participants

To ensure a more clear interpretation of the results (to focus on the variation in self-view), we controlled the ethnic background of the participants (cf. Matsumoto & Kupperbusch, 2001). All 101 participants (81 women) in this study were European American college students. They were enrolled in an advanced course on personality and well-being and received course credit for participation. The majority of the students (96%) were 18–25 years old.

Measures

Allocentrism and idiocentrism. To measure dispositional differences in allocentric and idiocentric tendencies, participants were asked to complete Singelis's (1994) Independent and Interdependent Self-Construal Scale. The independent subscale consists of 12 items that measure thoughts, feelings, and actions reflective of the separateness and uniqueness of the self (e.g., "I enjoy being unique and different from others in many respects"). The interdependent subscale consists of 12 items that tap into the connectedness of the self with others (e.g., "I often have the feeling that my relationships with others are more important than my own accomplishments").

Although the idiocentric/allocentric tendencies were analyzed as a continuous individual difference variable, we also split the sample into two subgroups. A person was classified as an idiocentric ($n = 59$) if his or her Independent score was higher than the Interdependent score. Conversely, participants who had higher Interdependent than Independent self-construal scores were classified as allocentrics ($n = 42$). Five respondents who had identical scores on both subscales were dropped from the analyses. The reason for splitting the sample into two subgroups was simply to ease the comparison between the current outcomes with the previous cross-cultural findings (Schimmack et al., 2002; Suh et al., 1998).

Life satisfaction. Global life satisfaction was measured by the Satisfaction With Life Scale (Diener, Emmons, Larsen, & Griffin, 1985), which is a five-item measure that asks respondents to rate their satisfaction with life. The response scale ranges from *strongly disagree* (1) to *strongly agree* (7), yielding a possible total score ranging from 5 to 35. The alpha coefficient of the scale was 0.91 in the present sample. Further details about this measure are available in Pavot and Diener (1993).

Emotional experience. The emotional experience of the participants was assessed by asking how frequently they felt 8 pleasant emotions that represent two positive higher order affect categories (i.e., joy, love), as well as 16 unpleasant emotions belonging to four negative affect categories (i.e., fear, anger, sadness, and shame–guilt). Diener, Smith, and Fujita (1995) provide a detailed discussion of the theoretical background and the factor structure of these emotion categories.

Participants indicated how frequently they experienced each of the discrete emotions during the previous month on a 7-point scale ranging from *never* (1) to *always* (7). The scores of the eight emotions of the joy and love categories were averaged and used as a measure of pleasant affect. Similarly, scores of the fear, anger, sadness, and shame–guilt categories were averaged to yield an unpleasant affect score. The mean alpha of the two pleasant emotion categories was 0.83, and the mean alpha of the four unpleasant emotion categories was 0.88. A more concise measure of emotional experience was created by subtracting the unpleasant affect score from the pleasant affect score (i.e., affect balance). This affect balance score was used as the emotion score in the regression analyses.

Social appraisal. In an exploratory study, we asked college students to list the most significant persons in their lives. Virtually everyone mentioned his or her parents. Based on this finding, participants were asked to rate on a 7-point scale (*terrible* to *delighted*) how their father and mother would evaluate their lives. The two ratings (father, mother) were averaged to obtain a single social appraisal score.

Results and Discussion

Within each subgroup, regression analysis was conducted to examine the relative weight of affect versus social appraisal in predicting life satisfaction. The standardized beta values of affect ($\beta = 0.51$) and social appraisal ($\beta = 0.34$) were both significant ($p < 0.01$) in predicting the life satisfaction of allocentric participants ($R^2 = 0.47$, $p < 0.001$). In contrast, the life satisfaction of idiocentrics was predicted ($R^2 = 0.43$, $p < 0.001$) significantly by affect ($\beta = 0.64$, $p < 0.001$) but not by social appraisal ($\beta = 0.07$, *ns*). Figure 1 offers a visual summary of

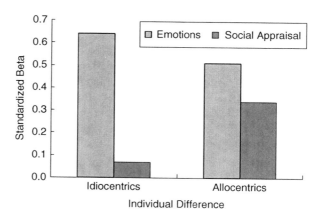

Fig. 1 Relative weight of emotions and social appraisal in predicting life satisfaction: individual difference

the standardized beta weights of the two predictors within each group. The current individual difference findings are strikingly similar to the patterns reported by Suh et al. (1998) at the cross-cultural level, between collectivistic and individualistic groups.

We further examined the data at a continuous individual difference level, conducting a regression analysis on the entire sample. For each individual, we obtained a single self-construal score by subtracting the person's Independent from his or her Interdependent self-construal score. We obtained a combined self-construal score for two reasons. First, conceptually, our focal interest was on the relative salience between the independent and the interdependent self-views within each individual, rather than on the absolute strength of each self-construal. Also important, the combined score preserved statistical power in the analyses of the individual difference result. In short, a higher score on this measure indicated greater salience of the Interdependent rather than the Independent self.

When the main effects were controlled for, the Self-Construal × Social Appraisal interaction was significant ($\beta = 0.20$, $p = 0.01$), but the Self-Construal × Affect interaction was not ($\beta = -0.09$, ns). In other words, those who viewed themselves in highly relational terms were more likely to use social appraisal information in evaluating their lives. The use of affective cues, on the other hand, did not systematically vary across individuals. The result indicates that individual difference in self-construal predicted the degree to which social (rather than affective) information is used in the life satisfaction judgments. This is an interesting finding that could not have been detected at a cultural level of analysis.

Overall, the current results are congruent with the prediction that the life satisfaction patterns at the individual difference level would resemble the findings at the cultural level (Suh et al., 1998). Also, in an unpublished study, we have replicated this phenomenon at an ethnic-group level between Asian Americans and European Americans (Suh & Diener, 2003). Collectively, these findings lend further credence to the idea that self-construal plays a pivotal role in weighing the affective versus social information in evaluating one's life. When the person's independence from others is central, how others view one's life seems to be of marginal concern. Attention in this case is directed primarily inward to the affective experiences. When the relational aspects of the self are salient, however, life satisfaction judgments are formed on a more balanced ground—on emotions as well as on social appraisal information. Whether the perceived social appraisal rating actually corresponds with the thoughts of others is an interesting question in itself (cf. Felson, 1993). The focal interest of this study, however, is more in the degree of attention people devote to the social appraisal than in accuracy of this information. What is found in this study is a positive association between the salience of the relational self and the degree of attention people pay to social appraisal in evaluating their lives.

The strongly converging pattern of results found across different conceptual levels (between cultures, between ethnic groups, individual difference) is very encouraging. Yet we conducted another study to overcome two limitations. First, thus far, all of the findings on this phenomenon are based on correlational data.

The inherent limits of correlational data (e.g., third-variable problem, ambiguous causal direction) apply to these findings. In Study 2, we tested the causal link from self-construal to the use of emotion/social cues in a controlled laboratory setting. Another issue concerns the content of the self-construal scale used in this study. We believe that the degree to which the self is conceived as an independent, separate being or as a common, relational being leads to the present difference in life satisfaction judgment patterns. Recently, however, several articles (e.g., Brewer & Chen, 2007; Hardin, Leong, & Bhagwat, 2004; Levine et al., 2003) have indicated that besides the independent/relational self-representation dimension, the Singelis (1994) scale also includes factors (e.g., esteem for group, behavioral consistency, orientation toward groups) that may confound our current interpretation. Given this multidimensional nature of the Singelis scale, we explicitly manipulated independent versus interdependent self-construal using a priming paradigm in Study 2.

Study 2: Priming Effects

Despite relatively stable individual differences in the self-concept, the relational and the independent aspects of identity coexist in all individuals (e.g., Reid & Deaux, 1996; Sedikides & Brewer, 2001). Furthermore, recent studies have demonstrated that situational cues can lead to "frame switching" between the different self-construal modes (Hong et al., 2000; Trafimow et al., 1991). Given the situational malleability of self-construal, would the findings of Study 1 replicate if the relational or the independent aspects were primed rather than simply measured? Would the consequences of the use of emotion/social information mirror those shaped by relatively stable factors, such as culture or personality?

In Study 2, we experimentally primed either the relational or the unique aspects of the self and examined its consequences on life satisfaction judgments. If self-construal indeed holds the key in causing the divergent life satisfaction judgment patterns, logically, the previous satisfaction judgmental patterns should emerge once again. In addition to providing a conceptual replication of the earlier findings, the current study will provide data that can speak more directly about the causal direction between self-construal and information use. To verify the robustness of the priming effect, we conducted the experiment in two cultural settings—in the United States and also in Korea.

Participants

The U.S. sample consisted of 77 students (37 women) enrolled in an introductory psychology course. The mean age of this American sample was 18.9, and the sample was predominantly White. In Korea, 137 college students (59 women) participated in this study for course credit. The mean age of this culturally homogeneous Korean sample was 20.5.

Measures

Priming procedure. Participants were randomly assigned to either the independent-self or the relational-self prime conditions developed by Trafimow et al. (1991) and validated in later studies (Trafimow & Finlay, 1996; Ybarra & Trafimow, 1998). Two forms of questionnaires were randomly distributed to the participants in both cultures. Those who received the independent-self form were asked, on the cover sheet, to "think of what makes you different from your family and friends" for 3 min. Those who received the relational-self form, on the other hand, were instructed to "think of what you have in common with your family and friends." Except for this difference, the questionnaire was identical across the two conditions. In the United States, 37 participants received the independent-self prime questionnaire, and 40 students completed the relational-self prime form. In Korea, 69 and 68 participants were assigned, respectively, to the independent- and the relational-self conditions.

Scales. Measures of life satisfaction and affect balance were identical to those described in Study 1. In the United States, the alpha coefficient was 0.86 for the life satisfaction measure and 0.75 for positive affect as well as for negative affect. In Korea, the alphas were 0.76 for life satisfaction, 0.91 for positive affect, and 0.82 for negative affect. As in Study 1, an affect balance score was calculated by subtracting the negative affect mean from the positive affect mean. More information about the cross-cultural validity of the current well-being measures is available in Diener, Suh, Smith, and Shao (1995), Shao (1993), and Suh (1994).

To obtain a social appraisal measure, participants were first asked to list the three most important persons in their lives (see also Suh, 2002). Next, using a 7-point scale ranging from *terrible* (1) to *delighted* (7), the participants indicated how they think their overall life is evaluated by each of the three significant others they listed. The mean of these three ratings was used as the social appraisal score. Overall, the Americans ($M = 5.84$, $SD = 0.70$) believed that their lives were viewed more positively ($p < 0.001$, $\eta^2 = 0.051$) by significant others than did the Korean sample ($M = 5.38$, $SD = 1.11$).

Results and Discussion

A regression analysis was conducted separately for each cultural group. Among the U.S. participants, a striking difference was found between the priming conditions in the relative weight placed on emotions and social appraisal in the judgment of life satisfaction (see Fig. 2). When the unique individuality of the self was primed (left graphs), life satisfaction was predicted primarily by emotions. The beta weight of emotions was significant ($\beta = 0.51$, $p < 0.01$), but social appraisal ($\beta = 0.05$, *ns*) was not. On the other hand, in the relational-self prime condition, both emotions ($\beta = 0.38$) and social appraisal ($\beta = 0.33$) accounted for a significant amount ($p < 0.05$) of the predicted life satisfaction variance. These outcomes closely mirror the differences found between idiocentric and allocentric individuals in Study 1.

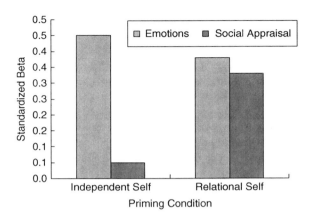

Fig. 2 Relative weight of emotions and social appraisal in predicting life satisfaction: priming effects among americans

The priming effects among the Koreans also appeared in the direction consistent with our prediction. As illustrated in Fig. 3, in the unique-self prime condition, only affect ($\beta = 0.36$, $p < 0.05$) significantly contributed to the prediction of life satisfaction (cf. social appraisal $\beta = -0.03$, ns). Conversely, when the relational aspects of the self were primed, only social appraisal significantly predicted life satisfaction ($\beta = 0.45$, $p < 0.001$). In contrast to the U.S. sample, the beta weight of affect was only marginally significant ($\beta = 0.19$, $p = 0.08$).

These priming results offer the first powerful empirical evidence supporting the argument that the salience of the relational versus the independent self creates different cognitive approaches in life satisfaction judgments. It is important to note that these experimental findings support the causal direction proposed throughout this research. Among collectivistic (Korean) as well as individualistic (American) cultural members, changes in self-perspective led to predicted patterns of information use. Also, the effects of the priming manipulations suggest that self-representations

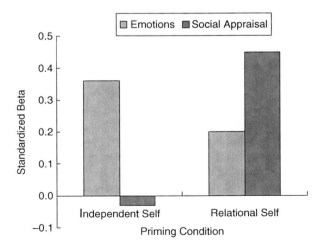

Fig. 3 Relative weight of emotions and social appraisal in predicting life satisfaction: priming effects among koreans

about unique, independent versus relational aspects of identity (rather than other dimensions tapped in existing self-measures) play a key role in producing this self-judgmental pattern.

In retrospect, it would have been interesting if we had included a control condition (no priming) in this research. Without a control condition to compare against, it is difficult to know precisely how atypical the relational-prime and the unique-prime outcomes are from the culture's typical state of affairs. For example, even though the relational-prime induces greater reliance of social appraisal in both cultures, the effect seems to be more extreme in Korea than in the United States. We hope these interesting issues (e.g., teasing apart the chronic cultural tendency versus priming effects) are addressed more systematically in future research.

Perhaps one of the more provocative implications of this study is that it seems to take relatively little (e.g., priming) to override the chronic information-processing habits shaped by stable factors, such as culture or personality. The American participants, contrary to the culturally ingrained cognitive habits, evaluated themselves significantly on social terms when the relational aspects of the self were primed. Similarly, Korean participants relied exclusively on emotional cues when the unique individuality of the self was highly accessible. Does this imply that cultural behaviors are more fragile and malleable than most have assumed? Our short answer is "not necessarily." This is an important theoretical issue that we address in the next section.

General Discussion

On what types of information are evaluations of one's life based? According to the current research, the answer depends on how the person conceptualizes herself or himself. At times, people draw a sharp boundary between the self and others, whereas at other times, they try to absorb the thoughts and experiences of others into the self-construal process. The present findings collectively demonstrate that this self-construal process, regardless of the specific cause (personality, priming effect), predicts the type of information used in global self-evaluations. When the distinct separateness of the self is salient, overall life is appraised prominently on the basis of internal emotions. When the self is viewed largely in relation to others, other people's appraisals, in addition to emotions, seem to become important in evaluating one's life.

Particularly notable is the fact that this pattern of results is found across various construct levels. This self-judgmental pattern, previously observed between cultures (Schimmack et al., 2002; Suh et al., 1998) and between ethnic groups (Suh & Diener, 2003) was replicated between personality types (Study 1) and in two separate priming studies (Study 2). The only common denominator across these studies was the difference in self-view; other factors, such as the study methods and the reasons underlying the self-view difference, varied considerably. Hence, the converging results lend strong support to the idea that the self plays a crucial role in the selection of internal/social information. Especially, the experimental data in

Study 2 offered critical support for this interpretation. In sum, we believe that a solid empirical link exists between self-construal and the use of information in life satisfaction judgments.

Our findings have significant implications for subjective well-being (Diener, Suh, Lucas, & Smith, 1999) researchers. Researchers in the field have recognized that global life satisfaction judgments are seldom outcomes of exhaustive cognitive calculations but more often a swift evaluation derived from a heuristic cue (Schwarz & Strack, 1999). What heuristic cue offers a reasonable summary of one's overall life? "Affect" has been a popular answer in the field (Schwarz & Clore, 1983). Present findings partly support this idea. In all but one case (the relational-self prime condition in Korea), participants consulted their emotions when evaluating their lives. However, when it comes to the question of whether emotion information alone is sufficient for making the satisfaction judgment, the answer seems to vary as a function of the dominant self-construal mode.

Another important issue prompted by this research concerns the malleability versus the stability of cultural behavior. Both in Korea and in the United States, priming manipulations had clearly visible effects on the self-judgment process. It illustrates that psychological dispositions shaped by cultures are still very flexible and sensitive to external input. However, we should not overstate the malleability of cultural behavior on the basis of the current priming findings. The priming effects experimentally induced in Study 2 are qualitatively different from the impact culture has on psychological behavior in several respects. Obviously, the priming effects are transient and momentary, whereas the cultural influences are enduring. Another important difference is the scope of the two effects. The self-construal that was manipulated in this study is only one specific slice of the infinite psychological tendencies molded by cultural forces. When we say that a person has become completely acculturated (if this is possible), for instance, we mean much more than whether the person defines himself or herself primarily in independent or relational terms.

The final, but perhaps the most crucial, distinction between priming versus cultural influence concerns the naturalness of the effect. Culture affects human behavior in such a thorough and inconspicuous manner that people usually need to be reminded of its influence. As we know, Durkheim used the metaphor of invisible air to illustrate this subtle but omnipresent power of culture. This idea is important for putting the current priming studies in proper perspective. In a sense, the relational-self prime is the type of situation that seems to occur naturally and on a constant basis in more collectivistic societies. The independent-self prime conditions, on the other hand, are the ones that are more likely to be created on a regular basis in individualistic cultures. Although priming is a powerful method for testing the conceptual links of a theory of cultural influence, we should not lose sight of the fact that the priming manipulations lack a critical feature of cultural influence—its regularity and naturalness.

In closing, we propose several future research possibilities that stem from the current findings. Besides life satisfaction, what other types of judgments or decisions are influenced by the differential use of affective and social information? For instance, as a function of the self-view, are other types of evaluations, such as judgments of morality, major life decisions, or impressions of other people, constructed more on either affective or on social cues? For instance, in one of our ongoing studies, Americans reported that the "essence" of a person is mostly hidden beneath the visible layer of the self, whereas East Asians emphasized the relatively visible, overt features of the self, such as appearance, gestures, and mannerisms (Suh, Park, & Park, 2006). Such different lay beliefs about the defining qualities of the person may have developed from cultural differences in the chronic amount of attention paid to the inner, private versus the overt, social dimensions of the self. There might be many other intriguing cultural and individual differences in judgments about the self, others, or the world that stem from the differential attention to these covert/social aspects of the self.

One final question this research triggers is whether relying more on affective or social cues makes a difference in the mean level of life satisfaction. Cultures that rely more on affective information tend to report higher mean levels of life satisfaction (Diener & Suh, 1999). Quite interesting, a similar phenomenon is also observed at the individual difference level. Among individuals, those who are particularly happy and enjoy high self-esteem are more likely than others to rely on internal, subjective cues than on external, social standards in their self-evaluation (e.g., Lyubomirsky & Ross, 1997; Wayment & Taylor, 1995). One possible explanation is that internal cues are more ambiguous and thus easier to reinterpret in a self-serving manner than are external, social cues (Updegraff & Suh, 2007). It seems worth examining, at the cross-cultural level, whether the type of information used in life satisfaction is also systematically related with mean cultural differences in subjective well-being (Suh, 2007).

Acknowledgments We are grateful to Michael Robinson, Jerry Clore, Harry Triandis, and Myungho Cha for their help and comments during the various phases of this research.

References

Brewer, M. B., & Chen, Y. (2007). Where (who) are collectives in collectivism? Toward conceptual clarification of individualism and collectivism. *Psychological Review, 114*, 133–151.
Diener, E., Emmons, R. A., Larsen, R. J., & Griffin, S. (1985). The Satisfaction With Life Scale. *Journal of Personality Assessment, 49*, 71–75.
Diener, E., Smith, H., & Fujita, F. (1995). The personality structure of affect. *Journal of Personality and Social Psychology, 69*, 130–141.
Diener, E., & Suh, E. M. (1999). National differences in subjective well-being. In D. Kahneman, E. Diener, & N. Schwarz (Eds.), *Well-being: The foundations of hedonic psychology* (pp. 434–450). New York: Russell Sage.
Diener, E., Suh, E. M., Lucas, R., & Smith, H. (1999). Subjective well-being: Three decades of progress. *Psychological Bulletin, 125*, 276–302.
Diener, E., Suh, E. M., Smith, H., & Shao, L. (1995). National differences in reported subjective well-being: Why do they occur? *Social Indicators Research, 34*, 7–32.
Felson, R. B. (1993). The (somewhat) social self: How others affect self-appraisals. In J. Suls (Ed.), *Psychological perspectives on the self: The self in social perspective* (pp. 1–26). Hillsdale, NJ: Lawrence Erlbaum.

Gardner, W. L., Gabriel, S., & Lee, A. Y. (1999). "I" value freedom, but "we" value relationships: Self-construal priming mirrors cultural differences in judgment. *Psychological Science, 10,* 321–326.

Hardin, E. E., Leong, F. T. L., & Bhagwat, A. A. (2004). Factor structure of the self-construal scale revisited. *Journal of Cross-Cultural Psychology, 35,* 327–345.

Hong, Y., Benet-Martinez, V., Chiu, C., & Morris, M. W. (2003). Boundaries of cultural influence: Construct activation as a mechanism for cultural differences in social perception. *Journal of Cross-Cultural Psychology, 34,* 453–464.

Hong, Y., Morris, M. W., Chiu, C., & Benet-Martinez, V. (2000). Multicultural minds: A dynamic constructivist approach to culture and cognition. *American Psychologist, 55,* 709–720.

Kashima, E., & Hardie, E. A. (2000). The development and validation of the Relational, Individual, and Collective Self-Aspects (RIC) scale. *Asian Journal of Social Psychology, 3,* 19–48.

Leung, K., Bond, M. H., de Carrasquel, S. R., Munoz, C., Hernandez, M., Murakami, F., et al. (2002). Social axioms: The search for universal dimensions of general beliefs about how the world functions. *Journal of Cross-Cultural Psychology, 33,* 286–302.

Levine, T. K., Bresnahan, M. J., Park, H. S., Lapinski, M. K., Wittenbaum, G. M., Shearman, S. M., et al. (2003). Self-construal scales lack validity. *Human Communication Research, 29,* 210–252.

Lyubomirsky, S., & Ross, L. (1997). Hedonic consequences of social comparison: A contrast of happy and unhappy people. *Journal of Personality and Social Psychology, 76,* 988–1007.

Markus, H. R., & Kitayama, S. (1991). Culture and self: Implications for cognition, emotion, and motivation. *Psychological Review, 98,* 224–253.

Matsumoto, D. (1999). Culture and self: An empirical assessment of Markus and Kitayama's theory of independent and interdependent self-construal. *Asian Journal of Social Psychology, 2,* 289–310.

Matsumoto, D., & Kupperbusch, C. (2001). Idiocentric and allocentric differences in emotional expression, experience, and the coherence between expression and experience. *Asian Journal of Social Psychology, 4,* 113–131.

Matsumoto, D., Weissman, M. D., Preston, K., Brown, B. R., & Kupperbusch, C. (1997). Context-specific measurement of individualism–collectivism on the individual level: The individualism–collectivism interpersonal assessment inventory. *Journal of Cross-Cultural Psychology, 28,* 743–767.

Matsumoto, D., & Yoo, S. H. (2006). Toward a new generation of cross-cultural research. *Perspectives on Psychological Science, 1,* 234–250.

Oyserman, D., Coon, H. M., & Kemmelmeier, M. (2002). Rethinking individualism and collectivism: Evaluation of theoretical assumptions and meta-analyses. *Psychological Bulletin, 128,* 3–72.

Pavot, W., & Diener, E. (1993). Review of the Satisfaction With Life Scale. *Psychological Assessment, 5,* 164–172.

Reid, A., & Deaux, K. (1996). Relationship between social and personal identities: Segregation or integration? *Journal of Personality and Social Psychology, 71,* 1084–1091.

Sato, T., & McCann, D. (1998). Individual differences in relatedness and individuality: An exploration of two constructs. *Personality and Individual Differences, 24,* 847–859.

Schimmack, U., Radhakrishnan, P., Oishi, S., Dzokoto, V., & Ahadi, S. (2002). Culture, personality, and subjective well-being: Integrating process models of life satisfaction. *Journal of Personality and Social Psychology, 82,* 582–593.

Schwarz, N., & Clore, G. (1983). Mood, misattribution, and judgments of well-being: Informative and directive functions of affective states. *Journal of Personality and Social Psychology, 45,* 513–523.

Schwarz, N., & Strack, F. (1999). Reports of subjective well-being: Judgmental processes and their methodological implications. In D. Kahneman, E. Diener, & N. Schwarz (Eds.), *Well-being: The foundations of hedonic psychology* (pp. 61–84). New York: Russell Sage.

Sedikides, C., & Brewer, M. B. (Eds.). (2001). *Individual self, relational self, collective self.* Philadelphia: Psychology Press.

Shao, L. (1993). *Multilanguage comparability of life satisfaction and happiness measures in mainland Chinese and American students*. Unpublished master's thesis, University of Illinois at Urbana-Champaign.

Singelis, T. M. (1994). The measurement of independent and interdependent self-construals. *Personality and Social Psychology Bulletin, 20,* 580–591.

Suh, E. (1994). *Emotion norms, values, familiarity, and subjective well-being: A cross-cultural examination*. Unpublished master's thesis, University of Illinois at Urbana-Champaign.

Suh, E. M. (2002). Culture, identity consistency, and subjective well-being. *Journal of Personality and Social Psychology, 86,* 1378–1391.

Suh, E. M. (2007). Downsides of an overly context-sensitive self: Implications from the culture and subjective well-being research. *Journal of Personality, 75,* 1321–1343.

Suh, E. M., & Diener, E. (2003). *Ethnic group differences in life satisfaction judgment patterns*. Unpublished data, University of California, Irvine.

Suh, E., Diener, E., Oishi, S., & Triandis, H. C. (1998). The shifting basis of life satisfaction judgments across cultures: Emotions versus norms. *Journal of Personality and Social Psychology, 74,* 494–512.

Suh, E. M., Park, E., & Park, J. (2006). *Essence of the person—inside or outside? Cultural differences in the weighting of visible and invisible personality cues*. Manuscript in preparation, Yonsei University.

Trafimow, D., & Finlay, K. A. (1996). The importance of subjective norms for a minority of people: Between-subjects and within-subjects analyses. *Personality and Social Psychology Bulletin, 22,* 820–828.

Trafimow, D., Triandis, H. C., & Goto, S. G. (1991). Some tests of the distinction between the private self and the collective self. *Journal of Personality and Social Psychology, 60,* 649–655.

Triandis, H. C. (1989). Self and social behavior in differing cultural contexts. *Psychological Review, 96,* 269–289.

Triandis, H. C., Chan, D. K. S., Bhawuk, D. P. S., Iwao, S., & Sinha, J. B. P. (1995). Multimethod probes of allocentrism and idiocentrism. *International Journal of Psychology, 30,* 461–480.

Triandis, H. C., Leung, K., Villareal, M., & Clack, F. L. (1985). Allocentric and idiocentric tendencies: Convergent and discriminant validation. *Journal of Research in Personality, 19,* 395–415.

Updegraff, J. A., & Suh, E. M. (2007). Happiness is a warm abstract thought: Self-construal abstractness and subjective well-being. *Journal of Positive Psychology, 2,* 18–28.

Wayment, H., & Taylor, S. E. (1995). Self-evaluation processes: Motives, information use, and self-esteem. *Journal of Personality, 63,* 729–757.

Ybarra, O., & Trafimow, D. (1998). How priming the private self or collective self affects the relative weights of attitudes and subjective norms. *Personality and Social Psychology Bulletin, 24,* 362–370.

The Dynamics of Daily Events and Well-Being Across Cultures: When Less Is More

Shigehiro Oishi, Ed Diener, Dong-Won Choi, Chu Kim-Prieto and Incheol Choi

Abstract The authors examined cultural and individual differences in the relation between daily events and daily satisfaction. In a preliminary study, they established cross-cultural equivalence of 50 daily events. In the main study, participants in the United States, Korea, and Japan completed daily surveys on the 50 events and daily satisfaction for 21 days. The multilevel random coefficient model analyses showed that (a) the within-person association between positive events and daily satisfaction was significantly stronger among Asian American, Korean, and Japanese participants than among European American participants and (b) the within-person association between positive events and daily satisfaction was significantly weaker among individuals high in global life satisfaction than among those low in global life satisfaction. The findings demonstrate a weaker effect of positive events on daily well-being among individuals and cultures high in global well-being.

Throughout the course of a typical day, people experience various events, some positive and others negative. A professor might give a brilliant lecture and receive a standing ovation from his students in the morning but return to his office in the afternoon to find out that his latest paper was rejected for publication. To what degree might a positive event such as giving an excellent lecture mitigate the damaging effect of a negative event such as rejection? Conversely, to what extent do negative events nullify the impact of positive events on daily satisfaction? The present research examined cultural and individual differences in the relation between daily events and daily satisfaction. Specifically, we sought to answer three fundamental questions: (a) How many positive events must be experienced to mitigate a negative event? (b) Are there individual and/or cultural differences in the number of positive events needed to nullify the effect of one negative event? and (c) What are the factors underlying these individual and cultural differences, ifthey do in fact exist?

S. Oishi (✉)
Department of Psychology, University of Virginia, P.O. Box 400400, Charlottesville, VA 22904-4400, USA
e-mail: soishi@virginia.edu

E. Diener (ed.), *Culture and Well-Being: The Collected Works of Ed Diener*, Social Indicators Research Series 38, DOI 10.1007/978-90-481-2352-0_8, © Springer Science+Business Media B.V. 2009

Answers to these questions will illuminate the process of adaptation to daily life events and shed light on the dynamic interplay between positive and negative daily experiences, bolstering the critical building blocks of recent theorizing and research on well-being (Diener & Oishi, 2005; Fredrickson & Losada, 2005; Kahneman, Krueger, Schkade, Schwarz, & Stone, 2004; Lyubomirsky, Sheldon, & Schkade, 2005; Myers, 2000; Wilson & Gilbert, 2005).

Life Events and Well-Being

Previous research on life events has uncovered important processes underlying how quickly people adapt to major life events, such as winning the lottery (Brickman, Coates, & Janoff-Bulman, 1978), the death of a spouse (Lehman, Wortman, & Williams, 1987; Lucas, Clark, Georgellis, & Diener, 2003; W. Stroebe, M. Stroebe, Abakoumkin, & Schut, 1996), and experiencing disability (Brickman et al., 1978), as well as to daily events, such as getting an A on an exam or receiving an unexpected gift (Seidlitz & Diener, 1993). It has also been shown that certain types of events are easier to adjust to than others (Janoff-Bulman, 1992; Weinsten, 1982). In addition, previous research on personality and coping styles has demonstrated that individuals vary not only in their reactivity to life events (Bolger & Zuckerman, 1995; Carver et al., 1993; Caspi et al., 2003; Peterson, Seligman, & Vaillant, (1988); Stone, Kennedy-Moore, & Neale, 1995) but also in the degree to which they actively create certain life events (Headey & Wearing, 1989; Seidlitz & Diener, 1993; Suh, Diener, & Fujita, 1996; Suls & Martin, 2005). The research on life events, adaptation, and well-being has thus far tended to examine either the effects of positive events on overall well-being without considering the nullifying effect of negative events, or the effect of negative events without considering the mitigating effect of positive events. With recent research (e.g., Folkman & Moskowitz, 2000; Fredrickson & Levenson, 1998) demonstrating the important mitigating power of positive affect, the next step is to determine the equilibrium point—that is, the number of positive life events one must experience to mitigate one negative event.

The Equilibrium Point

Fredrickson and Losada (2005) have recently extended Gottman's (1994) research on marital interactions and the critical ratio of positive versus negative interactions in order to document the emotional lives of flourishing versus languishing individuals. The researchers found that individuals who experienced at least 2.9 times more positive than negative emotions rated their lives to be satisfying, whereas those who had a positive-to-negative-emotion ratio of less than 2.9 to 1 rated their lives to be unsatisfying. Just as successful couples had five times more positive interactions than negative ones in Gottman's research, individuals, too, appear to need more positive than negative emotions to maintain a satisfying life.

Although Fredrickson and Losada (2005) were the first to explicitly examine the critical ratio of positive to negative emotions on overall well-being, several diary studies provide other relevant information. Lawton, DeVoe, and Parmelee (1995), for instance, examined daily events and affect among the elderly and found that the impact of negative events was 1.8 times stronger than that of positive ones.[1] Similarly, Nezlek & Gable (2001) reported that daily negative events were 2.25 times more strongly associated with participants' daily self-esteem than daily positive events (see also David, Green, Martin, & Suls, 1997; Nezlek & Plesko, 2003).

Beyond the realm of well-being research, there is a plethora of findings suggesting that the negative is more influential than the positive, observed in domains ranging from judgment and decision making (e.g., Kahneman & Tversky, 1979), person perception (e.g., Skowronski & Carlston, 1989), and psychophysiology (e.g., Cacioppo, Gardner, & Berntson, 1999; Ito, Larsen, Smith, & Cacioppo, 1998) to food (Rozin & Royzman, 2001) and marriage (see Gottman, 1994; Baumeister, Bratslavsky, Finkenauer, & Vohs, 2001; Rozin & Royzman, 2001; see also Taylor, 1991, for an excellent review).

Individual and Cultural Differences in the Equilibrium Point

Whereas the primacy of negative experiences over positive ones has been well documented across a variety of domains, individual differences in the degree of negative experience potency have rarely been examined (for exceptions, see Gable, Reis, & Elliot, 2000; Nezlek & Gable, 2001; Nezlek & Plesko, 2003). To our knowledge, moreover, cultural differences have never been examined. This absence of systematic investigation into individual and cultural differences in the relative impact of positive versus negative events on well-being may be due to the fact that no appropriate theoretical model exists. Thus, in order to put forward a systematic, theory-based investigation into individual and cultural differences in this area, we propose a frequency model of life events and well-being. Like Baumeister et al. (2001), we first postulate that the impact of a positive event should be larger for individuals or societies that experience positive events infrequently than for individuals or societies that experience positive events frequently. We propose that those who experience positive events frequently become accustomed to them, come to expect their frequent occurrence, and consequently pay less attention to them (cf. Kahneman & Thaler, 2006). Thus, a new positive event does not have the same import that it might for someone who does not experience positive events as frequently. In addition, people adapt more quickly to an event that can be easily explained (e.g., an expected event) than to an event that cannot be easily explained (e.g., a surprising event; Wilson, Centerbar, Kermer, & Gilbert, 2005). To the extent that

---

[1] The ratios reported here were computed using the regression coefficients reported in Lawton et al. (1995) and Nezlek and Gable (2001).

positive events are less expected for people who experience them less frequently, positive events should have a greater impact on the well-being of these individuals.

The frequency model points to an intriguing divergence between global and daily satisfaction. The frequent experience of positive events has repeatedly been shown to be associated with high global well-being (Diener, Sandvik, & Pavot, 1991; Schimmack, 2003). However, if our speculation is correct, this very factor is, ironically, also associated with the diminished effect of a positive event on daily satisfaction. In other words, individuals who experience positive events frequently are higher in global life satisfaction but benefit less on a day-to-day basis from the experience of a single positive event, as compared with those low in global life satisfaction. In more formal terms, we expect that global well-being is related to a declining benefit of positive events for daily satisfaction. That is, the within-person association between daily positive events and daily satisfaction should be weaker for individuals high in global life satisfaction and stronger for those low in global life satisfaction.

Projecting to the group level, we predict that a cultural group with higher levels of global well-being should benefit less on a day-to-day basis from the experience of a positive event as compared with a group with lower levels of global well-being. On average, the within-person association between daily positive events and daily satisfaction should be smaller in groups with higher levels of global well-being than in groups with lower levels of global well-being. Previous research in this regard has consistently found that Koreans, Japanese, and Asian Americans report lower levels of global life satisfaction than do European Americans (see Diener, Oishi, & Lucas, 2003, for a review). Moreover, it has been shown that North Americans expect more positive events to happen to them in the future than do Japanese (e.g., Chang & Asakawa, 2003; Heine & Lehman, 1995). Extrapolating from these findings, we anticipate that the benefit of a positive event on daily satisfaction will be higher for Koreans, Japanese, and Asian Americans than for European Americans.

In summary, we present the frequency model of life events and well-being and investigate a new set of questions about the interplay between positive and negative events across cultures. Before testing our main research questions, however, we first conducted a preliminary study to test the equivalence of 50 daily events in the United States, Japan, and Korea. Once the cross-cultural equivalence of these daily events was established, we conducted the main study, a 21-day diary study in the United States, Japan, and Korea. We chose the daily method for the several reasons. First, this method reduces memory biases, which are often present in research on life events and well-being (Kahneman et al., 2004; Reis & Gable, 2000). Second, many of the central theoretical questions regarding affective adaptation are, by nature, within-person phenomena (e.g., "How many positive events must an individual experience to mitigate a negative event?"), and the daily diary method provides an ideal test for such questions (Bolger, Davis, & Rafaeli, 2003; Tennen, Affleck, & Armeli, 2005). Finally, most cross-cultural research in the past has examined either mean differences (e.g., "Which nation is more satisfied?") or differences in the magnitude of between-person correlations (e.g., "Is the size of the correlation between self-esteem and life satisfaction different across cultures?"; for exceptions, see Mesquita & Karasawa, 2002; Oishi, Diener, Scollon, & Biswas-Diener, 2004; Watson, Clark, & Tellegen, 1984). In this regard, previous cross-cultural research has not sufficiently tested the effect of real-life contexts, including actual life events, on well-being.

Contextual effects are best detected when the same individual is observed on numerous occasions (Baltes, Reese, & Nesselroade, 1977; Lazarus, 2000). Several prominent psychologists have argued that the pattern of variation within an individual should serve as the basic building block of personality psychology (Allport, 1961; Fleeson, 2001; Mischel & Shoda, 1995; Nesselroade, 1984; Zevon & Tellegen, 1982). We echo this sentiment by arguing that scientific theories regarding culture and well-being should also be built from the bottom up, starting with the within-individual processes (see Oishi, 2004, for a brief theoretical discussion on this issue). The investigation of how the frequency of positive and negative events relates to the daily fluctuations in an individual's satisfaction, and how the pattern of these within-person associations might differ across cultural groups, will provide a valuable vantage point for understanding the processes of adaptation to life events and well-being across cultures.

Preliminary Study

We conducted a preliminary study with two goals in mind. The first goal was to test and establish cross-cultural equivalence of daily events used in the main daily diary study. This was an important first step because if positive events were perceived more positively and negative events were perceived less negatively in Culture A than in Culture B, participants in Culture A would be more likely to overcome a negative event with fewer positive events than would participants in Culture B. In other words, cultural differences in positivity–negativity ratings of daily events used in the main study could create artificial cultural differences in the number of positive events required to mitigate one negative event. The second goal of the preliminary study was to test and establish equivalence of the strength of positive and negative events. If the negative events included were extremely negative and the positive events were mildly positive, this would necessarily result in a negativity bias (i.e., more than one positive event would be required to overcome one negative event). To avoid this pitfall, we needed to establish that the positivity of positive events was equivalent in strength to the negativity of negative events included in the main study.

Method

Participants. Participants were 139 college students in the United States, Korea, and Japan. Specifically, the sample included 29 European American students (18 women, 11 men) and 44 Asian American students (27 women, 17 men) at California State University, East Bay; 36 Korean students (23 women, 13 men) at Yonsei

University and Seoul National University in Korea; and 30 Japanese students (18 women, 12 men) at Kansei Gakuin University in Japan.

Procedure. Participants were recruited in class or via e-mail. Potential participants contacted the researcher at each research site via e-mail and then were given the Web address of the questionnaire. They completed the Web survey at their own convenience. Participation was voluntary, and no compensation was given. Students at California State University, East Bay, completed the questionnaire in English, Korean students completed the questionnaire in Korean, and Japanese students completed the questionnaire in Japanese. All survey materials had been translated from English into Japanese and Korean by an experienced translator. The final versions of the materials were then tested for equivalence by psychologists in the respective cultures. Minor adjustments in wording were made to make the questionnaire and survey questions as clear as possible.

Participants were asked to indicate how good or bad each of the 50 events would be if it happened on a typical day, using a 7-point scale (1 = *extremely bad*, 4 = *neither bad nor good*, 7 = *extremely good*). We chose the 50 events from a review of the literature on life events by Seidlitz and Diener (1993), who had compiled a list of 80 events. Our research team, which includes one Japanese, one Korean, and two Asian Americans, examined these events and selected 25 positive and 25 negative events that appeared to occur commonly in Korea and Japan as well as in the United States. Of these, 13 positive and 13 negative events were used in the analyses in the main study; these are listed in the Appendix. In addition to the events in the Appendix, the original 50 events included "went to a concert, play, movie, or other artistic event," "went to a talk, seminar, or public meeting on a topic of interest," "went for a walk," "went to an athletic or sporting event," "attended a religious service (because I wanted to)," "engaged in spiritual reading or meditation," "engaged in creative art or craft work for leisure," "read an interesting article or book," "I improved my character," "did homework," "received a personal letter, phone call, or e-mail message," "I felt good physically and emotionally," "almost got run over, or hit someone while driving," "spilled food or drink on oneself or someone," "had an unexpected expense over $30 that I personally had to pay," "self or immediate family member was victim of a nonviolent crime," "received an unfairly low grade on a quiz, test, homework, or paper," "food I ate was not of satisfactory quality," and "performed poorly in a sports event."

Results and Discussion

Are positivity and negativity of daily events equivalent across cultures? We first computed the mean positivity-negativity ratings for each cultural group separately for the original 25 positive and 25 negative events and for the 13 positive and 13 negative events used in the main analyses (see Table 1). One-way analysis of variance (ANOVA) showed no cultural group differences in positivity ratings of the 25 positive events, $F(3, 135) = 0.35$, *ns*, or on the 13 positive events, $F(3, 135) = 0.10$, *ns*. One-way ANOVA also showed no cultural group differences in negativity of the 25 negative events, $F(3, 135) = 1.75$, $p = 0.16$, or the 13 negative events,

Table 1 Mean positivity–negativity ratings (and standard deviations) of daily events

Cultural group	Original 50 events		Final 26 events	
	Positive	Negative	Positive	Negative
European Americans	5.88 (0.50)	2.26 (0.50)	6.10 (0.51)	2.24 (0.51)
Asian Americans	5.81 (0.52)	2.26 (0.64)	6.15 (0.53)	2.25 (0.69)
Koreans	5.92 (0.49)	2.08 (0.40)	6.17 (0.52)	1.99 (0.40)
Japanese	5.84 (0.51)	2.04 (0.43)	6.13 (0.57)	1.99 (0.47)

Note. Mean ratings for the original 50 events (25 positive, 25 negative) and the 26 events used in the final analyses (13 positive, 13 negative). Ratings were made on a 7-point scale ($1 = extremely\ bad$, $4 = neither\ bad\ nor\ good$, $7 = extremely\ good$).

$F(3, 135) = 2.63$, $p = 0.06$. Because the cultural difference in the 13 negative events approached significance, we conducted post hoc tests with Bonferroni corrections. None of the six pairwise group comparisons, however, was close to significant ($ps > 0.22$). Thus, positivity-negativity of the daily events used in the main study did not differ across the four cultural groups.

Are positive events as positive as negative events are negative? Next, we tested whether positive events were perceived as positively as negative events were perceived negatively in our samples. We conducted a one-sample t test against the midpoint of the 7-point scale (4, *neither bad nor good*). As predicted, the mean positivity rating of the 25 positive events was significantly higher than the midpoint of 4 ($M_{dif} = 1.86$), $t(138) = 43.72$, $p < 0.001$, whereas the mean negativity rating of the 25 negative events was significantly lower than the midpoint of 4 ($M_{dif} = -1.84$), $t(138) = -42.08$, $p < 0.001$. The magnitudes of deviation from the midpoint were nearly identical, demonstrating the equivalence in strength of positivity-negativity of these 25 positive and 25 negative events. Similarly, the mean positivity rating of the 13 positive events was significantly higher than the midpoint of 4 ($M_{dif} = 2.14$), $t(138) = 47.82$, $p < 0.001$, whereas the mean negativity rating of the 13 negative events was significantly lower than the midpoint of 4 ($M_{dif} = -1.88$), $t(138) = -40.05$, $p < 0.001$. Again, the magnitudes of deviation from the midpoint were nearly symmetrical.

In sum, this study established the cross-cultural equivalence of daily events that were used in the subsequent main study, at least in terms of positivity and negativity. In addition, this study demonstrated that the positive events were as positive as the negative events were negative. With these two important assumptions supported, we moved on to the main daily dairy study.

Main Study

Method

Participants. Participants were 96 students (48 men, 47 women, 1 not specified) from Seoul National University in Seoul, South Korea; 45 students (11 men, 29 women, 5 not specified) from the International Christian University in Tokyo, Japan;

and 215 students from the University of Illinois at Urbana–Champaign (UIUC). Of the UIUC students, 109 (45 men, 64 women) identified themselves as European American, 101 (50 men, 51 women) identified themselves as Asian or Asian American, and 5 identified themselves as "other." To distinguish the Asians and Asian Americans at UIUC from the Koreans and Japanese in the present study, we use the term *Asian Americans* to refer to the former group in this article. Out of the 101 Asian Americans at UIUC, 38 were born in the United States and 63 were born outside of the United States; of the latter group, 45 had been in the United States for less than 2 years at the time of data collection.

Materials and Procedures

Participants met with a trained experimenter who spoke in the local language in the psychology office at each site. All materials had been translated from English into Japanese or Korean by an experienced translator. The final versions of the materials were then tested for equivalence by psychologists in the respective cultures. Minor wording adjustments were made to make the questionnaire and survey items as clear as possible.

Participants completed a short survey on global life satisfaction, assessed using the Satisfaction With Life Scale (SWLS; Diener, Emmons, Larsen, & Griffin, 1985). The SWLS consists of five items, including "The conditions of my life are excellent" and "I am satisfied with my life" ($\alpha = 0.82$ for European Americans, 0.86 for Asian Americans, 0.83 for Koreans, and 0.85 for Japanese). Participants indicated their agreement with the five statements on a 7-point scale (1 = *strongly disagree* to 7 = *strongly agree*). SWLS scores range from 5 to 35. Consistent with previous research (E. Diener, M. Diener, & C. Diener, 1995; Diener, Suh, Smith, & Shao, 1995; Oishi, 2002), significant cultural differences in global life satisfaction were found, $F(3, 322) = 10.40$, $p < 0.01$. Post hoc tests using Bonferroni adjustments indicated that European Americans were more satisfied with their lives ($M = 25.61$, $SD = 5.10$) than were Asian Americans ($M = 21.96$, $SD = 6.67$), Koreans ($M = 21.93$, $SD = 5.67$), and Japanese ($M = 20.46$, $SD = 5.93$). There were no significant differences between Asian Americans, Koreans, and Japanese.

After completing the SWLS, participants were given the instructions for responding to a daily Web survey, which they completed during the following 21 days. The first two questions of the daily diary survey were concerned with daily life satisfaction: "How was today?," measured on a 7-point scale (1 = *terrible* to 7 = *excellent*), and "How satisfied were you with your life today?," measured on a 7-point scale (1 = *very dissatisfied* to 7 = *very satisfied*). We combined responses on these items into a daily satisfaction score ($\alpha = 0.91$ for European Americans, 0.93 for Asian Americans, 0.94 for Koreans, and 0.88 for Japanese).

Next, participants were presented with a list of 50 events and asked to indicate how many of the events had happened to them that day. Because about half of the events did not correspond to another event of the opposite valence, we included in the following analyses only the 26 events that could be placed into pairs with events of opposite valence (see Appendix for the complete list). Selecting only these corresponding events (e.g., "got complimented" vs. "got ignored") made the positive–negative event ratio more meaningful. It should be noted, however, that the key findings of individual and cultural differences were very similar when we used the entire list of 50 events.[2] Because there were a few outliers who reported having experienced a particular event 1,000 times on a given day, we capped the daily frequency of each event at 20 (for over 99% of the participants, the frequency reported was already less than 20). The daily positive and negative event scores were computed by summing the daily frequencies of the 13 positive and 13 negative events. We also computed the average daily positive (FreqPos) and negative events (FreqNeg) over the 3-week period, which indicated individual differences in chronic level of positive and negative events (see Table 2 for descriptive statistics).

To ensure that participants completed the surveys every day, an experimenter checked the database each morning and sent an e-mail reminder to participants who had not yet completed the survey. Participants were allowed to complete each day's survey before noon on the following day; Kahneman et al. (2004) found that retrospective reports about the previous day's life events and affect are highly associated with concurrent reports. At the end of the daily diary study, participants returned to the psychology office, completed a brief survey, and received $25 in the United States or the equivalent amount in won in Korea or yen in Japan.

Table 2 Number of average daily positive and negative events

Event type and group	M	SD
Positive events		
European Americans	14.51[a]	8.77
Asian Americans	10.57[b,c]	8.23
Koreans	6.61[d]	3.71
Japanese	7.21[c,d]	4.24
Total	10.23	7.69
Negative events		
European Americans	4.14[a]	3.67
Asian Americans	3.10[a]	2.79
Koreans	2.79[b]	2.06
Japanese	3.72[a]	2.73
Total	3.40	2.95

Note. Means that share an alphabet superscript did not differ from one another. Means that do not share a superscript differed from one another, according to post hoc tests with Bonferroni adjustments, at the overall p value of 0.05.

---

[2] When we used the 50-item list of events, the positive–negative event impact ratio was 2.40:1 for European Americans, 1.43:1 for Asian Americans, 1.35:1 for Koreans, and 1.18:1 for Japanese. When only interpersonal events from the original 50 events were included, the positive–negative event impact ratio was 2.37:1 for European Americans, 1.72:1 for Asian Americans, 1.63:1 for Koreans, and 1.58:1 for Japanese. The key individual-difference findings on the overall frequency of positive and negative events and global life satisfaction were almost identical, regardless of whether we used the original 50 events or the 26 paired events.

Only participants with 10 or more daily surveys were included in the following analyses, to ensure reliable estimates of the within-person analyses (20 participants, or 5.7%, failed to provide a sufficient amount of data), resulting in 332 participants (100 European Americans, 98 Asian Americans, 94 Koreans, and 39 Japanese). Data provided by 3 Japanese participants were discarded because the participants had typed their responses in *hiragana* mode, which was not properly recognized in the database. Compliance was excellent. The average number of daily reports completed ranged from 18.97 among European Americans to 20.38 among Japanese.

Results and Discussion

We first test the main hypotheses regarding cultural differences in within-person association between daily events and daily satisfaction, followed by individual differences. Then, we examine cultural and individual differences simultaneously. Next, we examine a time-lag relation between daily events and daily satisfaction. Finally, we address other important issues, such as outliers, response styles, and acculturation.

Are there cultural differences in the negativity bias? We tested our main research questions on cultural differences in the within-person association between daily events and daily satisfaction with multilevel random coefficient models using the Hierarchical Linear Modeling (HLM) program (Version 5.02; Raudenbush, Bryk, Cheong, & Congdon, 2001). The Level 1 (within-person) model was as follows:

$$Y_{ij} = \beta_{0j} + \beta_{1j} \times (\text{positive event}) + \beta_{2j} \times (\text{negative event}) + r_{ij},$$

where Y_{ij} is daily satisfaction for person j on day i, β_{0j} is a random coefficient representing the intercept for person j (here, the average daily satisfaction over 21 days for person j because predictors were centered around each individual's mean), β_{1j} is a random coefficient for positive events, β_{2j} is a random coefficient for negative events, and r_{ij} represents error. Because both positive and negative events were centered around each individual's mean, coefficients for daily events described the relations between the daily deviations from each person's mean number of positive and negative events and deviations from that person's mean daily satisfaction.

Cultural differences in the average within-person association between daily events and satisfaction were tested at Level 2. The Level 2 (or between-person) model was specified as follows:

$$\beta_{0j} = \gamma_{00} + \gamma_{01} \times (\text{Code 1}) + \gamma_{02} \times (\text{Code 2}) + \gamma_{03} \times (\text{Code 3}) + u_{0j}$$
$$\beta_{1j} = \gamma_{10} + \gamma_{11} \times (\text{Code 1}) + \gamma_{12} \times (\text{Code 2}) + \gamma_{13} \times (\text{Code 3}) + u_{1j}$$
$$\beta_{2j} = \gamma_{20} + \gamma_{21} \times (\text{Code 1}) + \gamma_{22} \times (\text{Code 2}) + \gamma_{23} \times (\text{Code 3}) + u_{0j},$$

where each of the Level 1 variables was predicted by three dummy codes representing four different cultural groups: In Dummy Code 1, Asian Americans were coded as 1 and the rest were coded as 0; in Dummy Code 2, Koreans were coded as 1 and the rest were coded as 0, and in Dummy Code 3, Japanese were coded as 1 and the rest were coded as 0. This set of dummy codes allowed us to use European Americans as the reference group (i.e., Dummy Code 1 tested the difference between Asian Americans and European Americans; Dummy Code 2 tested the difference between Koreans and European Americans; Dummy Code 3 tested the difference between Japanese and European Americans). Before conducting this analysis, we checked for gender differences in the within-person association between daily events and daily satisfaction. Because no gender differences were found, we did not include gender in subsequent analyses.

Table 3 shows the results of the HLM analysis. γ_{00} indicates that the average daily satisfaction for European Americans was 4.718. The average daily satisfaction of Asian Americans was significantly lower than that of European Americans, as indicated by the significant γ_{01}. Although European Americans reported a higher level of general life satisfaction, as measured by the SWLS, than did Japanese and Koreans, there were no differences between European Americans and Koreans or between European Americans and Japanese in the average daily satisfaction, as indicated by the nonsignificant γ_{02} and γ_{03} (see Oishi, 2002, for similar findings).

The second section of Table 3 illustrates critical information with regard to cultural differences in the size of the average within-person association between daily positive events and daily satisfaction. Consistent with our prediction, a one-unit increase in daily positive event (i.e., each positive event) was associated with a greater increase in daily satisfaction for Asian Americans, Koreans, and Japanese than for European Americans (as indicated by the significant γ_{11}, γ_{12}, and γ_{13} in Table 3). Specifically, one positive event was associated with a 0.068-point increase in daily satisfaction for European Americans, as compared with a 0.094-point increase for Asian Americans, a 0.132-point increase for Koreans, and a 0.129-point increase for Japanese.

The last section of Table 3 illustrates the cultural similarities and differences in the average within-person association between daily negative events and daily satisfaction. γ_{21} and γ_{23} were nonsignificant, suggesting that the strength of the within-person association between negative events and daily satisfaction did not differ between Asian Americans and European Americans or between Japanese and European Americans. γ_{22}, however, was significant, indicating that the strength of association between daily negative events and daily satisfaction was stronger for Koreans than for European Americans. On a day when Koreans experienced one more negative event than usual, their daily satisfaction was 0.174 points lower than usual, whereas on a day when European Americans experienced one more negative event than average, their daily satisfaction was 0.130 points lower than average.

On the basis of the HLM analysis above, we computed the relative power of positive versus negative events on daily satisfaction. For European Americans, the unstandardized coefficient was 0.068 for positive events and −0.130 for negative events, indicating that negative events were 1.91 times more strongly associated with daily satisfaction than were positive events. The corresponding unstandardized coefficients were 0.094 and −0.123 for Asian Americans, indicating that one

Table 3 Hierarchical linear modeling analysis of daily life events and daily satisfaction

Predictor	Unstandardized coefficient	SE	t	p
For INTERCEPT1, β_0				
INTERCEPT2, γ_{00}	4.718	0.087	54.43	0.000
Dummy Code 1, γ_{01}	−0.277	0.123	−2.24	0.025
Dummy Code 2, γ_{02}	−0.116	0.124	−0.93	0.352
Dummy Code 3, γ_{03}	−0.223	0.163	−1.37	0.175
For positive event slope, β_1				
INTERCEPT2, γ_{10}	0.068	0.006	10.89	0.000
Dummy Code 1, γ_{11}	0.026	0.009	2.84	0.005
Dummy Code 2, γ_{12}	0.064	0.010	6.27	0.000
Dummy Code 3, γ_{13}	0.061	0.014	4.44	0.000
For negative event slope, β_2				
INTERCEPT2, γ_{20}	−0.130	0.011	−11.44	0.000
Dummy Code 1, γ_{21}	0.070	0.017	0.42	0.675
Dummy Code 2, γ_{22}	−0.044	0.017	−2.55	0.011
Dummy Code 3, γ_{23}	0.008	0.022	0.35	0.726

Note. Dummy Code 1: Asian Americans were coded as 1, others as 0. Dummy Code 2: Koreans were coded as 1, others as 0. Dummy Code 3: Japanese were coded as 1, others as 0. Approximate degree of freedom is 328.

negative event was only 1.31 times more strongly associated with daily satisfaction than one positive event. For Koreans, the unstandardized coefficients for positive and negative events were 0.132 and −0.174, indicating that the power of a negative event was 1.32 times stronger than that of a positive event. Finally, for Japanese, the unstandardized coefficients for positive and negative events were 0.123 and −0.123, meaning that a negative event had exactly the same degree of association with daily satisfaction as did a positive event. In other words, it took roughly two positive events (e.g., receiving two compliments) to offset one negative event (e.g., getting ignored once) for European Americans, whereas just one positive event neutralized a negative event for Japanese.

A closer look at the frequency effect: Individual differences. Next, we moved on to test our individual-difference hypothesis. The first postulate of our frequency model predicts that the size of the within-person association between daily positive (or negative) events and daily satisfaction should be larger among individuals who experience fewer positive (or negative) events. We tested this idea using the following two-level HLM model:

Level 1 (within person):

$$Y_{ij} = \beta_{0j} + \beta_{1j} \times (\text{positive event}) + \beta_{2j} \times (\text{negative event}) + r_{ij},$$

Level 2 (between person):

$$\beta_{0j} = \gamma_{00} + \gamma_{01} \times (\text{FreqPos}) + \gamma_{02} \times (\text{FreqNeg}) + r_{0j}$$
$$\beta_{1j} = \gamma_{10} + \gamma_{11} \times (\text{FreqPos}) + r_{1j}$$
$$\beta_{2j} = \gamma_{20} + \gamma_{21} \times (\text{FreqNeg}) + r_{2j},$$

where FreqPos and FreqNeg indicate the average frequency of daily positive and negative events, respectively, for each participant over the 21-day period. As expected, our analysis showed that individuals who experienced more positive events over the course of 21 days had a higher mean level of daily satisfaction, $\gamma_{01} = 0.065$, $SE = 0.0060$, $t = 10.92$, $p < 0.001$, and individuals who experienced more negative events overall had a lower mean level of daily satisfaction, $\gamma_{02} = -0.134$, $SE = 0.0155$, $t = -8.64$, $p < 0.001$. As was the case in the previous analysis, daily positive events were positively associated with daily satisfaction, $\gamma_{10} = 0.1035$, $SE = 0.0038$, $t = 26.89$, $p < 0.001$, and daily negative events were negatively associated with daily satisfaction, $\gamma_{20} = -0.1505$, $SE = 0.0067$, $t = -22.46$, $p < 0.01$.

Most important, and consistent with our frequency model, the association between daily positive events and daily satisfaction was significantly smaller for individuals who experienced more positive events overall, $\gamma_{11} = -0.0033$, $SE = 0.00039$, $t = -8.59$, $p < 0.001$. Again, in accordance with our hypothesis, the negative association between daily negative events and daily satisfaction was weaker for individuals who experienced a higher overall frequency of negative events, $\gamma_{21} = 0.0103$, $SE = 0.0017$, $t = 6.16$, $p < 0.001$. In short, the degree to which positive events were associated with daily satisfaction was smaller for individuals high in overall frequency of positive events, whereas the degree to which negative events were associated with decreased daily satisfaction was smaller for individuals high in overall frequency of negative events.

A closer look at global life satisfaction and daily satisfaction. Next, we tested the more general idea that individuals higher in global life satisfaction would benefit less from a given positive event in terms of their daily satisfaction. Global life satisfaction was significantly associated with the overall frequency of positive events ($r = 0.30$, $p < 0.01$) but unrelated to the overall frequency of negative events ($r = -0.04$, *ns*). The Level 1 (within-person) HLM model was exactly the same as the previously presented model. At Level 2 (between-person), Level 1 variables were predicted by the grand-centered SWLS score.

Consistent with previous research (e.g., Oishi, Schimmack, & Diener, 2001), individuals high in global life satisfaction had higher levels of daily satisfaction than those low in global life satisfaction, $\gamma_{01} = 0.063$, $SE = 0.007$, $t = 9.02$, $p < 0.001$. With regard to our prediction, the within-person association between daily positive events and daily satisfaction was, as expected, significantly smaller for individuals with higher levels of global life satisfaction than for those low in global life satisfaction, $\gamma_{11} = -0.0024$, $SE = 0.00067$, $t = -3.58$, $p < 0.001$. It is also worth noting that the within-person association between daily negative events and daily satisfaction was even more negative for individuals with higher levels of global life satisfaction, $\gamma_{21} = -0.00276$, $SE = 0.00108$, $t = -2.54$, $p < 0.05$. In other words, the daily satisfaction of individuals higher in global life satisfaction covaried with negative events more strongly than that of individuals lower in global life satisfaction, whereas it covaried with positive events less strongly than that of individuals lower in global life satisfaction.

A plausible alternative explanation for our individual-difference findings is that the within-person association between daily positive events and daily satisfaction is smaller among individuals high in global life satisfaction or high in overall frequency of positive events because their daily satisfaction fluctuates less. We examined the possibility of limited variability in the daily satisfaction of this group by computing a within-person standard deviation of daily satisfaction. The within-person variability index was not correlated with global life satisfaction ($r = -0.02$, ns) or with the overall frequency of daily positive events ($r = -0.01$, ns), a finding that rules out this alternative explanation.

Simultaneous examination of cultural and individual differences. Next, we examined the aforementioned cultural and individual differences simultaneously. Specifically, we tested the model in which overall frequency of positive and negative events, global life satisfaction, and three culture dummy variables were included at Level 2 to test whether the previously obtained individual and cultural differences were independent of each other. As in the initial analyses, overall daily satisfaction was higher among individuals with high global life satisfaction, $t = 6.43$, $p < 0.01$; those who experienced many positive events during the 21-day period, $t = 9.48$, $p < 0.01$; and those who experienced fewer negative events, $t = -8.08$, $p < 0.01$. Once these individual-difference variables were entered, the difference in average daily satisfaction between European Americans and Asian Americans disappeared, $t = -0.03$, $p = 0.98$. When global life satisfaction and overall frequency of daily events were controlled, Korean and Japanese participants had higher average daily satisfaction than European Americans, $ts > 2.87$, $ps < 0.01$.

Most central to our hypotheses, the within-person association between daily positive events and daily satisfaction remained significantly stronger among Japanese and Koreans than among European Americans, $ts > 2.72$, $ps < 0.01$, even when global life satisfaction and overall frequency of daily events were included in the analysis. In addition, the within-person association between daily positive events and daily satisfaction remained significantly smaller among those who experienced more positive events during the 21-day period than others, $t = -5.99$, $p < 0.01$. In contrast, the difference in the within-person association between daily positive events and daily satisfaction between European Americans and Asian Americans originally observed became nonsignificant, $t = 1.44$, $p = 0.15$. In addition, once the overall frequencies of positive and negative events were controlled, the within-person association between daily positive events and daily satisfaction was not different across individuals, depending on the level of global life satisfaction, $t = -1.09$, $p = 0.28$. With regard to the within-person association between daily negative events and daily satisfaction, all of the significant effects from the original analyses remained significant. Namely, the association was smaller among those who experienced more negative events overall than others, $t = 5.44$, $p < 0.01$, and larger among those high in global life satisfaction than those low in global life satisfaction, $t = -2.33$, $p < 0.05$. In short, the key differences between European Americans and Koreans/Japanese remained substantial even after controlling for individual differences in global life satisfaction and the overall frequency of positive and negative events. In addition, the frequency effect at the between-individual level also remained sizable after controlling for cultural differences. Thus, the individual differences and cultural differences we observed were largely independent of one another.

Time-lag analyses. In addition, we conducted three time-lag analyses in order to delineate (a) cultural differences in the temporal relations between daily events and satisfaction, (b) individual differences in the frequency effects, and (c) individual differences in global life satisfaction. The Level 1 (within-person) model was as follows:

$$Y_{ij} = \beta_{0j} + \beta_{1j} \times (\text{day } t \text{ positive event}) + \beta_{2j}$$
$$\times (\text{day t negative event}) + \beta_{3j} \times (\text{day t} - 1 \text{ positive event})$$
$$+ \beta_{4j} \times (\text{day } t - 1 \text{ negative event}) + \beta_{5j}$$
$$\times (\text{day } t - 1 \text{ satisfaction}) + r_{ij},$$

where Y_{ij} was day t satisfaction. In the first time-lag model, which tested cultural differences, each of the Level 1 variables (β_{0j} to β_{5j}) was predicted by the same set of dummy codes used in previous analyses at Level 2. In essence, this model tested the degree to which daily changes in the number of positive and negative events predicted daily changes in satisfaction. Even after controlling for the previous day's satisfaction and events experienced, the results remained comparable to the original analysis. As seen in Table 4, the average within-person association between changes in daily positive events and changes in daily satisfaction was significantly stronger for Asian Americans, Koreans, and Japanese than for European Americans. In the latter group, daily changes in the frequency of negative events had 1.78 times more impact on daily satisfaction than did such changes in the frequency of positive events (i.e., it took 1.78 positive events to mitigate one negative event). In contrast, daily changes in the frequency of negative events had 1.35 times more impact on daily satisfaction for Asian Americans and 1.33 times more impact for Koreans. For Japanese, daily changes in the frequency of negative events had less impact (i.e., 0.94 times) on daily satisfaction than did changes in the frequency of positive events. In sum, the time-lag analysis showed that Asian Americans, Koreans, and Japanese benefited more from daily positive events than did European Americans.

In the second time-lag model, the Level 2 predictors were the overall frequencies of positive and negative events, rather than cultural differences. The Level 1 model was identical to the one used in the previous analysis. This analysis revealed, again, that the degree to which daily changes in the frequency of positive events were associated with changes in daily satisfaction was weaker among individuals high in overall frequency of positive events, -0.0032, $SE = 0.000357$, $t = -8.95$, $p < 0.001$. The degree to which daily changes in the frequency of negative events were associated with changes in daily satisfaction was also weaker among individuals high in overall frequency of negative events, 0.010307, $SE = 0.001623$, $t = 6.37$, $p < 0.001$.

In the final time-lag model, the Level 2 predictors were global life satisfaction. Again, the Level 1 model was identical to the one used in the previous time-lag model. This analysis revealed, as hypothesized, that the magnitude of the

S. Oishi et al.

Table 4 Hierarchical linear modeling analysis of daily life events and daily satisfaction, controlling for previous day's events and well-being

Predictor	Unstandardized coefficient	SE	t	p
For INTERCEPT1, β_0				
INTERCEPT2, γ_{00}	4.718	0.086	54.442	0.000
Dummy Code 1, γ_{01}	−0.27	0.123	−2.244	0.025
Dummy Code 2, γ_{02}	−0.11	0.124	−0.933	0.351
Dummy Code 3, γ_{03}	−0.22	0.163	−1.356	0.175
For day t positive event slope, β_1				
INTERCEPT2, γ_{10}	0.068	0.005	11.480	0.000
Dummy Code 1, γ_{11}	0.023	0.008	2.682	0.008
Dummy Code 2, γ_{12}	0.062	0.009	6.372	0.000
Dummy Code 3, γ_{13}	0.059	0.013	4.417	0.000
For day t negative event slope, β_2				
INTERCEPT2, γ_{20}	−0.121	0.011	−10.720	0.000
Dummy Code 1, γ_{21}	−0.002	0.016	−0.168	0.867
Dummy Code 2, γ_{22}	−0.052	0.017	−3.049	0.003
Dummy Code 3, γ_{23}	0.001	0.021	0.061	0.952
For day $t-1$ positive event slope, β_3				
INTERCEPT2, γ_{30}	−0.014	0.003	−3.829	0.000
Dummy Code 1, γ_{31}	0.005	0.006	0.954	0.341
Dummy Code 2, γ_{32}	−0.001	0.007	−0.241	0.810
Dummy Code 3, γ_{33}	−0.002	0.010	−0.276	0.783
For day $t-1$ negative event slope, β_4				
INTERCEPT2, γ_{40}	0.0098	0.008	1.110	0.267
Dummy Code 1, γ_{41}	−0.015	0.013	−1.181	0.238
Dummy Code 2, γ_{42}	0.0000	0.013	0.004	0.996
Dummy Code 3, γ_{43}	−0.005	0.016	−0.334	0.738
For day $t-1$ well-being slope, β_5				
INTERCEPT2, γ_{50}	0.219	0.027	8.089	0.000
Dummy Code 1, γ_{51}	−0.003	0.036	−0.085	0.933
Dummy Code 2, γ_{52}	−0.081	0.036	−2.231	0.026
Dummy Code 3, γ_{53}	−0.071	0.045	−1.574	0.115

Note. Dummy Code 1: Asian Americans were coded as 1, others as 0. Dummy Code 2: Koreans were coded as 1, others as 0. Dummy Code 3: Japanese were coded as 1, others as 0. Approximate degree of freedom is 328.

within-person association between changes in the frequency of positive events and changes in daily satisfaction was significantly smaller among individuals high in global life satisfaction, -0.002431, $SE = 0.000643$, $t = -3.78$, $p < 0.001$, whereas the magnitude of the within-person association between changes in the frequency of negative events and changes in daily satisfaction was significantly larger among individuals high in global life satisfaction, -0.002774, $SE = 0.001073$, $t = 2.58$, $p = 0.01$.

Issues of outliers, response styles, and acculturation. Finally, we examined the issues of outliers, response styles, and acculturation. Analogous to putting the cap on reaction time data (Bargh & Chartrand, 2000), we capped the number of occurrences of each daily event at 20 in the aforementioned analyses. However, one might wonder whether this treatment still left many outliers in the data. We examined each participant's daily data separately, computing a skewness index and kurtosis for each individual's daily data. According to Curran, West, and Finch (1996), skewness greater than 2 and kurtosis greater than 7 should be considered outliers. Out of 332 participants, 21 (4 European Americans, 9 Asian Americans, and 8 Koreans) showed skewness greater than 2 and kurtosis greater than 7 on either positive or negative daily events. We reran the first HLM analysis with these individuals excluded. The results were almost identical to the original results: The within-person association between daily positive events and daily satisfaction was significantly larger among Asian Americans than among European Americans, $t = 3.28$, $p < 0.01$; among Koreans than among European Americans, $t = 4.20$, $p < 0.01$; and among Japanese than among European Americans, $t = 6.06$, $p < 0.01$. In addition, when outliers were excluded, the original frequency effect was again obtained. Namely, the within-person association between daily positive events and daily satisfaction was smaller among those who experienced more positive events overall than among those who experienced fewer positive events, $t = -8.78$, $p < 0.01$. Similarly, the within-person association between daily negative events and daily satisfaction was also smaller among those who experienced more negative events overall than others, $t = 6.35$, $p < 0.01$. Likewise, when outliers were excluded, the within-person association between daily positive events and daily satisfaction was smaller among individuals high in global life satisfaction than those low in global life satisfaction, $t = -3.71$, $p < 0.01$, whereas the within-person association between daily negative events and daily satisfaction was larger among those high in global life satisfaction than among those low in global life satisfaction, $t = -2.57$, $p = 0.01$.

Next, the findings reported above could possibly be due to individual and cultural differences in response styles. If response styles were responsible for our findings, then we should obtain similar cultural and individual differences with different content used as the dependent variable, as long as the response format is the same. At the end of the daily survey, we included an item regarding participants' satisfaction with today's weather, rated on the same 7-point scale used for the daily satisfaction item. Thus, we reran the first HLM analysis reported above after changing the dependent variable from daily satisfaction to daily weather satisfaction. Unlike in the original analysis on daily satisfaction, there were no differences between European Americans and Koreans or Asian Americans in the degree to which daily positive events were associated with daily weather satisfaction, $|t|s < 0.97$, $ps > 0.34$. Although daily positive events were more strongly associated with daily weather satisfaction among Japanese than among European Americans, $t = 2.57$, $p = 0.01$, daily negative events were also marginally more strongly associated with daily weather satisfaction among Japanese than among European Americans, $t = -1.85$, $p = 0.06$. We also reran the two individual-difference analyses reported after the first cultural difference analyses. Unlike in the original analyses, the overall frequency of daily positive events did not moderate the within-person relation between daily positive events and daily weather satisfaction, $t = -1.65$, $p = 0.10$, nor did the overall frequency of daily negative events moderate the within-person association between daily negative events and daily weather satisfaction, $t = 0.40$, $p = 0.69$. Similarly, the degree to which daily positive events were associated with daily weather satisfaction did not differ across individuals depending on the level of global life satisfaction, $t = -0.84$, $p = 0.40$, nor did the degree to which daily negative events were associated with weather satisfaction differ across individuals depending on the level of global life satisfaction, $t = -0.36$, $p = 0.72$. These analyses suggest that the alternative explanation for our findings based on individual and cultural differences in response styles is not viable.

Finally, we examined whether there was an acculturation effect among the Asian American sample. Specifically, we tested whether the 38 Asian Americans born in the United States would show different patterns than the 63 Asian Americans born outside of the United States. We reran the first HLM analysis reported above with the following change: The Level 2 predictor was the dummy code, in which Asian Americans born outside of the United States were coded as 0 and Asian Americans born in the United States were coded as 1. There were no differences in either the degree to which daily positive events were associated with daily satisfaction, $t = -1.07$, $p = 0.28$, or the degree to which daily negative events were associated with daily satisfaction, $t = 1.49$, $p = 0.14$. It took 1.39 positive events to counteract 1 negative event among Asian Americans born outside of the United States, whereas it took 1.19 positive events among U.S.-born Asian Americans. Thus, U.S.-born Asian Americans were no more similar to European Americans than were foreign-born Asian Americans in our study.

General Discussion

The present research used the daily diary method to examine individual and cultural differences in the equilibrium point of daily satisfaction. As predicted, the association between positive life events and daily satisfaction was stronger among Asian Americans, Koreans, and Japanese than among European Americans. Whereas it took nearly two positive events (e.g., getting complimented and getting an A) to mitigate one negative event (e.g., getting ignored) for European Americans, it took only about 1.3 positive events to have the same mitigating effect for Asian Americans and Koreans and only one positive event to mitigate the negative event for Japanese (see Fig. 1). Furthermore, in support of the frequency model of life events and well-being, we found systematic individual differences in the relative impact of positive versus negative life events on daily satisfaction in terms of both overall frequency and global life satisfaction. Finally, time-lag analyses replicated the aforementioned individual and cultural differences. This is the first study to demonstrate individual and cultural differences in the number of positive events required to counteract one negative event. It should be noted that we found support for our predictions after having established cross-cultural equivalence of the daily events used in the main diary study as well as equivalence in strength of positive and negative events in the preliminary study. Thus, our findings cannot be explained by cultural differences in positivity or negativity of the daily events used in our study. Moreover, we found similar individual and cultural differences when the original 50 events were

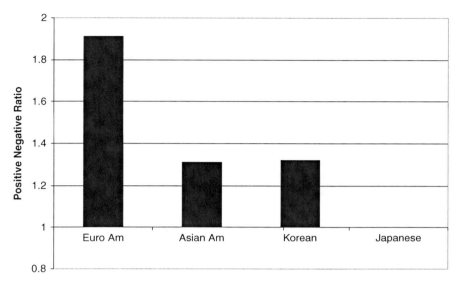

Fig. 1 The ratio of positive to negative events needed to maintain daily satisfaction equilibrium for each cultural group. The higher the ratio is, the more positive events are required, relative to negative events, to maintain the same level of daily satisfaction. Euro Am = European American; Asian Am = Asian American

included and when only interpersonal events were included (see Footnote 2). Thus, our findings were not limited to one particular kind of daily events.

Why Are There So Many "Happy" People but So Few "Very Happy" People?

Previous research has shown that although most people are above neutral in terms of well-being (E. Diener & C. Diener, 1996), very few people report being very happy, and those who do rarely stay that way for a long time (Diener & Seligman, 2002). The explanation for these findings has remained a mystery; however, the present findings offer a possible solution. As global life satisfaction increases, the potency of each negative event increases with it, so that more positive events are needed to mitigate each negative event. Unfortunately, many negative events, such as power outages, flat tires, and flight delays, are unavoidable. Because satisfied individuals already experience many positive events, moving to "very satisfied" by improving the positive–negative event ratio is very difficult. Even if one manages to increase the frequency of positive events he or she experiences, this increase is accompanied by an even stronger negativity bias. The bias is so strong toward the highest end of well-being that it is virtually impossible to reach that point, let alone stay there. What is more, because people often spend much effort and energy on getting over a negative event, they may not have sufficient energy or resources to surpass their prior level of well-being (Taylor, 1991).

Divergent Processes in Culture and Well-Being

The evidence presented in this article contradicts data gathered in previous research on culture and well-being, which has generally converged on the notion that European Americans pay more attention to positive emotions, as well as to other positive aspects of life, than do East Asians (Diener, Scollon, Oishi, Dzokoto, & Suh, 2000; Oishi, 2002; Oishi & Diener, 2003; Schimmack, Radhakrishnan, Oishi, Dzokoto, & Ahadi, 2003; Wirtz, 2004). Suh, Diener, Oishi, and Triandis (1998), for instance, showed that the frequency of positive emotion is less strongly associated with life satisfaction for people in collectivist cultures such as Korea and Japan. Additionally, Oishi (2002) demonstrated that although both the most and the least satisfying days contributed to overall weekly satisfaction for Asians, only the most satisfying day influenced overall satisfaction for European Americans. Likewise, European Americans evaluated their overall experiences as more satisfying than did Asians, even when there were no corresponding cultural differences in average daily satisfaction or actual experience (Oishi, 2002; Oishi & Diener, 2003; Wirtz, 2004). On the contrary, the current study suggests that it is Asians' daily satisfaction that is more susceptible to the power of a positive event.

To make sense of this paradox, one must consider both the type of well-being judgment under study and the role of novelty. In the context of evaluating a single day, novel or unexpected events should have a stronger impact than expected or frequently experienced events. However, in the context of evaluating a longer period of time, or life in general, memories of specific events are not always accessible, and individuals fall back on more general beliefs and expectancies about life (Kashima, 2000; Kim-Prieto, Diener, Tamir, Scollon, & Diener, 2005; Robinson & Clore, 2002; see Taylor, 1991, for the application of the mobilization–minimization hypothesis to memory of emotional experiences).

By examining (a) the within-person process as opposed to interindividual differences and (b) daily judgments (short-term) as opposed to global (long-term) judgments of well-being (cf. Diener & Fujita, 2005; Oishi et al., 2001), the present research provides a more complex, but also more complete, picture of culture and well-being. On average, European Americans hold more positive attitudes toward their lives and themselves (Chang & Asakawa, 2003; Heine & Lehman, 1995) and enjoy a higher level of global life satisfaction and self-esteem than Asian Americans, Japanese, or Koreans (Diener, Suh, Smith, Shao, 1995; Oishi & Sullivan, 2005). In terms of daily satisfaction, however, Asian Americans, Japanese, and Koreans benefit more from each positive event that happens to them. Asian Americans, Japanese, and Koreans, whose attitudes and expectations are not as positive as European Americans', might be amplifying the impact of each positive event. Given the present findings, although it may be good to have positive global expectations of happiness and life satisfaction in general, such expectations may undermine the impact of specific positive experiences on daily satisfaction. In this sense, less is sometimes more.

Before closing, we should note several limitations of the current research. First, although we identified intriguing counterintuitive phenomena, the underlying mechanisms at play are not yet fully identified. One important goal for future research is to explore the positive–negative ratio in terms of events that vary in novelty, controllability, and internal versus external causes. Second, the 13 positive events and 13 negative events that we chose to focus on in our analyses might not be exactly equivalent in terms of their meanings across cultures. In addition, the specific number of positive events required to nullify the detrimental effect of one negative event is likely to change, depending on specific events used (see Footnote 2 for examples). Furthermore, although the life events we included in the daily survey were quite diverse, by providing participants with a fixed list, we have overlooked the experience of events that were not included in the survey. Although we made sure that these events were meaningful to every cultural group we examined, the list of daily events was based on research conducted in the United States. Thus, in the future it will be important to test the current hypotheses using ideographic events generated by participants themselves. Finally, cultural differences in overall frequency of positive and negative events might be due to cultural differences in reporting styles. Asian Americans, Koreans, and Japanese might not have registered the same mildly flattering comment from a friend as a compliment, whereas European Americans might have. This might have contributed in part to our findings, although reporting styles cannot fully explain cultural differences in the key variables, as the differences between European Americans and Koreans/Japanese in the key within-person association between positive events and daily satisfaction remained significant when the overall frequency of positive and negative events were statistically controlled.

Conclusion

In accordance with the frequency model of life events and well-being, we found that the potency of positive events was stronger for Asian Americans, Japanese, and Koreans than for European Americans. We also found systematic individual differences in the power of positive events on daily satisfaction in terms of both overall frequency and global life satisfaction. In sum, the underlying processes of the frequency model were supported at both the individual and cultural levels of analysis, showing that less is sometimes more. Furthermore, we discovered intriguing divergence between global and daily satisfaction: Experiencing many positive events may be good for global happiness, but it could also reduce the impact of each positive event on daily happiness. The present findings suggest that the quest for greater happiness is not a straightforward one, in part because of the paradoxical interplay of daily events, daily satisfaction, and global well-being.

Acknowledgments This research was supported by National Institute of Mental Health Grant R01-MH16-849-01 to Ed Diener and Shigehiro Oishi. We thank Kaoru Nishimura and Naoko Ooi, along with their graduate students at the International Christian University, and Hidefumi Hitokoto for their help with data collection in Japan; Sang Hee Park, JeeHyun Chung, Hyekyung Park, Nang Yeon Lim, and Minkyung Koo for their help with data collection in South Korea; and Will Tov and Maya Tamir for their help with data management at the University of Illinois at Urbana–Champaign. We also thank Tim Wilson, Jon Haidt, Christie Scollon, Jerry Clore, Jesse Graham, Margarita Krochik, Patrick Seder, Jaime Kurtz, Kate Ranagath, Janetta Lun, Gary Sherman, and Minkyung Koo for their invaluable comments on earlier versions of this article.

Appendix

Daily life events

Positive events

1a. Received an A on a quiz, test, homework, or paper
2a. Got complimented
3a. Received a gift

3b. Lost something valuable/Dropped something valuable and broke it (vase, clock, etc.)

4a. Had fun
5a. My friends were understanding and supportive of me
6a. I was supportive of someone who needed me
7a. I learned much in school

4b. Had hassles
5b. A friend did something that made me disappointed or ashamed of him/her
6b. Said something to someone I deeply regretted afterwards
7b. Missed a class or an appointment/Was late for a class or appointment

8a. I impressed my friends
9a. I got along well with people around me
10a. Worked out

8b. Had an embarrassing moment
9b. Had an argument with someone

10b. Had a headache, stomach ache, or a small cut

11a. My relationship with boyfriend/girlfriend or spouse was good
12a. I made a new friend
13a. Had a meal with friends

11b. Was turned down asking someone out on a date

12b. Missed being with my family
13b. Was stood up

Negative events

1b. Received a D on a quiz, test, homework, or paper
2b. Got ignored/Was called by a derogatory name

References

Allport, G. (1961). *Patterns and growth in personality*. New York: Holt, Rinehart & Winston.
Baltes, P. B., Reese, H. W., & Nesselroade, J. R. (1977). *Life-span developmental psychology: Introduction to research methods*. Monterey, CA: Brooks/Cole.
Bargh, J. A., & Chartrand, T. L. (2000). The mind in the middle: A practical guide to priming and automaticity research. In H. T. Reis & C. M. Judd (Eds.), *Handbook of research methods in social and personality psychology* (pp. 251–285). New York: Cambridge University Press.

Baumeister, R. F., Bratslavsky, E., Finkenauer, C., & Vohs, K. D. (2001). Bad is stronger than good. *Review of General Psychology, 4*, 323–370.

Bolger, N., Davis, A., & Rafaeli, E. (2003). Diary methods: Capturing life as it is lived. *Annual Review of Psychology, 54*, 579–616.

Bolger, N., & Zuckerman, A. (1995). A framework for studying personality in the stress process. *Journal of Personality and Social Psychology, 69*, 890–902.

Brickman, P., Coates, D., & Janoff-Bulman, R. (1978). Lottery winners and accident victims: Is happiness relative? *Journal of Personality and Social Psychology, 36*, 917–927.

Cacioppo, J. T., Gardner, W. L., & Berntson, G. G. (1999). The affect system has parallel and integrative processing components: Form follows function. *Journal of Personality and Social Psychology, 76*, 839–855.

Carver, C. S., Pozo, C., Harris, S. D., Noriega, V., Scheier, M. F., Robinson, D. S., et al. (1993). How coping mediates the effect of optimism on distress: A study of women with early stage breast cancer. *Journal of Personality and Social Psychology, 65*, 375–390.

Caspi, A., Sugden, K., Moffitt, T. E., Taylor, A., Craig, I. W., Harrington, H., et al. (2003, July 18). Influence of life stress on depression: Moderation by a polymorphism in the 5-HTT gene. *Science, 301*, 386–389.

Chang, E. C., & Asakawa, K. (2003). Cultural variations on optimistic and pessimistic bias for self versus a sibling: Is there evidence for self-enhancement in the West and for self-criticism in the East when the reference group is specified? *Journal of Personality and Social Psychology, 84*, 569–581.

Curran, P. J., West, S. G., & Finch, J. F. (1996). The robustness of test statistics to nonnormality and specification error in confirmatory factor analysis. *Psychological Methods, 1*, 16–29.

David, J. P., Green, P. J., Martin, R., & Suls, J. (1997). Differential roles of neuroticism, extraversion, and event desirability for mood in daily life: An integrative model of top-down and bottom-up influences. *Personality and Social Psychology Bulletin, 73*, 149–159.

Diener, E., & Diener, C. (1996). Most people are happy. *Psychological Science, 7*, 181–185.

Diener, E., Diener, M., & Diener, C. (1995). Factors predicting the subjective well-being of rations. *Journal of Personality and Social Psychology, 69*, 851–864.

Diener, E., Emmons, R. A., Larsen, R. J., & Griffin, S. (1985). The Satisfaction With Life Scale. *Journal of Personality Assessment, 49*, 71–75.

Diener, E., & Fujita, F. (2005). *Hedonism revisited: Life satisfaction is more than the sum of pleasant days.* Manuscript under review, University of Illinois at Urbana–Champaign.

Diener, E., & Oishi, S. (2005). The nonobvious social psychology of happiness. *Psychological Inquiry, 16*, 162–167.

Diener, E., Oishi, S., & Lucas, R. E. (2003). Culture, personality, and well-being. *Annual Review of Psychology, 54*, 403–425.

Diener, E., Sandvik, E., & Pavot, W. (1991). Happiness is the frequency, not the intensity, of positive versus negative affect. In F. Strack & M. Argyle (Eds.), *Subjective well-being: An interdisciplinary perspective* (pp. 119–139). Elmsford, NY: Pergamon Press.

Diener, E., Scollon, C. K. N., Oishi, S., Dzokoto, V., & Suh, E. M. (2000). Positivity and the construction of life satisfaction judgments: Global happiness is not the sum of its parts. *Journal of Happiness Studies, 1*, 159–176.

Diener, E., & Seligman, M. E. P. (2002). Very happy people. *Psychological Science, 13*, 81–84.

Diener, E., Suh, E., Smith, H., & Shao, L. (1995). National differences in reported subjective well-being: Why do they occur? *Social Indicators Research, 34*, 7–32.

Fleeson, W. (2001). Toward a structure- and process-integrated view of personality: Traits as density distributions of states. *Journal of Personality and Social Psychology, 80*, 1011–1027.

Folkman, S., & Moskowitz, J. T. (2000). Positive affect and the other side of coping. *American Psychologist, 55*, 647–654.

Fredrickson, B. L., & Levenson, R. W. (1998). Positive emotions speed recovery from the cardiovascular sequelae of negative emotions. *Cognition & Emotion, 12*, 191–220.

Fredrickson, B. L., & Losada, M. F. (2005). Positive affect and the complex dynamics of human flourishing. *American Psychologist, 60*, 678–686.

Gable, S. L., Reis, H. T., & Elliot, A. J. (2000). Behavioral activation and inhibition in everyday life. *Journal of Personality and Social Psychology, 78*, 1135–1149.

Gottman, J. M. (1994). *What predicts divorce? The relationship between marital processes and marital outcomes.* Hillsdale, NJ: Erlbaum.

Headey, B., & Wearing, A. (1989). Personality, life events, and subjective well-being: Toward a dynamic equilibrium model. *Journal of Personality and Social Psychology, 57*, 731–739.

Heine, S. J., & Lehman, D. R. (1995). Cultural variation in unrealistic optimism: Does the West feel more invulnerable than the East? *Journal of Personality and Social Psychology, 68*, 595–607.

Ito, T. A., Larsen, J. T., Smith, N. K., & Cacioppo, J. T. (1998). Negative information weighs more heavily on the brain: The negativity bias in evaluative categorizations. *Journal of Personality and Social Psychology, 75*, 887–900.

Janoff-Bulman, R. (1992). *Shattered assumptions: Toward a new psychology of trauma.* New York: Free Press.

Kahneman, D., Krueger, A. B., Schkade, D. A., Schwarz, N., & Stone, A. A. (2004, December 3). A survey method for characterizing daily life experience: The day reconstruction method. *Science, 306*, 1776–1780.

Kahneman, D., & Thaler, R. H. (2006). Anomalies-utility maximization and experienced utility. *Journal of Economic Perspectives, 20*, 221–234.

Kahneman, D., & Tversky, A. (1979). Prospect theory: An analysis of decision under risk. *Econometrica, 47*, 263–291.

Kashima, Y. (2000). Maintaining cultural stereotypes in the serial reproduction of narratives. *Personality and Social Psychology Bulletin, 26*, 594–604.

Kim-Prieto, C., Diener, E., Tamir, M., Scollon, C., & Diener, M. (2005). Integrating the diverse definitions of happiness: A time-sequential framework of subjective well-being. *Journal of Happiness Studies, 6*, 261–300.

Lawton, M. P., DeVoe, M. R., & Parmelee, P. (1995). Relationship of events and affect in the daily life of an elderly population. *Psychology and Aging, 10*, 469–477.

Lazarus, R. S. (2000). Toward better research on stress and coping. *American Psychologist, 55*, 665–673.

Lehman, D. R., Wortman, C. B., & Williams, A. F. (1987). Long-term effects of losing a spouse or child in a motor vehicle crash. *Journal of Personality and Social Psychology, 52*, 218–231.

Lucas, R. E., Clark, A. E., Georgellis, Y., & Diener, E. (2003). Reexamining adaptation and the set point model of happiness: Reactions to changes in marital status. *Journal of Personality and Social Psychology, 84*, 527–539.

Lyubomirsky, S., Sheldon, K. M., & Schkade, D. (2005). Pursuing happiness: The architecture of sustainable change. *Review of General Psychology, 9*, 111–131.

Mesquita, B., & Karasawa, M. (2002). Different emotional lives. *Cognition & Emotion, 16*, 127–141.

Mischel, W., & Shoda, Y. (1995). A cognitive–affective system theory of personality: Reconceptualizing situations, dispositions, dynamics, and invariance in personality structure. *Psychological Review, 102*, 246–268.

Myers, D. G. (2000). The funds, friends, and faith of happy people. *American Psychologist, 55*, 56–67.

Nesselroade, J. R. (1984). Concepts of intraindividual variability and change: Impressions of Cattell's influence on lifespan developmental psychology. *Multivariate Behavioral Research, 19*, 269–286.

Nezlek, J. B., & Gable, S. L. (2001). Depression as a moderator of relationships between positive daily events and day-to-day psychological adjustment. *Personality and Social Psychology Bulletin, 27*, 1692–1704.

Nezlek, J. B., & Plesko, R. M. (2003). Affect- and self-based models of relationships between daily events and daily well-being. *Personality and Social Psychology Bulletin, 29*, 584–596.

Oishi, S. (2002). Experiencing and remembering of well-being: A cross-cultural analysis. *Personality and Social Psychology Bulletin, 28*, 1398–1406.

Oishi, S. (2004). Culture *in* personality: A neo-Allportian view. *Journal of Research in Personality, 38*, 68–74.

Oishi, S., & Diener, E. (2003). Culture and well-being: The cycle of action, evaluation and decision. *Personality and Social Psychology Bulletin, 29*, 939–949.

Oishi, S., Diener, E., Scollon, C. N., & Biswas-Diener, R. (2004). Cross-situational consistency of affective experiences across cultures. *Journal of Personality and Social Psychology, 86*, 460–472.

Oishi, S., Schimmack, U., & Diener, E. (2001). Pleasures and subjective well-being. *European Journal of Personality, 15*, 153–167.

Oishi, S., & Sullivan, H. W. (2005). The mediating role of parental expectations in culture and well-being. *Journal of Personality, 73*, 1267–1294.

Peterson, C., Seligman, M. E. P., & Vaillant, G. E. (1988). Pessimistic explanatory style is a risk factor for physical illness: A thirty-five-year longitudinal study. *Journal of Personality and Social Psychology, 55*, 23–27.

Raudenbush, S., Bryk, A., Cheong, Y. F., & Congdon, R. (2001). *HLM5: Hierarchical linear and nonlinear modeling*. Chicago: Scientific Software International.

Reis, H. T., & Gable, S. L. (2000). Event-sampling methods. In H. T. Reis & C. M. Judd (Eds.), *Handbook of research methods in social and personality psychology* (pp. 190–222). New York: Cambridge University Press.

Robinson, M. D., & Clore, G. L. (2002). Belief and feeling: Evidence for an accessibility model of emotional self-report. *Psychological Bulletin, 128*, 934–960.

Rozin, P., & Royzman, E. B. (2001). Negativity bias, negativity dominance, and contagion. *Personality and Social Psychology Bulletin, 5*, 296–320.

Schimmack, U. (2003). Affect measurement in experience sampling research. *Journal of Happiness Studies, 4*, 79–106.

Schimmack, U., Radhakrishnan, P., Oishi, S., Dzokoto, V., & Ahadi, S. (2002). Culture, personality, and subjective well-being: Integrating process models of life satisfaction. *Journal of Personality and Social Psychology, 82*, 582–593.

Seidlitz, L., & Diener, E. (1993). Memory for positive versus negative life events: Theories for the differences between happy and unhappy persons. *Journal of Personality and Social Psychology, 64*, 654–663.

Skowronski, J. J., & Carlston, D. E. (1989). Negativity and extremity biases in impression formation: A review of explanations. *Psychological Bulletin, 105*, 131–142.

Stone, A. A., Kennedy-Moore, E., & Neale, J. M. (1995). Association between daily coping and end-of-day mood. *Health Psychology, 14*, 341–349.

Stroebe, W., Stroebe, M., Abakoumkin, G., & Schut, H. (1996). The role of loneliness and social support in adjustment to loss: A test of attachment versus stress theory. *Journal of Personality and Social Psychology, 70*, 1241–1249.

Suh, E., Diener, E., & Fujita, F. (1996). Events and subjective well-being: Only recent events matter. *Journal of Personality and Social Psychology, 70*, 1091–1102.

Suh, E., Diener, E., Oishi, S., & Triandis, H. C. (1998). The shifting basis of life satisfaction judgments across cultures: Emotions versus norms. *Journal of Personality and Social Psychology, 74*, 482–493.

Suls, J., & Martin, R. (2005). The daily life of the garden-variety neurotic: Reactivity, stressor exposure, mood spillover, and maladaptive coping. *Journal of Personality, 73*, 1485–1510.

Taylor, S. E. (1991). Asymmetrical effects of positive and negative events: The mobilization–minimization hypothesis. *Psychological Bulletin, 110*, 67–85.

Tennen, H., Affleck, G., & Armeli, S. (2005). Personality and daily experience revisited. *Journal of Personality, 73*, 1465–1484.

Watson, D., Clark, L. A., & Tellegen, A. (1984). Cross-cultural convergence in the structure of mood: A Japanese replication and a comparison with U.S. findings. *Journal of Personality and Social Psychology, 47*, 127–144.

Weinsten, N. D. (1982). Community noise problems: Evidence against adaptation. *Journal of Environmental Psychology, 2,* 87–97.

Wilson, T. D., Centerbar, D. B., Kermer, D. A., & Gilbert, D. T. (2005). The pleasures of uncertainty: Prolonging positive moods in ways people do not anticipate. *Journal of Personality and Social Psychology, 88,* 5–21.

Wilson, T. D., & Gilbert, D. T. (2005). *Making sense: A model of affective adaptation.* Manuscript under review, University of Virginia, Charlottesville.

Wirtz, D. R. (2004). *Focusing on the good versus focusing on the bad: An analysis of East–West differences in subjective well-being.* Unpublished doctoral dissertation, University of Illinois at Urbana–Champaign.

Zevon, M., & Tellegen, A. (1982). The structure of mood change: Idiographic/nomothetic analysis. *Journal of Personality and Social Psychology, 43,* 111–122.

Norms for Experiencing Emotions in Different Cultures: Inter- and Intranational Differences

Michael Eid and Ed Diener

Abstract Within- and between-nations differences in norms for experiencing emotions were analyzed in a cross-cultural study with 1,846 respondents from 2 individualistic (United States, Australia) and 2 collectivistic (China, Taiwan) countries. A multigroup latent class analysis revealed that there were both universal and culture-specific types of norms for experiencing emotions. Moreover, strong intranational variability in norms for affect could be detected, particularly for collectivistic nations. Unexpectedly, individualistic nations were most uniform in norms, particularly with regard to pleasant affect. Individualistic and collectivistic nations differed most strongly in norms for self-reflective emotions (e.g., pride and guilt). Norms for emotions were related to emotional experiences within nations. Furthermore, there were strong national differences in reported emotional experiences, even when norms were held constant.

The cross-cultural perspective has a long tradition in research on emotions. More than 100 years ago, Charles Darwin (1872/1970) based the theoretical considerations in his book *The Expression of the Emotions in Man and Animals* to a large degree on reports he had received from people living in different cultures of the world. Since that time, cross-cultural comparisons have become the most important ethological research strategy for proving the assumption that there are universal, biologically determined programs, particularly for the expression of emotions. Reviewing the results of this ethological research paradigm, Grammer and Eibl-Eibesfeldt (1993) came to the conclusion that there is a universal human system not only for producing emotions but also for understanding the expression of emotions.

From the perspective of cross-cultural anthropology and psychology, however, the biological perspective is not sufficient for a full understanding of the experience and expression of emotions and must be complemented by consideration of the cultural context in which emotions are experienced, expressed, and perceived (e.g., Kitayama & Markus, 1995; Markus & Kitayama, 1991; Matsumoto, 1996;

M. Eid (✉)
Habelschwerdter Allee 45 – Raum JK 27/207 14195 Berlin
e-mail: eid@zedat.fu-berlin.de

E. Diener (ed.), *Culture and Well-Being: The Collected Works of Ed Diener*, Social Indicators Research Series 38, DOI 10.1007/978-90-481-2352-0_9,
© Springer Science+Business Media B.V. 2009

Mesquita & Ellsworth, 2001; Mesquita & Frijda, 1992; Scherer, 1994, 1997; Scherer & Wallbott, 1994; Scherer, Wallbott, & Summerfield, 1986; Shaver, Wu, & Schwartz, 1992; Wallbott & Scherer, 1988). If we follow Triandis's (1997) definition of a *cultural syndrome* as a "shared set of beliefs, attitudes, norms, values, and behavior organized around a central theme and found among speakers of one language, in one time period, and in one geographic region" (p. 443), it is necessary to identify cultural syndromes that are related to the experience, expression, regulation, and socialization of emotions.

According to Frijda and Mesquita (1995), cultural influences on the emotion process are mediated to a large extent by the significance an emotion has for an individual. Frijda and Mesquita distinguished among three aspects of emotion that are culturally influenced. First, they considered social consequences of emotions that regulate the *expression* and *suppression* of emotions. Second, they stressed the importance of norms for *experiencing* different emotions. Third, they discussed social–cohesive functions of emotions. Several ethnographic studies have shown that there are strong cultural differences in the social consequences of emotions, particularly in how the expression of emotions is valued. The expression of anger, for example, is strongly disapproved of by the Utku Eskimos (Briggs, 1970), whereas the Kaluli are expected and even encouraged to show their anger (Schieffelin, 1983; for further examples, see Mesquita & Frijda, 1992).

There are strong cultural differences in *display rules* (Ekman & Friesen, 1969; Izard, 1980) that are learned during the socialization process (Saarni, 1999). There are also cultural differences in the norms for experiencing different emotions. Hochschild (1983), for example, discussed the role of *feeling rules*, social norms that prescribe how people should feel in specific situations (e.g., on a wedding day, at a funeral). In addition to *situational* feeling rules, norms for the experience of emotions can also be present in a society in the form of *generalized* expectations. This means that emotions can differ in their desirability and perceived appropriateness across situations. The emotional climate of nations can be characterized by generalized norms for experiencing different emotions and the fact that these norms are subject to historical change (Stearns, 1994; Stearns & Lewis, 1998).

Most of the research on cultural differences in emotions has focused on the first aspect, the social consequences of emotion manifestations and how they regulate the expression versus suppression of emotions. Mesquita and Frijda (1992), however, reviewed evidence that there are cultural similarities and differences in all components of the emotion process (i.e., antecedent events, event coding, appraisal, physiological reaction patterns, action readiness, emotional behavior, and regulation). In explaining cultural differences in these components, not only are the norms for the expression of emotions relevant but also the norms for the experience of emotions. For example, people who value positive emotions might be more alert to positive events, might seek situations that provoke positive emotions, might appraise positive events in a more positive way, might stay in positive situations longer, and might try to maintain their positive feelings or even enhance them. However, people who think that positive feelings are inappropriate are likely to avoid situations that cause positive feelings, might not be able to appraise positive situations in a positive way, might withdraw from positive situations much earlier, and might even try to dampen positive feelings. On the other hand, people who think that negative emotions (e.g., anger) are appropriate might seek anger-provoking situations when they assume that these situations would be helpful (e.g., for clarifying conflicts, for asserting their goals). These people might be more prone to appraise situations with respect to the situation's potential for hindering their goal, they might not withdraw from anger situations, and they might try to maintain their anger as long as they think this would be necessary for asserting their goals. However, people who believe that the experience of anger is inappropriate might avoid anger-provoking situations. They might not focus on components of a situation that hinder a personal goal when appraising a situation, and they might try to withdraw from an anger situation early and try to suppress or dampen their anger reaction. Hence, norms for the experience of emotions might have a strong influence on the regulation of one's emotions.

Moreover, values and norms for experiencing emotions might be important not only for an individual emotional episode but also for regulating emotions in other people. People who think that the experience of positive emotions (e.g., pride) is inappropriate are likely to disapprove of those emotional experiences in other people. This might be particularly important for the socialization process (Saarni, 1999). Parents who think that specific emotions are inappropriate are likely to raise their children in such a way that the children learn to avoid specific emotional situations and emotional reactions, to develop a specific appraisal style, and to regulate their emotions in such a way that they maintain a "correct" emotional life. Parents who think that specific emotions are positive are likely to encourage their children to feel and express these emotions and to reward emotional behavior that is in line with their own emotional norms. Saarni (1999) pointed out that parents are expected to socialize their children to behave and feel according to normative beliefs about desirable and appropriate emotional behavior. There are several ethnographic studies that are in accord with these assumptions (for an overview, see Ulich & Mayring, 1992). Finally, knowledge of norms for experiencing emotions might be very important for cross-cultural communication and the relationships of people in different cultures.

We owe much of our knowledge of cultural influences on emotions to ethnographic and anthropological studies. These studies have produced interesting insights into cultural specificities, but they are limited in several ways. First, they are single-case studies that focus on one culture that is described in detail. These studies do not discuss whether there are cross-cultural differences in emotional norms and how these cross-cultural differences are explained. Second, these studies often refer to small groups, and the generalizability of the results might be questionable. Third, they focus on aspects of emotion that are typical for a culture. How strong within-culture differences are compared with cross-cultural differences is not analyzed.

If we take a cross-cultural perspective, at least two questions are important: (a) Which cultures should differ in values and norms for experiencing emotions (according to theoretical models), and why? and (b) Can cross-cultural differences in values and norms be empirically confirmed (according to empirical studies)?

Values and Norms for Experiencing Emotions

Cultural differences in values and norms for experiencing emotions can be predicted from cultural differences in self-construals. In cross-cultural psychology, two prototypical self-construals, the independent and the interdependent self-construal, have been distinguished by several authors (e.g., Gardner, Gabriel, & Lee, 1999; Markus & Kitayama, 1991; Triandis, 1989). The independent self consists of a configuration of inner attributes (e.g., dispositions, motives, and values) that make an individual unique from others. In cultures where an *independent self* is predominant, people are expected to become independent from others and to pursue and assert individual goals. People with an individual self focus on their own attributes, abilities, and preferences and tend to express these attributes in public and in private. The personality pattern that characterizes the independent self is also named *idiocentrism* (Triandis, 1997). Cultures in which idiocentrism is the predominant personality pattern are called *individualistic* cultures (Triandis, 1997). Hence, people with an independent self are found in individualistic (e.g., Western) cultures more often than in collectivistic ones (e.g., Eastern cultures).

The *interdependent (relational) self*, on the other hand, is characterized by the belief that the self cannot be separated from others or from the social context. The self is part of all-embracing social relationships, and people with an interdependent self focus on and are regulated by the emotions, thoughts, and actions of other people. The personality pattern characterizing the interdependent self is also called *allocentrism* (Triandis, 1997). In *collectivistic* cultures, in which this construal of the self is predominant, the social norm is to maintain harmony with others, to meet social obligations, and to support the goals of others who are in a social relationship with oneself. Thus, in contrast to individualistic cultures, the norm is not to become independent from others but to fulfill one's social duties.

Lee, Aaker, and Gardner (2000) showed that differences in self-construals are accompanied by differences in regulatory focus (approach vs. avoidance). Lee et al. (2000) defined regulatory focus as "the extension of the basic hedonic principle of approach and avoidance to allow for distinct self-regulatory strategies and needs" (p. 1122). People with independent self-construals are promotion focused. They focus more strongly on information that is relevant for approaching their own aspirations and wishes. Moreover, they place more emphasis on positive than on negative information regarding themselves. People with an interdependent self, on the other hand, are more prevention focused. They place more attention on information that prevents them from violating social norms. Furthermore, they emphasize negative information regarding themselves.

Differences in self-construal and regulatory focus might be strongly related to norms for experiencing emotions. In particular, it can be expected that there are strong cultural differences in *self-conscious* or *self-reflective* emotions—emotions that reflect on the individual's own doing (Tangney & Fischer, 1995) and that are, therefore, important for self-regulation. Self-conscious emotions that indicate that personal goals have been successfully approached might be more important and desirable for people with independent self-construals, who are more promotion focused. Therefore, the self-conscious emotions that arise from succeeding by one's own efforts (e.g., pride) are highly valued in individualistic societies. However, self-conscious emotions that indicate that one's controllable actions are wrong or insufficient (negative information regarding oneself) might be more important and desirable for people with interdependent self-construals, who are more prevention focused. Consequently, the self-conscious emotions that are caused by violating social norms and by failing to fulfill social obligations (e.g., guilt) are likely to be more highly valued in collectivistic societies. Cross-cultural differences in norms for emotions might be less important for other emotions that are not self-conscious in nature and that arise more from external causes than from internal, controllable sources (e.g., anger, worry, joy).

There have been few empirical cross-cultural studies on norms for experiencing emotions. Most cross-cultural studies on emotions refer to cross-cultural differences in the frequency, intensity, or expression of emotions (see, e.g., Kitayama, Markus, & Matsumoto, 1995; Stipek, 1998; Stipek, Weiner, & Li, 1989). These studies allow only indirect and, therefore, limited conclusions about how emotions are generally valued in these cultures. For example, people might think that positive emotions are very desirable. If they are not able to seek positive situations or to react to positive events with positive emotions, however, they will not feel positive emotions frequently or intensely. Thus, norms and feelings are distinct components of the emotion process, and, consequently, variables characterizing the feeling of emotions are only indirect indicators of norms and attitudes. In the following, the results of some previous studies on norms for affect are summarized.

Stipek (1998) compared the value of pride between Chinese and Americans. She found that for the Chinese, pride is more acceptable for achievements that benefit others than for achievements that are due to personal accomplishments. Sommers (1984) explored the values of different emotions by asking six questions, but only with small samples. Sommers found that there were strong cross-cultural similarities with respect to the emotions of love, happiness, and joy, which were considered desirable in all cultures. Also, hate, terror, and rage were considered as dangerous and destructive in all cultures. Furthermore, guilt, frustration, fear, shame, and embarrassment were consistently considered aversive. Cross-cultural differences were shown with respect to specific emotions. The Americans valued enthusiasm very strongly, the Greeks highly valued respect, and the West Indians valued pride. The Chinese considered more negative emotions to be useful and constructive than did the three other nations.

Although they give valuable insights into the norms for emotions, previous studies are limited in two ways. First, they have often focused either on a limited number of emotions and nations or on small samples. Second, differences between cultures have typically been analyzed by comparing mean values (or other statistics) between the cultures without testing whether the assumption of measurement equivalence across cultures was fulfilled. Comparing means, for example, presumes that individuals use the scales in the same way (assumption of measurement invariance). This means that there are not individual response styles such as the preference for one response category (e.g., the middle one) or the avoidance of response categories (e.g., the extreme ones). If individual response styles are present, mean values can only be compared if the response styles are equally distributed in the different cultures. The absence of interindividual differences in response styles can be statistically tested in the framework of item response theory by demonstrating that the item parameters do not differ between individuals or subgroups of individuals (e.g., Drasgow & Kanfer, 1985). The assumption that all individuals use the scales in the same way, however, can be questioned with regard to two issues: (a) Several analyses that have been undertaken during the past years have shown that this assumption is often not fulfilled even within individual cultures (e.g., Eid & Rauber, 2000; Rost, Carstensen, & von Davier, 1997). (b) Moreover, as Leung and Bond (1989) pointed out, it is possible that different response styles exist between the varying cultures (see also Bond, 1996). Consequently, the measurement invariance assumption must be tested within each culture as well as between different cultures to ensure that these mean differences are not of an artificial nature. Previous studies on norms for emotions, however, have not tested whether the assumption of measurement invariance holds. One aim of the present study is to test whether the same norm structure can be found in different cultures (the problem of structural equivalence in cross-cultural psychology; van de Vijver & Leung, 1996, 1997).

In cross-cultural psychology, several methods have been applied to test the assumptions of measurement and structural equivalence (for an overview, see van de Vijver & Leung, 1996, 1997). Most typically, these assumptions have been tested by dimensional models such as confirmatory factor analysis or latent trait models of item response theory. Dimensional models, however, are not appropriate for testing the measurement equivalence of norms for emotions in the present research context. Dimensional models assume that all individuals and items can be ordered on a continuum. This assumption is very strong if we consider norms for emotions. It is very reasonable that, within cultures, individuals differ in the types of emotions that they consider desirable and undesirable. For example, there might be people who think that anger is desirable but guilt is not, and there might be people for whom the opposite is true. These differences in norm patterns can be adequately assessed in a typological model. A typological model is also important from an emotion regulatory standpoint. Following Tangney, Wagner, Fletcher, and Gramzow's (1992) research, for instance, it can be hypothesized that people who rate anger as an unacceptable emotion and guilt as an acceptable one tend to ascribe negative events to themselves, whereas for people with the opposite rating pattern, it is expected that they tend to blame other people for negative events. These individual profiles, however, are not visible if we compare means across cultures. A mean structure that, for example, implies that anger is not acceptable in a country yet guilt is acceptable does not indicate how uniform this difference is within cultures. Cross-cultural researchers have hitherto been frustrated by the fact that they want to examine cultural differences but recognize that very large variations also exist within cultures. To answer this challenge and interweave cultural and individual differences, we suggest the use of *multigroup latent class analysis* (e.g., Lazarsfeld & Henry, 1968; McCutcheon, 1987). This type of analysis is able to address issues of scale equivalence as well as within-nation variability.

Latent class analysis is a procedure for categorical response variables and is based on four assumptions (e.g., Clogg, 1995; Eid, 2001; Langeheine & Rost, 1988). It is first assumed that a population is not homogeneous; rather, it is composed of subpopulations. These subpopulations are called latent classes because they are not directly observable. Each individual in the population can and must belong to only one subpopulation; that is, the classes are disjunctive and exhaustive. The membership of a population is not known a priori, and only the membership probabilities (assignment probabilities) and the class sizes can be estimated. Second, all of the people belonging to the same class are homogeneous with respect to the class conditional response probabilities for the various categories of items. Third, the class structure holds for all items analyzed. Fourth, local stochastic independence is assumed. This means that the responses on items are independent, given latent class membership (hence, local independence). This assumption implies that the class structure explains all associations between the observable responses. In the framework of latent class analysis, measurement invariance exists when the response probabilities of the latent classes do not differ between the various cultures.

The typological combination of norms for different affects is theoretically more interesting than the simple comparison of mean values across cultures. Consequently, a typological approach that considers different rating patterns within a culture and between cultures is an appropriate starting point for the analysis of inter- and intra-cultural differences. If we compare typological structures across cultures, however, we have to ensure that the typological structures (measurement model) are identical in different cultures (measurement invariance). Thus, we need a typological model whose cross-cultural generalizability (measurement invariance) can be statistically tested. Multigroup latent class analysis is an appropriate model for testing typological structures between cultures. Compared with other methodological approaches that are traditionally applied in cross-cultural psychology, latent class analysis has a further strong methodological advantage. In methods traditionally applied in cross-cultural psychology, it is typically assumed that the parameters of a model (e.g., factor loadings) are the same for all individuals of a culture. This means that a culture has to be homogeneous and that heterogeneity is only allowed for individuals belonging to different cultures. If the assumption of measurement equivalence (e.g., assumption of equal factor loadings) across cultures must be rejected, this means that individuals from different cultures cannot be compared, for instance, with respect to a mean score. One strong advantage of latent class analysis is that the assumption of homogeneous cultures is not made. Moreover, there might be subgroups within one culture that differ with respect to the parameters of a model. These subgroups might exist in different cultures, but there might be subgroups that are so culture specific that they do not occur in other cultures. Thus, latent class analysis is able to detect universal types that exist in all cultures and culture-specific types that exist only in specific cultures. For example, there might be (universal) patterns of norms for emotions that can be found in all nations but also patterns of norms for emotions that are so specific that they can be found only in single nations. The assumption of measurement invariance would then hold only for the universal types (subgroups) that can be found in all cultures. Culture-specific classes, however, reveal structural differences between cultures and indicate individuals who are most typical for the uniqueness of a culture. For researchers interested in indigenous aspects of a culture, these people might be of major interest. The capability of latent class analysis to detect universal and culture-specific classes goes far beyond other statistical models for cross-cultural comparisons. Although multigroup latent class analysis appears to be perfectly suited for cross-cultural emotion psychology, as far as we know this type of analysis has not been used in this field until now (for other applications of multigroup latent class analysis in sociology and political sciences, see McCutcheon, 1998; McCutcheon & Hagenaars, 1997; McCutcheon & Nawojczyk, 1995). In the following, we show how latent class analysis can be used to analyze and test cross-cultural differences in emotion norms in a much stronger way than is possible by comparing mean values.

In addition to this methodological aim, we pursue four more substantive aims. The first aim is to analyze whether explicitly measured norms differ between individualistic and collectivistic cultures in the way predicted by the cultural differences in self-construals and regulatory focus that we outlined earlier. Differences in the cultures should primarily be found for the self-evaluative emotion pride. Collectivistic countries should differ notably from individualistic countries in such a way that types (latent classes) that are characterized by the undesirability of pride occur more frequently. Concerning the negative emotions, types for which guilt is undesirable should be found more frequently in the individualistic nations (i.e., the United States and Australia) than in collectivistic ones. On the other hand, types with the opposite tendencies should be found more often in collectivistic countries.

Our second aim is to analyze whether norms for emotions are related to the frequency and intensity of emotions and whether these relations can be consistently found in different cultures. As we outlined above, there might be only a weak relation between norms and the experience of feelings, but this question has not been sufficiently explored with empirical data.

Our third aim is to scrutinize whether there are cross-cultural differences in the intensity and frequency of reported emotional experiences if we compare people who have the same norms but belong to different cultures. This is another as yet unexplored question. These analyses go beyond traditional studies, which compare the intensity and frequency of emotions between cultures without measuring norms. The intensity and frequency of emotions between cultures might be partly or totally due to differences in the norms for emotions. However, if we correct for differences in the norms, we can compare individuals who are homogeneous with respect to what emotions they consider desirable. If there are cross-cultural differences in the intensity and frequency of emotions between people who have the same norm, this might be more indicative of cross-cultural differences in regulation abilities, genetic differences, or life circumstances that influence emotional feelings.

Method

Participants

We analyzed four subsamples of a large study on emotions in 41 countries (Suh, Diener, Oishi, & Triandis, 1998). In the following, we refer to the subsamples of college students from the United States ($N = 443$), Australia ($N = 292$), Taiwan

(N = 553), and the People's Republic of China (N = 558). We selected these four countries on the basis of the following criteria: First, the countries investigated should differ in their individualistic versus collectivistic orientation. According to Harry Triandis's judgments (personal communication, May 1, 1993), the countries can be classified in the following way on a 10-point individualism scale, where 10 = most individualistic and 1 = least individualistic: United States = 10 points, Australia = 9 points, Taiwan = 5 points, and China = 2 points. Second, the subsamples must be sufficiently large to perform latent class analyses. The design of the larger study is described in detail by Suh et al. (1998).

Materials

The participants were required to complete a questionnaire that contained items for assessing their life satisfaction, experience of emotions, and personality. Chinese and Taiwanese students completed a Mandarin Chinese version of the questionnaire. The English questionnaire was translated into Chinese by a native Chinese-speaking bilingual scientist. A retranslation was performed by a native Chinese-speaking bilingual scientist with a Ph.D. in psychology. The retranslation was compared with the original version by three native English-speaking people and was rated on a 7-point scale (1 = *totally incorrect*, 7 = *completely correct*). The retranslation was rated a 6 by two people and a 7 by one person.

One of the questions dealt with the norms for emotions. It read, "In the following question we would like you to indicate how appropriate or desirable it is to experience certain emotions. Please use the following scale to give your answer to each emotion."[1] The following emotions were presented: joy, affection, pride, contentment, anger, fear, sadness, and guilt. The theoretical background for selecting these emotions was described by Diener, Smith, and Fuijta (1995). The statements could be answered on 7-point scales with the following response categories: *extremely desirable and appropriate, desirable and appropriate, slightly desirable and appropriate, neutral (neither desirable nor undesirable), slightly undesirable and inappropriate, undesirable and inappropriate*, and *extremely undesirable and inappropriate*.

The frequency of emotions was assessed by the following instruction: "Using the scale below, indicate how often you feel each of the emotions listed below. Put a number from 1 to 7 to accurately reflect how much of the time when you are awake you feel that emotion. How much of the time during the past month have you felt

---

[1] One reviewer argued that "appropriate" and "desirable" might not have the same meaning. In a recently conducted German study (Mohiyeddini & Eid, 2001), we assessed norms for emotions by separate scales, including an *appropriate* item and a *desirable* item. We found that the associations between the appropriateness judgments and the desirability judgments were very high for the different emotions (median of the coefficients of contingency for the two items = 0.77), showing that respondents do not differentiate much between the concepts.

each emotion?" The same list of emotions was given. The participants rated each emotion on a seven-category response scale ranging from *never* (1) to *always* (7).

The intensity of emotions was assessed by the instruction, "Now use the scale below to indicate the intensity of these emotions WHEN YOU DO FEEL THEM. That is, when you do experience this emotion, no matter how rarely, typically how INTENSE is your emotional experience?" The intensity of each emotion from the emotion list described above was rated on a 7-point scale ranging from *none—I never experienced it* (1) to *extremely intense* (7).

Procedure

In the first step, the items measuring norms for affect were analyzed by latent class analysis. The multiculture (multigroup) latent class models were analyzed with the computer program PANMARK (van de Pol et al., 1996). To reduce the cells of the multidimensional contingency table, we used two strategies: First, the three desirable and the three undesirable categories of the norm items were reduced to one category each. Thus, response variables with three categories underlie the latent class analyses. Second, the positive emotions of joy, affection, pride, and contentment were analyzed separately from the negative emotions of anger, fear, sadness, and guilt. The positive and negative emotions were analyzed separately because of past evidence that the two are based on systems that show some degree of independence (e.g., Cacioppo & Gardner, 1999).

To analyze the class structure, we first determined, separately for each nation, the common minimal class number for all the participating nations that provided a satisfactory model fit. Then we conducted a multigroup latent class analysis including all nations. We compared several solutions using four different goodness-of-fit criteria: the likelihood ratio test, the Pearson chi-square test, the Cressie-Read test, and the Aknike information criterion (AIC; for a description of these statistics, see Read & Cressie, 1988). Because of sparse tables, we applied the bootstrapping methodology and used 300 bootstrapping analyses (see Langeheine, Pannekoek, & van de Pol, 1996). In the case of sparse tables, the *p* values of the test statistics might not be valid because the assumption that the test statistics are distributed according to a chi-square distribution might be violated. Bootstrapping analysis cures this problem because the distributions of the test statistics can be estimated, and therefore the estimation of the *p* values is more valid (Langeheine et al., 1996). We report the original *p* values that were estimated on the basis of the assumption that the test statistics are distributed according to a chi-square distribution. In addition, we also report the bootstrapping *p* values. However, we interpret only the bootstrapping *p* values because we have sparse tables. To test the assumption of measurement invariance, we restricted all response probabilities to be equal across nations. We evaluated the fit of the restricted models by four criteria. First, the models should not have been rejected by any of the three tests (likelihood ratio test, Pearson chi-square test, Cressie-Read test) using a bootstrapping alpha of 0.05. Second, we considered the likelihood ratio difference test. This means that we calculated the differences between the values of the likelihood ratio test of the unrestricted models and the values of the likelihood ratio test of the models with measurement invariance. Because we have sparse tables we applied Holt and Macready's (1989) recommendation and considered likelihood ratio difference tests as significant if the probability value was smaller than 0.01. Because PANMARK does not provide bootstrapping results for likelihood ratio difference tests, we used traditional p values for these tests. Third, we made the decision even more rigorous by comparing the restricted solutions with the unrestricted ones. If there was any hint that relaxing the strong assumption of total measurement invariance would lead to a more appropriate model, we analyzed a model with relaxed measurement invariance assumptions (partial measurement invariance) and tested this model against the unrestricted one. Fourth, we compared the AIC values of all models considered and chose the model with the lowest AIC value. Hence, we used a very conservative test strategy to ensure that the models we selected represented true cross-cultural consistencies and variations and that we did not overlook substantive cultural differences.

To analyze whether and how the latent classes of respondents differ in their frequency and intensity of experienced emotions, we applied the following strategy. First, all participants were assigned to the latent norm classes for which their assignment probabilities were maximum. Because PANMARK does not calculate the individual assignment probabilities, we used the computer program LEM (Vermunt, 1993) for these analyses. Then, differences between classes and differences between nations were analyzed by analysis of variance and the Kruskal–Wallis test, because the assumption of equal variances between cells was violated in some cases (see below).

Results

Latent Class Analyses of the Norm Items

The goodness-of-fit coefficients for the different latent class models are given in Table 1. We first consider the unrestricted analyses. The latent class analyses revealed that a five-class structure for positive emotions and a six-class structure for negative emotions showed a good model fit for all nations. In these analyses, no restrictions about the nations were added, which means that the response probabilities can differ between nations. For both positive and negative emotions, a model with perfect measurement invariance (equal response probabilities between all nations) shows appropriate fit coefficients for the positive emotions but is inappropriate for the negative emotions. A detailed inspection of the results revealed that the perfect measurement invariance assumption for all nations might be too strong. Rather, a model in which the measurement invariance hypothesis in one class of the Chinese population was removed was superior to a model with perfect measurement invariance but not significantly worse than the unrestricted model according to the criteria described in the Method section. Because this was also true for positive emotions,

Table 1 Goodness-of-fit coefficients for different latent class models

Model	df	Likelihood ratio test			Pearson chi-square test			Cressie–Read test			Akaike information criterion
		Value	p	p(B)	Value	p	p(B)	Value	p	p(B)	
Positive emotions											
No measurement invariance	144	102.75	1.00	1.00	102.78	1.00	1.00	96.02	1.00	1.00	12,813.28
Measurement invariance	264	258.40	0.59	0.27	314.45	0.02	0.36	271.24	0.37	0.31	12,728.93
Partial measurement invariance	256	219.65	0.95	0.67	316.29	0.01	0.60	250.37	0.59	0.61	12,706.19
Negative emotions											
No measurement invariance	108	145.59	0.01	1.00	128.91	0.08	1.00	130.04	0.07	1.00	18,042.92
Measurement invariance	252	354.29	< 0.01	0.05	331.19	<0.01	0.10	327.73	<0.01	0.07	17,963.61
Partial measurement invariance	244	321.50	<0.01	0.32	298.94	0.01	0.35	295.83	0.01	0.32	17,946.83

Note. $p(B)$ represents the probability values calculated on the basis of 300 nonnaive bootstrapping analyses.

we accepted a solution with partial measurement invariance for both types of affect. The model with partial measurement invariance assumes that there is perfect measurement invariance between Australia, Taiwan, and the United States. Furthermore, all classes in the Chinese population, with the exception of one class, showed measurement invariance with the three other nations. However, there was one class for both types of affect that was specific to China.

Positive emotions. Before the results of the positive emotions are presented, we would like to reiterate how our theoretical considerations about cultural differences in self-evaluative emotions are related to our data set. We expected that differences in the cultures should primarily be found for the self-evaluative emotion pride. The collectivistic country, China, should differ notably from both the individualistic countries, the United States and Australia, in such a way that types (latent classes) that are characterized by the undesirability of pride occur more frequently. The prevalence rate of these types in Taiwan should lie between the rate for China and both the other countries, because with regard to the individualism–collectivism variable, Taiwan can be classified between China and the other two countries.

The latent class solution for the positive emotions is illustrated in Table 2. The rows refer to the five different classes. The first four classes are based on the measurement invariance hypothesis for all the countries, Class 5a is invariant for the United States, Australia, and Taiwan, and Class 5b is specific to China. In the last row, the concentration coefficient is given. We come to this coefficient later. The first four columns contain the response probabilities of the three categories for the four emotions: desirable and appropriate, neutral, and undesirable and inappropriate. For example, the response probabilities for joy in Class 1 indicate that people belonging to this class think (with a probability of 1.00) that joy is desirable and appropriate. For Class 2, the probability is maximum (0.74) for the category *neutral* and smaller for the categories *desirable/appropriate* (0.19) and *undesirable/inappropriate* (0.09). Hence, people belonging to this class can be characterized as people with a neutral attitude to joy. The response probabilities for the other emotions and classes can be interpreted analogously. The last four columns indicate the relative class sizes in the four nations. A class size of 0.00 means that the class does not exist in a nation as a result of the empirical analysis. The empty cell in Row 5a indicates that the measurement invariance assumption has been relaxed for China and that the probabilities in the Chinese sample were not restricted to be equal to the other nations. The probability of Class 5 in China is presented in a separate row to make sure that Class 5 in China refers to a different response pattern. Therefore, the empty cell in Row 5a indicates that the size of Class 5 in China can be found in another row. Conceptually, a value of 0.00 and an empty cell mean the same thing, namely that the pattern does not exist in a nation.

How can the classes be characterized and how are they distributed across the different nations? Class 1 consists of people who rated all positive emotions as desirable and appropriate because the probability for the category *desirable and appropriate* is close to 1. Eighty-three percent of the Australian sample and 83% of the American sample belong to this class, but only 9% of the Chinese sample and 32% of the Taiwanese sample do so. Class 2 consists of people who rated all

Table 2 Norms for positive emotions: conditional response probabilities, class sizes, and concentration coefficients

Class and response category	Conditional response probabilities				Class sizes			
	Joy	Affection	Pride	Contentment	AU	US	CH	TW
1								
D/A	1.00	1.00	0.92	0.99				
N	0.00	0.00	0.04	0.01	0.83	0.83	0.09	0.32
UD/IA	0.00	0.00	0.04	0.00				
2								
D/A	0.19	0.11	0.00	0.05				
N	0.74	0.89	0.83	0.90	0.00	0.01	0.09	0.06
UD/IA	0.08	0.00	0.17	0.05				
3								
D/A	0.81	0.77	0.55	0.54				
N	0.11	0.16	0.45	0.24	0.00	0.14	0.32	0.00
UD/IA	0.09	0.08	0.00	0.22				
4								
D/A	0.79	0.72	0.08	0.36				
N	0.10	0.17	0.00	0.16	0.03	0.03	0.34	0.06
UD/IA	0.11	0.11	0.92	0.48				
5a								
D/A	0.96	0.92	0.41	0.90				
N	0.04	0.06	0.34	0.11	0.14	0.00		0.57
UD/IA	0.01	0.02	0.25	0.00				
5b								
D/A	0.13	0.00	0.20	0.19				
N	0.24	0.24	0.16	0.27			0.16	
UD/IA	0.64	0.76	0.64	0.54				
CON					0.29	0.29	0.74	0.56

Note. Concentration (CON; Wickens, 1989) = 1 − sum of the squared probabilities. The minimum concentration in this analysis (five categories of the latent class variable) was zero, and the maximum concentration was 0.80. AU = Australia; US = the United States; CH = China; TW = Taiwan; D/A = desirable and appropriate; N = neutral; UD/IA = undesirable and inappropriate.

the emotions as neutral. This class is small in all nations, indicating that people have a (positive or negative) attitude toward the pleasant emotions. The sizes of this class are significantly different from zero in China and Taiwan but trivial in the two other nations. Class 3 is characterized by the high desirability of joy and affection. Pride and contentment are also to some extent desirable, yet people belonging to this class are rather indifferent with respect to these emotions. Thirty-two percent of the Chinese sample and 14% of the American sample belong to this class. For the other countries, this class is not of importance. Class 4 differs from Class 3 essentially in that the emotion of pride is explicitly rated as undesirable and inappropriate, whereas contentment tends to be rated rather indifferently. This class is most representative of the Chinese sample, because 34% of that sample can be classified here. Class 5 differs in its response probabilities between China and the three other nations. Class 5a, which is not found in China but is found in all other nations, is characterized by a high desirability of joy, affection, and contentment, whereas pride is rated rather indifferently. This class is prototypical for Taiwan, with more than half of the Taiwanese sample belonging to this class. Class 5a looks very similar to Class 3 in profile, but the two classes differ in the numerical values of the response probabilities, in particular for the category *desirable and appropriate*. The Chinese-specific class, Class 5b, stands out because all of the assessed emotions are rated as undesirable and inappropriate, with 16% of the Chinese sample thinking that positive emotions are undesirable.

How can these results be interpreted with respect to our theoretical considerations? Concerning the positive emotions, pride is the most relevant. Class 4 can be interpreted as a typical collectivistic pattern in which pride is considered undesirable. After all, one third of the Chinese sample belongs to this group, thus supporting the assumption that collectivistic cultures consider pride more undesirable than do individualistic ones. Class 5a also points in this direction with its indifference with respect to pride. This class is typical for Taiwan, which is currently on its way from being a collectivistic country to being an individualistic country. In general, the analyses confirm that the classes are differentiated principally with respect to pride.

In the last row in Table 2, the concentration coefficients are given for each nation. The concentration coefficients were calculated on the basis of the class sizes (probabilities of the latent classes). The concentration coefficient is a measure for the variability of probabilities (see Wickens, 1989). It is zero if one latent class has a probability of 1 and, consequently, all other classes have a probability of zero. It is maximum if all latent classes have the same probabilities. Hence, the larger the concentration is, the larger is the within-nation heterogeneity. The concentration coefficients show that the heterogeneity is very large in China and relatively small in Australia and the United States, with Taiwan in between. This result indicates that the individualistic nations of Australia and the United States are very homogeneous nations with respect to norms for positive emotions, whereas the more collectivistic nations of China and Taiwan are rather heterogeneous.

Negative emotions. Concerning the negative emotions, we expected that in the individualistic nations (the United States and Australia), types of people for whom guilt is undesirable should be found more frequently than in China. On the other hand, types with the opposite tendencies should be found more often in China. The relative frequencies in Taiwan should once again lie between those of the individualistic countries and that of China. No predictions were formulated with respect to the other emotions.

The results of the latent class analyses with respect to anger, fear, sadness, and guilt are shown in Table 3. Class 1 identifies a group that rates all of the negative emotions as desirable and appropriate. This class is approximately the same size (with a class size of about 22%) for all four nations. Class 2 is characterized by the fact that all four emotions are considered undesirable and inappropriate. This class is the largest in the United States, Australia, and Taiwan, with class sizes between 35 and 44%. This class, however, is comparatively small in China (14%). Thus, there are rather few people in China who think that negative emotions are generally undesirable and inappropriate. In Class 3, the modal response probability for all emotions

Table 3 Norms for Negative Emotions: Conditional Response Probabilities, Class Sizes, and Concentration Coefficients

Class and response category	Conditional response probabilities				Class sizes			
	Anger	Fear	Sadness	Guilt	AU	US	CH	TW
1								
D/A	0.82	0.89	0.94	0.74				
N	0.10	0.09	0.06	0.18	0.24	0.22	0.22	0.21
UD/IA	0.08	0.01	0.00	0.08				
2								
D/A	0.06	0.00	0.00	0.05				
N	0.08	0.16	0.11	0.09	0.35	0.44	0.14	0.41
UD/IA	0.86	0.84	0.89	0.86				
3								
D/A	0.11	0.12	0.00	0.03				
N	0.60	0.71	0.90	0.76	0.03	0.06	0.12	0.17
UD/IA	0.29	0.16	0.10	0.21				
4								
D/A	0.32	0.04	0.64	0.68				
N	0.19	0.34	0.35	0.32	0.08	0.05	0.14	0.11
UD/IA	0.49	0.62	0.01	0.00				
5								
D/A	0.49	0.88	0.05	0.38				
N	0.15	0.00	0.21	0.21	0.03	0.09	0.15	0.04
UD/IA	0.36	0.12	0.74	0.42				
6a								
D/A	0.51	0.31	0.56	0.00				
N	0.20	0.26	0.12	0.08	0.27	0.13		0.06
UD/IA	0.29	0.43	0.32	0.92				
6b								
D/A	0.45	0.01	0.31	0.25				
N	0.27	0.40	0.00	0.20			0.23	
UD/IA	0.28	0.59	0.69	0.55				
CON					0.74	0.73	0.82	0.74

Note. Concentration (CON; Wickens, 1989) = 1 – sum of the squared probabilities. The minimum concentration in this analysis (six categories of the latent class variable) was zero, and the maximum was 0.83. AU = Australia; US = the United States; CH = China; TW = Taiwan; D/A = desirable and appropriate; N = neutral; UD/IA = undesirable and inappropriate.

is the neutral, middle category. This class is larger in both Asiatic countries than in the United States or Australia. In sum, the first three classes represent differences in the level of desirability (i.e., desirable, neutral, undesirable) that are similar for all negative emotions. The remaining classes, however, portray typological differences between specific emotions. In Class 4, guilt is rated as desirable and appropriate, whereas the modal value for anger is undesirable and inappropriate. Furthermore, sadness is considered desirable, whereas fear is undesirable. This class is comparably small in all countries, albeit somewhat larger in China and Taiwan than in the other two countries. Class 5 is characterized by the contrast between fear, which is desirable, and sadness, which is undesirable. It is relatively small in all the countries and is most common in China. Finally, Classes 6a and 6b point to a typical pattern for individualistic countries—that is, the undesirability of guilt. There are structural differences between China and the other three countries: Mainly, guilt is less undesirable in China than in the other countries, and sadness is somewhat undesirable in China yet moderately desirable in the other three countries. This class is seldom found in Taiwan, whereas it is relatively common in the other countries. In sum, there are strong national differences in the desirability of guilt. In China, the classes in which the probability of the undesirable category for guilt is close to 1 (Classes 2 and 6a) are comparatively sparsely occupied (14%) or do not exist, whereas 62% of Australians, 57% of Americans, and 47% of Taiwanese belong to these classes.

The concentration coefficients indicate that the national differences in heterogeneity are smaller for negative affect than for positive affect. The concentration coefficients are all rather large, showing that there is strong intranational heterogeneity with respect to norms for negative affect. Again, China is the nation with the largest intranational heterogeneity, with a concentration coefficient that is close to the maximum possible value.

In conclusion, regarding the results for positive and negative affect norms, it can be said that the self-conscious emotions pride and guilt differentiate between the nations most clearly. We return to this result in the Discussion.

Within-Nation Differences Between Classes

To analyze differences in the reported intensity and frequency of experienced emotions, we assigned all participants to the latent classes for which their assignment probabilities were maximum. The mean classification (assignment) probabilities for the different latent classes are given in Table 4. The mean classification probabilities can be interpreted as reliability coefficients (maximum value = 1.00). High values indicate high reliability. The mean classification probabilities in our study are rather large, showing that a reliable assignment was possible. Next, mean differences in the frequency and intensity of emotions between these classes were analyzed by analysis of variance. Because the assumption of equal variances between cells (tested by the Levene test) was violated in several analyses and because a violation of this assumption, in combination with unequal cell sizes, questions the validity of the F test (Stevens, 1996), we also tested differences between classes with the Kruskal–Wallis test, a nonparametric statistical test. With this test, differences in the mean ranks between classes were analyzed. We only report the mean values because most readers might be unfamiliar with mean ranks. The mean values, the correlation between norm classes and the frequency and intensity judgments, the F tests, and the Kruskal–Wallis tests for within-nation differences are given in Tables 5, 6, 7,

Table 4 Mean classification probabilities

Norm items	Class 1	Class 2	Class 3	Class 4	Class 5	Class 6
Positive affect	0.81	0.86	0.92	0.93	0.85	
Negative affect	0.89	0.88	0.81	0.73	0.79	0.79

Table 5 Frequency of positive emotions: within-nation mean differences

Emotion	Class 1	2	3	4	5	r	F(dfs)	L	χ^2(df)
Australia									
Joy	3.86	4.00		3.33	4.14	0.07	5.22 (3,284)		2.15 (3)
Affection	4.47	6.00		3.50	3.43	0.16	2.65* (3,283)		7.63 (3)
Pride	3.48	1.00		3.17	2.29	0.18	3.09* (3,283)		9.86* (3)
Contentment	4.02	3.00		2.67	3.29	0.18	2.76* (3,284)		8.06* (3)
China									
Joy	3.03	3.10	3.31	3.11	3.02	0.09	1.09 (4,531)		6.55 (4)
Affection	2.76	2.29	2.67	2.41	2.66	0.11	1.59 (4,533)	**	7.51 (4)
Pride	2.28	2.22	2.49	2.06	2.41	0.14	2.58* (4,533)	**	10.26* (4)
Contentment	2.24	2.18	2.43	2.06	2.49	0.22	2.41* (4,531)	**	8.14 (4)
Taiwan									
Joy	4.44	3.31	4.00	3.87	4.25	0.24	8.14** (4,526)		28.70** (4)
Affection	4.39	2.91	3.50	3.50	4.44	0.26	9.92** (4,528)	**	38.40** (4)
Pride	3.52	2.46	3.50	1.94	2.61	0.40	25.25** (4,528)	**	88.01** (4)
Contentment	3.90	2.97	4.00	2.63	3.66	0.23	7.63** (4,528)		30.57** (4)
United States									
Joy	4.09	2.00	3.85	3.90		0.13	2.51 (3,430)	*	7.05 (3)
Affection	4.42	4.00	3.70	4.50		0.14	3.07* (3,432)		9.61* (3)
Pride	4.04	1.00	3.59	3.20		0.18	4.67** (3,431)		11.68** (3)
Contentment	4.16	3.50	3.43	3.80		0.16	3.67* (3,432)		9.86** (3)

Note. Reported are the mean values (possible range = 1–7). Empty columns indicate that the class does not exist in a culture. r represents the correlation between the class variable and the dependent variable (calculated by the square root of η^2). The chi-square test we used was the Kruskal-Wallis test. The sample size for the chi-squares can be computed using the degrees of freedom of the F tests: $N = df_1 + df_2 + 1$. L = Levene test of equal error variances (asterisks indicate the significance of violations of the homogeneity assumption).
* $p < 0.05$; ** $p < 0.01$.

Table 6 Intensity of positive emotions: within-nation mean differences

Emotion	Class 1	2	3	4	5	r	F(dfs)	L	χ^2(df)
Australia									
Joy	4.89	3.00		3.83	4.29	0.18	3.16* (3,284)		7.08 (3)
Affection	4.99	5.00		4.00	4.00	0.17	2.74* (3,284)		7.07 (3)
Pride	4.03	2.00		3.17	2.43	0.22	4.93* (3,284)		13.63** (3)
Contentment	4.35	4.00		3.17	3.71	0.16	2.49 (3,284)		7.08 (3)
China									
Joy	3.90	3.43	3.84	3.63	3.41	0.14	2.76* (4,532)	**	11.75* (4)
Affection	3.55	2.90	3.54	3.23	3.02	0.14	2.91* (4,532)		11.05* (4)
Pride	3.09	2.75	3.15	2.51	2.78	0.18	4.59** (4,532)	*	18.86** (4)
Contentment	3.06	2.69	3.03	2.64	2.69	0.14	2.57* (4,530)		11.27* (4)
Taiwan									
Joy	5.12	3.77	5.00	3.88	4.81	0.32	14.74** (4,528)	*	49.44** (4)
Affection	4.77	3.51	4.00	4.13	4.59	0.23	7.60** (4,527)	**	34.37** (4)
Pride	4.07	2.83	3.00	2.38	3.01	0.41	26.89** (4,528)		90.76** (4)
Contentment	4.57	3.43	3.50	2.81	4.17	0.32	14.76** (4,528)		52.82** (4)
United States									
Joy	4.81	2.00	4.43	4.10		0.20	6.23** (3,432)		11.98** (3)
Affection	5.06	2.50	4.37	4.90		0.20	6.24** (3,431)		15.57** (3)
Pride	4.46	1.50	3.98	3.40		0.19	5.42** (3,431)	*	10.69* (3)
Contentment	4.43	3.50	3.35	3.70		0.25	9.33** (3,432)	*	21.99* (3)

Note. Reported are the mean values (possible range = 1–7). Empty columns indicate that the class does not exist in a culture, r represents the correlation between the class variable and the dependent variable (calculated by the square root of η^2). The chi-square test we used was the Kruskal-Wallis test. The sample size for the chi-squares can be computed using the degrees of freedom of the F tests: $N = df_{f1} + df_{f2} + 1$. L = Levene test of equal error variances (asterisks indicate the significance of violations of the homogeneity assumption).
* $p < 0.05$; ** $p < 0.01$.

Table 7 Frequency of negative emotions: within-nation mean differences

Emotion	Class						r	F(dfs)	L	χ^2(df)
	1	2	3	4	5	6				
Australia										
Anger	2.77	2.67	2.50	2.77	3.20	3.13	0.20	2.34* (5,284)	*	9.15 (5)
Fear	2.44	2.40	2.40	2.96	2.50	2.49	0.16	1.51 (5,283)		5.02 (5)
Sadness	2.88	2.87	2.90	2.77	3.40	2.93	0.07	0.30 (5,284)		0.53 (5)
Guilt	2.36	2.11	2.20	2.85	2.40	2.36	0.19	2.16 (5,284)	*	9.69 (5)
China										
Anger	2.50	2.26	2.38	2.37	2.54	2.50	0.08	0.64 (5,534)		7.19 (5)
Fear	2.63	2.31	2.57	2.47	2.91	2.22	0.16	2.71* (5,532)		14.70* (5)
Sadness	2.65	2.16	2.38	2.62	2.34	2.58	0.14	2.15 (5,534)	*	11.70* (5)
Guilt	2.27	1.89	2.00	2.26	2.04	2.22	0.10	1.19 (5,535)	**	2.78 (5)
Taiwan										
Anger	2.75	2.41	2.52	2.36	2.78	2.87	0.14	3.32** (5,523)		15.30** (5)
Fear	2.77	2.54	2.77	2.51	3.00	2.80	0.13	1.86 (5,525)		9.64 (5)
Sadness	2.59	2.62	2.65	2.30	2.61	3.40	0.16	2.87* (5,525)	*	11.85* (5)
Guilt	2.31	2.11	2.21	2.34	2.57	1.87	0.13	1.84 (5,525)		11.32* (5)
United States										
Anger	3.24	2.93	3.09	3.29	3.07	3.49	0.16	2.31* (5,420)		12.48* (5)
Fear	2.79	2.51	2.48	2.67	2.67	2.70	0.12	1.30 (5,422)		6.06 (5)
Sadness	3.06	3.01	2.96	2.95	2.86	2.97	0.04	0.19 (5,422)		1.49 (5)
Guilt	2.62	2.39	2.13	2.76	2.40	2.65	0.13	1.51 (5,422)		8.60 (5)

Note. Reported are the mean values (possible range = 1–7). Empty columns indicate that the class does not exist in a culture. *r* represents the correlation between the class variable and the dependent variable (calculated by the square root of η^2). The chi-square test we used was the Kruskal–Wallis test. The sample size for the chi-squares can be computed using the degrees of freedom of the *F* tests: $N = df_1 + df_2 + 1$. L = Levene test of equal error variances (asterisks indicate the significance of violations of the homogeneity assumption).

* $p < 0.05$; ** $p < 0.01$.

and 8. If the Levene test indicates that the equal variance assumption is violated, the results of the Kruskal–Wallis test should be interpreted. Moreover, it is important to note that some classes are very small in some nations (see Tables 2 and 3) and that, therefore, the F test should generally be interpreted cautiously. However, as the results show, the F test and the Kruskal–Wallis test led us to the same conclusion with respect to the significance of the results in many cases, showing cross-analyses consistency of the findings.

Positive emotional experience. Between-classes differences in the reported frequency and the intensity of emotions are given for all nations in Tables 5 and 6. In general, the correlations between the norm classes and the frequency and intensity judgments are low to medium sized when they are evaluated with respect to Cohen's (1988) classification of effect sizes. They are comparably large in Taiwan. The mean differences are significant in most cases, showing that differences in norms are related to differences in emotional experiences. Generally, the mean frequency and intensity values are larger in classes in which these emotions are considered desirable than in classes in which these emotions are considered neutral or undesirable. In particular, in the two collectivistic nations, the frequency and intensity values of pride are rather small in Class 4, in which all positive emotions are considered desirable with the exception of pride and contentment.

Negative emotional experiences. The results concerning the frequency and intensity of negative emotions across latent norm classes are less consistent across nations, and the correlations are also low to medium sized (see Tables 7 and 8). When we consider the Kruskal–Wallis test only, 10 out of 32 associations between norms and experience are significant. Moreover, with only one exception, significant associations were only found for the two collectivistic nations. This result shows that norms for positive emotions are more closely linked to emotional experiences than are norms for negative emotions.

Between-Nations Differences Within Classes

In the next step, we analyzed between-nations differences in the reported experience of affect within each of the latent classes. In these analyses, differences between nations in the norms for emotions are controlled. Thus, mean differences in the frequency and intensity of emotions between nations do not reflect differences in the desirability of emotions. The most interesting question regarding these analyses is whether individuals who do not differ in their attitudes toward emotions between nations do differ in the intensity and frequency of their emotions. The results of these analyses are given in Tables 9, 10, 11, and 12. The mean values on which these analyses are based are the mean values reported in Tables 5, 6, 7, and 8. Again, we only focus on the most interesting results.

Positive emotional experiences. Significant international differences were found for all classes, with the exception of Class 5a and Class 5b. Class 5a exists only in Australia and Taiwan, and within this class the two nations are not different. Class

Table 8 Intensity of negative emotions: within-nation mean differences

Emotion	Class						r	F(dfs)	L	χ^2(df)
	1	2	3	4	5	6				
Australia										
Anger	4.53	4.31	3.80	4.19	5.00	4.71	0.17	1.71 (5,284)		9.03 (5)
Fear	3.68	3.76	3.80	3.96	4.40	3.75	0.08	0.41 (5,284)		2.04 (5)
Sadness	4.50	4.29	4.60	4.52	4.40	4.51	0.08	0.34 (5,283)		2.02 (5)
Guilt	3.59	3.43	3.20	4.04	3.20	3.54	0.12	0.81 (5,283)		3.14 (5)
China										
Anger	3.44	2.51	2.98	2.93	3.04	3.10	0.20	4.30** (5,534)		20.41** (5)
Fear	2.94	2.15	2.90	2.80	2.86	2.49	0.20	4.30** (5,535)		23.55** (5)
Sadness	3.27	2.81	3.03	3.11	3.04	2.99	0.09	0.99 (5,533)		5.80 (5)
Guilt	2.91	2.41	2.71	2.91	2.55	2.74	0.11	1.45 (5,533)		8.34 (5)
Taiwan										
Anger	3.93	3.44	3.21	3.08	3.65	4.07	0.21	4.99** (5,525)	**	20.51** (5)
Fear	3.51	3.39	3.50	2.91	3.70	3.53	0.14	2.23 (5,525)		10.00 (5)
Sadness	3.61	3.69	3.31	2.96	3.65	4.53	0.20	4.38** (5,524)	*	21.39** (5)
Guilt	3.03	3.04	2.90	2.75	2.95	3.27	0.08	0.62 (5,524)		2.63 (5)
United States										
Anger	4.62	4.38	4.00	4.76	4.79	4.03	0.16	2.18 (5,421)		10.96 (5)
Fear	3.71	3.55	3.52	3.81	3.74	3.57	0.07	0.40 (5,422)		1.62 (5)
Sadness	4.29	4.16	3.61	4.00	4.00	4.14	0.10	0.97 (5,422)		5.63 (5)
Guilt	3.70	3.62	3.22	4.10	3.48	3.32	0.12	1.16 (5,420)		4.87 (5)

Note. Reported are the mean values (possible range = 1–7). Empty columns indicate that the class does not exist in a culture, r represents the correlation between the class variable and the dependent variable (calculated by the square root of η^2). The chi-square test we used was the Kruskal–Wallis test. The sample size for the chi-squares can be computed using the degrees of freedom of the F tests: $N = df_1 + df_2 + 1$. L = Levene test of equal error variances (asterisks indicate the significance of violations of the homogeneity assumption).
* $p < 0.05$; ** $p < 0.01$.

Table 9 Frequency of positive emotions: between-nations mean differences within different norm types (classes)

Emotion	r	F(dfs)	L	χ^2(df)
		Class 1		
Joy	0.30	31.08** (3, 977)		81.25** (3)
Affection	0.29	30.95** (3, 979)	**	75.05** (3)
Pride	0.32	38.28** (3, 978)	**	103.34** (3)
Contentment	0.35	44.92** (3, 980)	**	109.26** (3)
		Class 2		
Joy	0.19	1.08 (3, 85)		5.14 (3)
Affection	0.45	7.19** (3, 85)		16.78** (3)
Pride	0.22	1.45 (3, 84)		5.93 (3)
Contentment	0.33	3.59* (3, 85)		12.37** (3)
		Class 3		
Joy	0.20	4.16* (2, 195)		9.08* (2)
Affection	0.30	9.62** (2, 196)		24.96** (2)
Pride	0.32	11.02** (2, 196)		20.32** (2)
Contentment	0.31	10.25** (2, 195)		19.41** (2)
		Class 4		
Joy	0.23	2.60 (3, 199)		7.88* (3)
Affection	0.36	10.20** (3, 201)		22.04** (3)
Pride	0.25	4.57** (3, 201)		10.18* (3)
Contentment	0.32	7.40** (3, 199)		15.23** (3)
		Class 5a		
Joy	0.00	0.07 (1, 230)		0.09 (1)
Affection	0.11	2.83 (1, 231)		2.74 (1)
Pride	0.05	0.74 (1, 231)		0.56 (1)
Contentment	0.05	0.62 (1, 231)		1.12 (1)

Note. Reported are the mean values (possible range = 1–7). Empty columns indicate that the class does not exist in a culture, r represents the correlation between the class variable and the dependent variable (calculated by the square root of η^2). The chi-square test we used was the Kruskal–Wallis test. The sample size for the chi-squares can be computed using the degrees of freedom of the F tests: $N = df_1 + df_2 + 1$. L = Levene test of equal error variances (asterisks indicate the significance of violations of the homogeneity assumption).
* $p < 0.05$; ** $p < 0.01$.

5b could not be compared between nations because it exists only in China. The first interesting result concerning the frequency and intensity of positive emotions is that China has, in all classes with exception of Class 2 and for all positive emotions, the lowest mean value (see Tables 5 and 6). This shows that China is the nation with the lowest frequency and intensity of positive emotions even if we correct for national differences in the desirability of emotions. The mean values of the other nations depend on the latent classes. In general, Australia, Taiwan, and the United States are quite similar, with the exception of the frequency and intensity of pride in Class 4, the class in which pride is undesirable. In this class, the mean values of the

Table 10 Intensity of positive emotions: between-nations mean differences within different norm types (classes)

Emotion	r	F(dfs)	L	χ^2(df)
		Class 1		
Joy	0.26	23.71**(3, 980)		68.89**(3)
Affection	0.29	30.61** (3, 978)	**	58.48**(3)
Pride	0.26	23.13**(3, 979)	**	63.75**(3)
Contentment	0.29	30.03**(3, 980)		77.25**(3)
		Class 2		
Joy	0.25	1.96 (3, 85)		7.13 (3)
Affection	0.30	2.76*(3, 85)	**	8.03*(3)
Pride	0.16	0.79 (3, 85)		2.87 (3)
Contentment	0.31	3.12*(3, 85)		10.57*(3)
		Class 3		
Joy	0.22	4.97**(2, 196)		9.49**(2)
Affection	0.23	5.28**(2, 195)		9.36**(2)
Pride	0.21	4.67**(2, 196)		9.54**(2)
Contentment	0.09	0.84 (2, 195)		1.27 (2)
		Class 4		
Joy	0.09	0.51 (3, 199)		1.28 (3)
Affection	0.26	4.80**(3, 201)		12.71**(3)
Pride	0.16	1.83 (3, 200)	*	2.72 (3)
Contentment	0.18	2.27 (3, 201)		5.28 (3)
		Class 5a		
Joy	0.08	1.67 (1, 231)		2.09 (1)
Affection	0.07	1.20 (1, 231)		1.94 (1)
Pride	0.08	1.49 (1, 231)		1.47 (1)
Contentment	0.06	0.98 (1, 231)		1.78 (1)

Note. Reported are the mean values (possible range = 1–7). Empty columns indicate that the class does not exist in a culture. r represents the correlation between the class variable and the dependent variable (calculated by the square root of η^2). The chi-square test we used was the Kruskal–Wallis test. The sample size for the chi-squares can be computed using the degrees of freedom of the F tests: $N = df_1 + df_2 + 1$. L = Levene test of equal error variances (asterisks indicate the significance of violations of the homogeneity assumption).
* $p < 0.05$; ** $p < 0.01$.

frequency and intensity of pride are lower in Taiwan than in Australia and the United States. This is in line with the role pride plays in more collectivistic countries.

Negative emotional experiences. The results for the negative emotions are given in Tables 11 and 8.12. For the negative emotions, the national differences are rather strong for anger, and the differences are stronger for the intensity than for the frequency judgments. For the intensity judgements, the international differences are rather strong in Class 2, in which all negative emotions are considered undesirable, in Class 4, in which only sadness and guilt are desirable, and in Class 5, in which anger and fear are desirable but sadness and guilt are not. In general, China has the lowest mean values in the majority of classes. This result implies that, controlling for norms for negative affect, the Chinese report less frequent and less intense unpleas-

Table 11 Frequency of negative emotions: between-nations mean differences within different norm types (classes)

Emotion	r	F(dfs)	L	χ^2(df)
		Class 1		
Anger	0.26	9.78** (3, 408)	**	28.45** (3)
Fear	0.11	1.59 (3, 408)	**	8.47* (3)
Sadness	0.16	3.77 (3, 409)		13.95** (3)
Guilt	0.12	1.88 (3, 409)	**	14.79** (3)
		Class 2		
Anger	0.24	12.35** (3, 591)		49.63** (3)
Fear	0.08	1.18 (3, 593)	**	12.19** (3)
Sadness	0.25	13.20 (3, 594)		41.18** (3)
Guilt	0.17	5.83** (3, 595)		16.69** (3)
		Class 3		
Anger	0.21	2.93* (3, 191)		9.08* (3)
Fear	0.11	0.74 (3, 191)		5.15 (3)
Sadness	0.18	2.12 (3, 191)		7.74** (3)
Guilt	0.09	0.57 (3, 191)		9.26* (3)
		Class 4		
Anger	0.27	5.07** (3, 187)		16.03** (3)
Fear	0.13	1.12 (3, 188)		6.21 (3)
Sadness	0.19	2.38 (3, 188)		7.40 (3)
Guilt	0.16	1.77 (3, 188)		8.98* (3)
		Class 5		
Anger	0.20	2.00 (3, 136)		9.36* (3)
Fear	0.11	0.55 (3, 135)	**	1.43 (3)
Sadness	0.21	2.10 (3, 136)		5.91 (3)
Guilt	0.17	1.40 (3, 135)		7.37 (3)
		Class 6a		
Anger	0.16	1.80 (2, 134)		3.97 (2)
Fear	0.10	0.77 (2, 134)		1.44 (2)
Sadness	0.13	1.08 (2, 134)		1.60 (2)
Guilt	0.18	2.32 (2, 134)		9.26* (2)

Note. Reported are the mean values (possible range = 1–7). Empty columns indicate that the class does not exist in a culture. r represents the correlation between the class variable and the dependent variable (calculated by the square root of η^2). The chi-square test we used was the Kruskal–Wallis test. The sample size for the chi-squares can be computed using the degrees of freedom of the F tests: $N = df_1 + df_2 + 1$. L = Levene test of equal error variances (asterisks indicate the significance of violations of the homogeneity assumption).
* $p < 0.05$; ** $p < 0.01$.

ant emotions. Considering the frequency of the negative emotions, Taiwan is similar to Australia and the United States, but with respect to the intensity of negative emotions, there are stronger differences between Taiwan and the two individualistic countries. Hence, there is a tendency for people in the more individualistic countries of Australia and the United States to feel negative emotions more intensely than do people in the more collectivistic countries of China and Taiwan.

Table 12 Intensity of negative emotions: between-nations mean differences within different norm types (classes)

Emotion	r	F(dfs)	L	χ^2(df)
		Class 1		
Anger	0.31	14.59** (3, 409)		41.55** (3)
Fear	0.24	8.65** (3, 409)		29.06** (3)
Sadness	0.32	15.11** (3, 409)		42.02** (3)
Guilt	0.23	7.50** (3, 407)		21.46** (3)
		Class 2		
Anger	0.43	44.29** (3, 593)		111.76** (3)
Fear	0.35	28.24** (3, 594)	*	72.48** (3)
Sadness	0.31	20.73** (3, 593)		53.08** (3)
Guilt	0.26	14.87** (3, 594)		41.07** (3)
		Class 3		
Anger	0.24	4.07** (3, 190)		11.50** (3)
Fear	0.23	3.43* (3, 191)		10.40* (3)
Sadness	0.25	4.38** (3, 191)		10.54* (3)
Guilt	0.12	0.92 (3, 189)	*	4.84 (3)
		Class 4		
Anger	0.46	16.57** (3, 188)	*	36.25** (3)
Fear	0.34	8.36** (3, 188)		18.64** (3)
Sadness	0.37	9.90** (3, 187)		24.74* (3)
Guilt	0.34	7.99 (3, 188)		18.23** (3)
		Class 5		
Anger	0.49	14.39** (3, 137)		32.71** (3)
Fear	0.31	4.80** (3, 136)		14.89** (3)
Sadness	0.28	3.83* (3, 135)		11.78** (3)
Guilt	0.27	3.48* (3, 136)		13.75** (3)
		Class 6a		
Anger	0.23	3.99* (2, 134)		9.30* (2)
Fear	0.07	0.36 (2, 134)		0.91 (2)
Sadness	0.12	0.98 (2, 134)		2.20 (2)
Guilt	0.07	0.33 (2, 134)		0.71 (2)

Note. Reported are the mean values (possible range = 1–7). Empty columns indicate that the class does not exist in a culture. *r* represents the correlation between the class variable and the dependent variable (calculated by the square root of η^2). The chi-square test we used was the Kruskal–Wallis test. The sample size for the chi-squares can be computed using the degrees of freedom of the F tests: $N = df_1 + df_2 + 1$. L = Levene test of equal error variances (asterisks indicate the significance of violations of the homogeneity assumption).
* $p < 0.05$; ** $p < 0.01$.

Discussion

The analyses reveal a number of interesting insights into the structure of norms for emotions and the cross-cultural generalizability of this structure. We discuss the results in five areas: (a) the structure of norms for emotions, (b) intranational variability in norms for affect, (c) norms and emotional experiences, (d) between-nations differences in emotional experience, and (e) the use of latent class analysis in cross-cultural studies on emotions.

The Structure of Norms for Emotions

Considering the results of the norms for positive and negative emotions together, the main differences between nations can be found in pride and guilt. In more collectivistic cultures guilt is more important, whereas in individualistic cultures pride is of greater relevance. Hence, the results confirm our theoretical predictions that the group of emotions that are often prone to cross-cultural differences is the self-conscious or self-reflective emotions—emotions that reflect on the individual's own actions (see Tangney & Fischer, 1995). The approach-oriented, individualistic cultures think that self-reflective emotions about a person doing well are good, whereas the collectivistic, Confucian cultures in the Pacific Rim believe that self-reflective emotions that indicate that one's controllable actions are wrong or insufficient are desirable. This is in line with cultural differences in regulatory focus. For cultures that are promotion focused, pride is more important, whereas for cultures that are prevention focused, guilt is more desirable.

Generally, the results show that not all "positive" emotions are considered positive (i.e., desirable, appropriate) by most individuals. Furthermore, not all "negative" emotions are considered negative (i.e., undesirable, inappropriate) by most individuals. This finding has consequences for the concept of social desirability. In studies scrutinizing whether affect judgments are biased by a social desirability response style, it is typically assumed that positive emotions are considered desirable and negative emotions are considered undesirable. However, this basic assumption seems to be wrong. A stronger test for the assumption that affect judgments are (not) distorted by social desirability would be to take into account group differences in the desirability of emotions and analyze the influence of desirability judgments on affect judgments in different subgroups.

Intranational Variability in Norms for Affect

The nations in this study do not have one set of norms to which everyone adheres. Instead, the countries include people with a variety of views about the normativeness of emotions. The nations on average differ, but this disguises the fact that there is substantial variability in norms within the societies. Culture seems to influence the number of people adhering to a particular viewpoint, but the cultures are nevertheless heterogeneous enough that there are differences within them. Thus, cross-cultural researchers need to consider not only average cultural differences but also the variability within cultures.

These within-nation differences can be explained by two concepts of cross-cultural psychology: first, the distinction between idiocentrism and allocentrism, and, second, the distinction between tight versus loose cultures (e.g., Triandis, 1989). The concepts of idiocentrism and allocentrism reflect the distinction between individualism and collectivism and are concepts we can use to characterize nations on the individual level. Thus, within individualistic and collectivistic nations there can be idiocentric and allocentric individuals. However, in individualistic nations there should be more idiocentric individuals, and in collectivistic countries there should be more allocentric individuals. The latent class analyses revealed that most people of the two individualistic countries show an idiocentric norm pattern: In the two more collectivistic nations, both idiocentric and allocentric patterns can be found, although most of the people belong to the more allocentric patterns.

Nations differ not only in their collectivism and individualism but also in how loose or tight they are. Tight cultures are very homogeneous with respect to norms. In tight cultures, there is a high pressure on all individuals of a society to follow these norms. Loose cultures do not have such strong norms and tolerate more deviations. The concentration coefficient might be regarded as a measure of the tightness versus looseness of a nation regarding the variables under study. According to this coefficient, Australia and the United States are relatively tight nations with respect to norms for positive affect. In these nations, there might be pressure on individuals to be joyful, happy, and full of love and pride and to make use of their constitutional right to the pursuit of happiness. Deviations from this norm of happiness might have a strong impact, and being unhappy might be regarded as failing. People who are less happy are expected to correct their unhappiness by using, for instance, psychotherapy. It was unexpected that the individualistic nations are the most uniform with regard to pleasant affect norms. Although these nations are "loose" in terms of the norms for behavior, at the level of emotions they appear not to be loose. Rather, the desirability of happiness seems to be prescribed by the culture. Indeed, one justification for people "doing their own thing" is that everyone ought to be happy and, therefore, follow their own desires. Thus, allowing for more variability in individual behavior seems, ironically, to require a strong norm about the desirability of positive experiences.

The two more collectivistic nations seem to be looser countries with respect to norms for positive emotions. In particular, China, which was characterized as "a collectivistic, but 'relatively' loose country" by Triandis (1989, p. 511), shows a large variety in norm types. In China, people who are unhappy might also be accepted, because in China there are also individuals who think that positive emotions are undesirable. Pride is considered undesirable by a large number of people in the two more collectivistic countries, but there are still many people who think that feeling pride is acceptable. Thus, the norms for positive emotions (e.g., not to feel pride) seem not to be so strong that all individuals must follow them. This might be a sign that there is a movement to more diversity in these countries. For norms for negative emotions, the intranational variety differs less strongly between nations. All nations are relatively heterogeneous in their norms for experiencing unpleasant emotions, but China is nevertheless the most heterogeneous. From a methodological point of view, the results show that latent class analysis is an appropriate methodology to discover international differences in the tightness versus looseness of nations.

Norms and Emotional Experiences

In terms of emotional experiences, we found that there are low-to medium-sized correlations between norm classes and emotional experiences. For positive emotions, we found a consistent pattern such that the frequency and intensity of positive emotions are related to the norm classes in such a way that higher desirability goes along with respondents reporting more experience of this emotion. For negative affect, however, the results were much more inconsistent. We discuss the results for both types of affect separately. However, it should be noted that the variegated pattern of findings suggests that people do not automatically infer norms from their own emotional experiences.

For positive emotions, significant associations with respect to the frequency of emotions were predominantly found for pride and contentment. This is in line with the latent structure of the norm data because the classes differ mainly between the desirability of pride and contentment. The association between the desirability and frequency of positive emotions might point to the influence of emotion regulation. People who think that a positive emotion is desirable might seek that emotion more strongly than other people. On the other hand, if a person thinks, for example, that pride is undesirable, that person will avoid situations in which this emotion occurs. If those situations cannot be avoided, the person will appraise the situation in such a way that pride will not arise; if this is not possible, it is likely that the person will regulate this feeling downward. Hence, the association between the frequency of positive affect and norms for these emotions suggests that regulative behavior is effective. However, although individuals can and do seek such situations, no situation is perfectly under the control of individuals, and therefore the associations might not be very strong.

The associations between norm classes and emotional experiences, in particular emotion intensity, might also suggest the importance of socialization influences. If individuals have learned that specific emotions are desirable, they are free to feel these emotions intensely. However, if they have learned that specific emotions are undesirable or inappropriate, they might have learned to regulate this feeling downward.

Why are the results so different for negative emotions? One interesting result is that not only people who think that negative emotions are desirable but also people who think that negative emotions are undesirable feel them (moderately) frequently and intensely. One possible explanation for this phenomenon is that there might be two groups of people. One group of people may often experience negative emotions because, for them, negative emotions have a positive function, indicating that something is going wrong. These people might be able to use this indicator of negative emotions to cope with the situations that elicit these emotions. Additionally, there might be another group of people who frequently experience these emotions but are not able to regulate them—these people might be stuck with the emotions without making use of their function. These people might be genetically predisposed to negative affect and therefore experience it more often and believe that it is not appropriate because they find it to be aversive. These assumptions would predict that inter-individual differences in norms might be only weakly related to interindividual differences in emotional experiences. These assumptions, however, are speculative, and they indicate that the linkage between emotional norms and emotional experiences might be rather complex. However, this subject seems to be a very fascinating topic of future cross-cultural studies on emotions.

Between-Nations Differences in Emotional Experience

There appear to be differences in the experience of emotions across nations even when norms are held constant. Thus, it appears that factors such as genetics or life circumstances also influence emotional experiences beyond the influence of norms.

The most important result here is the finding that China consistently shows the lowest experiences in almost all norm classes. People in China also have the lowest frequency and intensity scores of both positive and negative affects. This result can be explained by the general value emotions have in China (for an overview, see Russell & Yik, 1996). Several authors, such as Klineberg (1938), Potter (1988), and Wu (1982), have pointed out that in China there is a general attitude to consider emotions as dangerous, irrelevant, or illness causing. Moreover, the moderation or suppression of emotions is generally highly valued in China. In particular, the value of a moderated emotional life might explain the relatively low scores of the Chinese even in the classes in which the emotions are considered desirable. An alternative explanation is that there are genetical differences in the physiology of emotional responses between different countries.

Another interesting result is that Taiwan is very similar to Australia and the United States with respect to almost all positive emotions, with the exception of pride. Regarding pride, Taiwan is more similar to China. Considering the frequency of negative emotions, Taiwan is similar to Australia and the United States, but with respect to the intensity of negative emotions there are stronger differences between Taiwan and the two individualistic countries. These results confirm the role of Taiwan as a nation that is historically and philosophically strongly linked to China but now is more oriented to individualistic values.

Latent Class Analysis in Cross-Cultural Studies on Emotions

The analyses show that latent class analysis is a helpful methodology to explore and test typological structures of emotion. With latent class analysis, it is possible to consider (a) categorical response variables, (b) intra- and international differences in individual profiles, and (c) universal and culture-specific norm types. Furthermore, it is possible to test the equivalence of structures across cultures in a strong way. The results reveal that the strong assumption of measurement invariance had to be rejected for the total sample but that there are subgroups of individuals that are equivalent across nations and subgroups that are culture specific. Comparing the nations by one statistic (e.g., the mean value), as is often done, obscures this cultural variety and complexity.

A model with universal and culture-specific norm classes fits the data very well. This clearly shows that there is structural equivalence and structural diversity between nations. It also demonstrates the advantage of latent class analysis in separating universal from culture-specific emotion patterns that go beyond "traditional" methods of cross-cultural psychology. Furthermore, the latent classes revealed that there are different typologies of norms. In particular, for negative emotions we found quite different norm patterns. One interesting result, for example, is that the desirability of anger contrasts sharply with the desirability of guilt. In classes in which anger is desirable, guilt is always undesirable, and in classes in which anger is undesirable, guilt is always desirable. A further interesting result is that there are classes in which all positive emotions are considered undesirable and all negative emotions are considered desirable. These different norm patterns demonstrate that a typological approach is superior to and more informative than a dimensional approach.

In the study of norms for emotions presented in this article, generalized norms for affect were analyzed. In future studies, it might be interesting to use latent class analysis for exploring the structure of situation-specific feeling rules and to scrutinize how strongly norms of emotions generalize across situations. Moreover, it might be useful to include more nations differing in individualism and collectivism.

References

Bond, M. H. (1996). Chinese values. In M. H. Bond (Ed.). *The handbook of Chinese psychology*. Hong Kong: Oxford University Press.

Briggs, J. L. (1970). *Never in anger: Portrait of an Eskimo family*. Cambridge, MA: Harvard University Press.

Cacioppo, J. T., & Gardner, W. L. (1999). Emotion. *Annual Review of Psychology, 50*, 191–214.

Clogg, C. (1995). Latent class models: Recent developments and prospects for the future. In G. Arminger, C. C. Clogg, & M. E. Sobel (Eds.), *Handbook of statistical modeling in the social sciences* (pp. 311–359). New York: Plenum.

Cohen, J. (1988). *Statistical power analysis for the behavioral sciences* (2nd ed.). Hillsdale, NJ: Erlbaum.

Darwin, C. (1970). *The expression of the emotions in man and animals*. Chicago: University of Chicago Press. (Original work published 1872)

Diener, E., Smith, H., & Fuijta, F. (1995). The personality structure of affect. *Journal of Personality and Social Psychology, 69*, 130–141.

Drasgow, F., & Kanfer, R. (1985). Equivalence of psychological measurement in heterogeneous populations. *Journal of Applied Psychology, 70*, 662–680.

Eid, M. (2001). Advanced statistical models for the study of appraisal and emotional reaction. In K. R. Scherer, A. Schorr, & T. Johnstone (Eds.), *Appraisal processes in emotion: Theory, methods, research* (pp. 319–330). New York: Oxford University Press.

Eid, M., & Rauber, M. (2000). Detecting measurement invariance in organizational surveys. *European Journal of Psychological Assessment, 16*, 20–30.

Ekman, P., & Friesen, W. V. (1969). The repertoire of nonverbal behavior Categories, origins, usage, and coding. *Semiotica, 1*, 49–98.

Frijda, N. H., & Mesquita, B. (1995). The social roles and functions of emotions. In S. Kitayama & H. R. Markus (Eds.), *Emotion and culture: Empirical studies of mutual influence* (pp. 51–87). Washington, DC: American Psychological Association.

Gardner, W. L., Gabriel, S., & Lee, A. (1999). "I" value freedom, but "we" value relationships: Self-construal priming mirrors cultural differences in judgment. *Psychological Science, 10*, 321–326.

Grammer, K., & Eibl-Eibesfeldt, I. (1993). Emotionspsychologie im Kulturenvergleich [Emotion psychology in cultural comparisons]. In A. Thomas (Ed.), *Kulturvergleichende Psychologie. Eine Einführung* (pp. 289–322). Göttingen, Germany: Hogrefe.

Hochschild, R. (1983). *The managed heart*. Berkeley, CA: University of California Press.

Holt, J. A., & Macready, G. B. (1989). A simulation study of the difference chi-square statistic for comparing latent class models under violation of regularity conditions. *Applied Psychological Measurement, 13*, 221–231.

Izard, C. E. (1980). Cross-cultural perspectives on emotion and emotion communication. In H. C. Triandis & W. Lonner (Eds.), *Handbook of cross-cultural psychology* (Vol. 3, pp. 185–221). Boston: Allyn & Bacon.

Kitayama, S., & Markus, H. R. (Eds.) (1995). *Emotion and culture: Empirical studies of mutual influence* (pp. 23–50). Washington, DC: American Psychological Association.

Kitayama, S., Markus, H. R., & Matsumoto, D. (1995). Culture, self, and emotion: A cultural perspective on "self-conscious" emotions. In J. P. Tangney & K. Fisher (Eds.), *Self-conscious emotions: The psychology of shame, guilt, embarrassment, and pride* (pp. 439–464). New York: Guilford Press.

Klineberg, O. (1938). Emotional expression in Chinese literature. *Journal of Abnormal and Social Psychology, 33*, 517–520.

Langeheine, R., Pannekoek, J., & van de Pol, F. (1996). Bootstrapping goodness-of-fit measures in categorical data analysis. *Sociological Methods and Research, 24*, 492–516

Langeheine, R., & Rost, J. (1988). *Latent trait and latent class models*. New York: Plenum.

Lazarsfeld, P. F., & Henry, N. W. (1968). *Latent structure analysis*. Boston: Houghton Mifflin.

Lee, A. Y., Aaker, J. L., & Gardner, W. L. (2000). The pleasures and pains of distinct self-construals: The role of interdependence in regulatory focus. *Journal of Personality and Social Psychology, 78*, 1122–1134.

Leung, K., & Bond, M. H. (1989). On the empirical identification of dimensions for cross-cultural comparisons. *Journal of Cross-Cultural Psychology, 20*, 133–151.

Markus, H. R., & Kitayama, S. (1991). Culture and the self: Implications for cognition, emotion, and motivation. *Psychological Review, 98*, 224–253.

Matsumoto, D. (1996). *Culture and psychology*. Pacific Grove, CA: Brooks/Cole.

McCutcheon A. L. (1987). *Latent class analysis*. Newbury Park, CA: Sage.

McCutcheon, A. L. (1998). Correspondence analysis used complementary to latent class analysis in comparative social research. In J. Blasius & M. Greenacre (Eds.), *Visualization of categorical data* (pp. 477–488). San Diego, CA: Academic Press.

McCutcheon, A. L., & Hagenaars, J. A. (1997). Comparative social research with multi-sample latent class models. In J. Rost & R. Langeheine (Eds.), *Applications of latent trait and latent class models in the social sciences* (pp. 266–277). Münster, Germany: Waxmann.

McCutcheon, A. L., & Nawojczyk, M. (1995). Making the break: Popular sentiment toward legalized abortion among American and Polish Catholic laities. *International Journal of Public Opinion Research, 7*, 232–252.

Mesquita, B., & Ellsworth, P. (2001). The role of culture in appraisal. In K. R. Scherer, A. Schorr, & T. Johnstone (Eds.), *Appraisal processes in emotion: Theory, methods, research* (pp. 233–248). New York: Oxford University Press.

Mesquita, B., & Frijda, N. H. (1992). Cultural variations in emotions: A review. *Psychological Bulletin, 112*, 179–204.

Mohiyeddini, C., & Eid, M. (2001). Norms for the expression and the experience of emotions. Unpublished raw data.

Potter, S. H. (1988). The cultural construction of emotion in rural Chinese social life. *Ethos, 16*, 181–208.

Read, T., & Cressie, N. (1988). *Goodness-of-fir statistics for discrete multivariate data.* New York: Springer.

Rost, J., Carstensen, C., & von Davier, M. (1997). Applying the mixed Rasch model to personality questionnaires. In J. Rost & R. Langeheine (Eds.), *Applications of latent trait and latent class models in the social sciences* (pp. 324–332). Münster, Germany: Waxmann.

Russell, J. A., & Yik, M. S. M. (1996). Emotion among the Chinese. In M. H. Bond (Ed.), *The handbook of Chinese psychology* (pp. 166–188). Hong Kong: Oxford University Press.

Saarni, C. (1999). *The development of emotional competence.* New York: Guilford.

Scherer, K. (1994). Evidence for both universality and cultural specificity of emotion elicitation. In P. Ekman & R. J. Davidson (Eds.), *The nature of emotion. Fundamental questions* (pp. 172–175). New York: Oxford University Press.

Scherer, K. (1997). The role of culture in emotion-antecedent appraisal. *Journal of Personality and Social Psychology, 73*, 902–922.

Scherer, K. R., & Wallbott, H. G. (1994). Evidence for universality and cultural variation of differential emotion response patterning. *Journal of Personality and Social Psychology, 66*, 310–328.

Scherer, K. R., Wallbott, H. G., & Summerfield, A. B. (Eds.). (1986). *Experiencing emotion: A cross-cultural study.* Cambridge, England: Cambridge University Press.

Schieffelin, E. D. (1983). Anger and shame in the tropical forest: An affect as a cultural system in Paua New Guinea. *Ethos, 11*, 181–191.

Shaver, P. R., Wu, S., & Schwartz, J. C. (1992). Cross-cultural similarities and differences in emotion and its representation. In M. S. Clark (Ed.), *Emotion: Review of personality and social psychology* (pp. 175–213). Newbury Park, CA: Sage.

Sommers, S. (1984). Adults evaluating their emotions: A cross-cultural perspective. In C. Z. Malatesta & C. Izard (Eds.), *Emotions in adult development* (pp. 319–338). Beverly Hills, CA: Sage.

Stearns, P. N. (1994). *American cool: Constructing a twentieth century emotional style.* New York: New York University Press.

Stearns, P. N., & Lewis, J. (1998). *An emotional history of the United States.* New York: New York University Press.

Stevens, J. (1996). *Applied multivariate statistics for the social sciences* (3rd ed.). Mahwah, NJ: Erlbaum.

Stipek, D. (1998). Differences between Americans and Chinese in the circumstances evoking pride, shame, and guilt. *Journal of Cross-Cultural Psychology, 29*, 616–629.

Stipek, D., Weiner, B., & Li, K. (1989). Testing some attribution-emotion relations in the People's Republic of China. *Journal of Personality and Social Psychology, 56*, 109–116.

Suh, E., Diener, E., Oishi, S., & Triandis, H. C. (1998). The shifting basis of life satisfaction judgments across cultures: Emotions versus norms. *Journal of Personality and Social Psychology, 74*, 482–493.

Tangney, J. P., & Fischer, K. (Eds.). (1995). *Self-conscious emotions: The psychology of shame, guilt, embarrassment, and pride.* New York: Guilford Press.

Tangney, J. P., Wagner, P., Fletcher, C., & Gramzow, R. (1992). Shamed into anger? The relation of shame and guilt to anger and self-reported aggression. *Journal of Personality and Social Psychology, 62*, 669–675.

Triandis, H. (1989). The self and social behavior in differing cultural contexts. *Psychological Review, 96*, 506–520.

Triandis, H. (1997). Cross-cultural perspectives on personality. In R. Hogan, J. Johnson, & S. R. Briggs (Eds.), *Handbook of personality psychology* (pp. 439–464). San Diego, CA: Academic Press.

Ulich, D., & Mayring, P. (1992). *Psychologie der Emotionen* [Psychology of emotions]. Stuttgart, Germany: Kohlhammer.

van de Pol, F., Langeheine, R., & de Jong, W. (1996). *PANMARK 3. Panel analysis using Markov chains—A latent class analysis program*. Voorburg, the Netherlands: Netherlands Central Bureau of Statistics.

van de Vijver, F., & Leung, K. (1996). Methods and data analysis of comparative research. In J. W. Berry, Y. H. Poortinga, & J. Pandey (Eds.), *Handbook of cross-cultural psychology* (2nd ed., Vol. 1, pp. 257–300). Chicago: Allyn & Bacon.

van de Vijver, F., & Leung, K. (1997). *Methods and data analysis for cross-cultural research*. Thousand Oaks, CA: Sage.

Vermunt, J. (1993). *LEM: Log-linear and event history analysis with missing data using the EM algorithm* (WORC Paper 93.09.015/7). Tilburg, the Netherlands: Tilburg University.

Wallbott, H. G., & Scherer, K. R. (1988). How universal and specific is emotional experience? Evidence from 27 countries. In K. R. Scherer (Ed.), *Facets of emotions* (pp. 31–56). Hillsdale, NJ: Erlbaum.

Wickens, T. D. (1989). *Multiway contingency table analysis for the social sciences*. Hillsdale, NJ: Erlbaum.

Wu, D. (1982). Psychotherapy and emotion in traditional Chinese medicine. In A. J. Marsella & G. M. White (Eds.), *Cultural conceptions of mental health and therapy* (pp. 285–301). Dordrecht, the Netherlands: Reidel.

Emotions Across Cultures and Methods

Christie Napa Scollon, Ed Diener, Shigehiro Oishi and Robert Biswas-Diener

Abstract Participants included 46 European American, 33 Asian American, 91 Japanese, 160 Indian, and 80 Hispanic students ($N = 416$). Discrete emotions, as well as pleasant and unpleasant emotions, were assessed: (a) with global self-report measures, (b) using an experience-sampling method for 1 week, and (c) by asking participants to recall their emotions from the experience sampling week. Cultural differences emerged for nearly all measures. The inclusion of indigenous emotions in India and Japan did not alter the conclusions substantially, although pride showed a pattern across cultures that differed from the other positive emotions. In all five cultural groups and for both pleasant and unpleasant emotions, global reports of emotion predicted retrospective recall even after controlling for reports made during the experience sampling period, suggesting that individuals' general conceptions of their emotional lives influenced their memories of emotions. Cultural differences emerged in the degree to which recall of frequency of emotion was related to experience sampling reports of intensity of emotions. Despite the memory bias, the three methods led to similar conclusions about the relative position of the groups.

A consistent and intriguing finding in the subjective well-being (SWB) literature is that individuals from Asian cultures tend to report lower levels of life satisfaction, less pleasant emotion, and greater negative emotion compared to North Americans (e.g., E. Diener, M. Diener, & C. Diener, 1995; Kitayama, Markus, & Kurokawa, 2000). Even within the United States, differences among ethnic groups mirror cross-national findings, with Asian Americans reporting lower SWB than European Americans (e.g., Okazaki, 1997, 2000; Schkade & Kahneman, 1998). Notably, however, most cross-cultural comparisons of emotion have been based on global measures or recalled reports of emotion, making it difficult to disentangle the meaning of cultural differences. Do cultural differences in global or retrospective reports reflect differences in everyday emotional experience? Or do cultures

C.N. Scollon (✉)
School of Social Sciences, Singapore Management University, 90 Stamford Rd., #04-71, Singapore 178903
e-mail: cscollon@smu.edu.sg

E. Diener (ed.), *Culture and Well-Being: The Collected Works of Ed Diener*, Social Indicators Research Series 38, DOI 10.1007/978-90-481-2352-0_10,
© Springer Science+Business Media B.V. 2009

differ in their memory for emotions, or both? Because global and retrospective reports of emotion are vulnerable to memory reconstruction (Kahneman, 1999), a deeper understanding of the emotional lives of individuals from different cultures requires a study of online emotion or measures of emotion as they occur (Flannery, 1999).

The aims of the present study were twofold. First, this research represents an exploratory effort at quantifying the frequency of specific emotions, including indigenous emotions, across cultures. Thus far, these topics have traditionally received treatment in ethnographic and retrospective self-report studies (Flannery, 1999), whereas the present study sought to document whether cultural differences exist in online or momentary reports of emotion compared to global and retrospective measures. Although this may be a straightforward descriptive goal, it is of fundamental importance because little is currently known about online emotional experience across cultures. Empirically establishing the base rates of specific emotions is necessary because it is possible for cultures to have identical antecedents and components of an emotion, and yet differ only in their frequency of experience (Flannery, 1999; Mesquita & Frijda, 1992). Because the present study used multiple measures, we were also able to examine whether the different measures converged on the same conclusions. This is an important question for the measurement of emotions within and between cultures, because the convergence and divergence of multiple measurement methods can help us understand the processes underlying cultural differences. For example, if Culture A scores higher than Culture B on a global measure of x, but there are no differences between A and B using an online measure of x, this would suggest that memory processes influence cultural differences in the global measures.

In addition, we explored the contribution of indigenous emotion terms to the measurement of emotion in two of our samples (Japan and India). The indigenous emotions address an important concern that often arises in culture and emotion research. Do indigenous emotion terms capture the emotional lives of non-Westerners in ways that the "standard" Western emotion terms do not? To answer this question, we used cluster analyses that included indigenous emotions to determine whether indigenous emotions form distinct clusters from the traditional clusters of pleasant and unpleasant affect that are often found in studies of Western emotions. We describe these indigenous emotions and the analyses in greater detail in the Method section.

Another objective was to move beyond the descriptive level and explore the influences on memory for emotion across cultures. This goal was guided by previous research showing that memory for emotion is a reconstructive process with systematic influences that can explain memory biases. One source that may guide memory for emotions is a person's self-concept. Diener, Larsen, and Emmons (1984), for instance, found that when asked to recall their emotions, individuals scoring high on trait measures of happiness overestimated the amount of positive emotion they had experienced, whereas unhappy individuals overestimated the amount of negative emotion they had experienced. Similarly, Feldman Barrett

(1997) found that neurotic individuals remembered more negative emotion, whereas extraverts remembered more positive emotion compared to their online reports. Other influences on memory have been identified, such as implicit theories (Ross, 1989), current appraisals (Levine, 1997), stereotypes (Robinson, Johnson, & Shields, 1998), and cultural theories (Oishi, 2002). However, in the present study, we chose to focus on the influence of self-concept across cultures.

Although past studies demonstrated that the self-concept influences memory for emotions, the present study extends this work by investigating whether this relation holds across cultures. To this end, we asked participants to record their emotions online and later asked them to recall their emotions from the online sampling period. We also included a global self-report measure of emotions that served as an approximation of the individual's emotional self-concept. If the self-concept contributes to emotional recall, we would expect there to be a sizable relation between the global measure and the recall measure, controlling for online experience.

The relation between online and recalled reports of emotion raises additional questions that have not been examined in previous research. For instance, is recalled frequency of emotion related to the online intensity of emotions?[1] Because intense emotions seem more memorable, we predicted that intensity would be associated with the recall of frequency of emotions. In addition, if some cultures value or attend to intense emotions more than others, emotion memory for individuals in those cultures may be more influenced by intense experiences.

Semantic Knowledge Use in the Recall of Large Time Frames

According to Robinson and Clore (2002a), individuals rely on different strategies for estimating their past emotional experience, depending on the frame of reference. In recalling short, discrete time frames such as momentary recall (e.g., "How happy were you in the past 30 minutes?"), individuals are able to draw on episodic knowledge. That is, they recall specific instances to inform their judgment of how happy they were. In contrast, when people recall longer, more abstract time frames (e.g., "How happy are you in general?" or "How happy were you in the past month?"), they abandon a retrieve-and-aggregate strategy, favoring instead the use of heuristic information or semantic knowledge (e.g., general beliefs about the self) to "fill in" where specific episodic memories are not accessible or are too difficult to retrieve or calculate (Robinson & Clore, 2002a).

In a series of reaction time studies, Robinson and Clore (2002b) found strong support for their model. Their studies capitalized on the fact that reliance on heuristic information is less effortful and allows for quicker responding in recall.

---

[1] We assessed emotion recall in terms of the frequency of various discrete emotions, but we could compute intensity and frequency from the online ratings. From the online reports, we defined frequency as how often people feel emotions, regardless of the strength; intensity was defined as the average intensity of emotion the people report on those occasions when they do feel them.

Importantly, if heuristic information is implicated in recalling longer, but not shorter, time frames, then speed of recall should reflect a curvilinear pattern, not a linear increase (e.g., greater time to recall longer time frames). Indeed, Robinson and Clore (2002b) found that participants were as quick at making recalled judgments about the past year as they were about the past hour. Robinson and Clore's (2002b) findings are important because they suggest that distortions in memory for emotion can be accounted for in systematic ways by identifying the heuristic sources of information (e.g., self-concept, implicit theories, or current appraisals) on which people rely.

Based on Robinson and Clore's (2002a, 2002b) theory and findings, in the present study we chose to treat retrospective reports of emotion that referenced the past month as a measure that approximates a person's self-concept. We do not claim that this measure captures all aspects of individuals' complex self-concepts. Indeed, one common conception of self-concept—self-esteem—is notably absent from our definition. However, we chose to focus on global beliefs about one's emotions as self-concept rather than self-esteem. We were interested in what influences memory for emotions; thus, it was appropriate and necessary to use a global measure that referenced emotions rather than global good feelings about the self. In fact, Christensen, Wood, and Feldman Barrett (2003) found that global self-esteem predicted memory for state self-esteem (controlling for online state self-esteem), but only in a few instances did global self-esteem predict memory for emotions. Our theoretical question was whether beliefs about one's own emotions influence the recall of them.

Predictions

Frequency of specific emotions across cultures. Past research has shown that Hispanic and European American cultures tend to emphasize good feelings, and individuals in these cultures are more likely to engage in self-enhancement, including the enhancement of positive feelings (Heine, Lehman, Markus, & Kitayama, 1999; Triandis, Marin, Lisansky, & Betancourt, 1984). This tendency is clearly reflected in the cultural norms for these groups. Hispanics and European Americans consider pleasant feelings to be much more desirable and appropriate than unpleasant emotions (e.g., Diener, Scollon, Oishi, Dzokoto, & Suh, 2000; Diener & Suh, 1999; M. Diener, Fujita, Kim-Prieto, & Diener, 2003). In contrast, Asian cultures emphasize pleasant and unpleasant feelings nearly equally (Diener & Suh, 1999).

An added dimension that has been studied by Kitayama and Markus and colleagues is social disengagement versus engagement. This dimension captures the degree to which an emotion affirms the identity of an individual as a distinct, separate entity (disengaged) versus the individual as part of a social group (engaged). Using retrospective reports, Kitayama et al. (2000) showed that Japanese indicated feeling more engaged emotions of positive and negative valence, whereas Americans reported feeling more engaged and disengaged positive emotions. Menon and Shweder (1994) have also noted the significance of the engagement dimension in India. For instance, Indians are more likely to view shame and happiness as more similar than shame and anger, because anger is an emotion that is divisive and separates people. On the other hand, North Americans consider anger and shame to be more similar because of valence.

In the present study, although we did not sample all of the same emotions as Kitayama et al. (2000), we were able to compare across cultures on two relevant emotions: pride and guilt. In many ways, pride serves as a prototypical disengaged, positive emotion because pride often results from accomplishing one's goals or affirming some internal attribute (e.g., "I am special"), which reinforces the separateness of the self from others (Kitayama, Markus, & Matsumoto, 1995).[2] In contrast, guilt serves as a prototypical engaged emotion because it strengthens the bonds between people (e.g., remorse leading to remedy leading to forgiveness); but guilt is also an unpleasant feeling. Accordingly, we expected Hispanics and European Americans to report more pride and less guilt than Asian Americans, Japanese, and Indians in global and retrospective reports because pride is pleasant and guilt is unpleasant. In fact, we expected European Americans and Hispanics to report overall higher levels of pleasant emotion and lower levels of unpleasant emotion (replicating previous studies). Because guilt is engaging and pride is disengaging, we expected Asian Americans, Japanese, and Indians to report more guilt and less pride. Given that this is the first study to our knowledge that uses online measures of specific emotions, predictions for online measures were more tentative. On one hand, Oishi (2002) found no cultural differences in online emotion between Asian Americans and European Americans, which might lead us to expect no cultural differences for the online measure. On the other hand, evidence from retrospective reports indicates clear differences in the frequency of experience of specific emotions, particularly pride and guilt, across cultures.

What influences memory? We hypothesized that self-concept would predict memory for emotions across cultures, even after controlling for online emotion. However, we did not have any theoretical formulations about how this process would vary by culture or specific emotion. We also predicted that intensity of emotions might be associated with the recall of frequency of emotions—especially for cultures that highly value one type of emotional experience over another. Because Hispanic and American cultural norms emphasize positive feelings, we predicted that intense pleasant experiences would be implicated in the recall of frequency of pleasant feelings for these groups, whereas intense negative experiences would not be implicated in recall of amount of unpleasant feelings. Because Asian cultures tend to equally value positive and negative (Diener & Suh, 1999), we predicted that either intensity information would have no relation to their recall of frequency, or intensity of pleasant and unpleasant feelings would equally predict memory.

---

[2] Of course it is possible for people to feel pride about others, but this is not the typical default sense of the word (see Kitayama et al., 2000).

Method

Participant Samples

We examined three cultural samples within the United States (European American, Asian American, and Hispanic) and two societies outside of the mainstream Western tradition (India and Japan). Through these five cultural groups, we hoped to have a diverse sample of subcultures within one Western nation, as well as two non-Western cultures. We studied college students so that each culture would be represented by individuals of approximately the same age, education, and relative income. Thus, these factors would not be confounded with culture. In addition, we included cultural groups that have largely been ignored in the culture and emotion literature. Latinos and Indians have received little attention (Biswas-Diener & Diener, 2001), despite the fact that India is the second largest nation in the world and is leading the world in population growth, and Latino Americans make up nearly 12% of the U.S. population and are on the verge of being the largest ethnic minority group in the United States.

A total of 416 college students participated in this study. Although small in comparison to some international surveys, our samples were quite respectable by the standards of experience sampling studies. Some participants did not have experience sampling data due to technical failures; others did not complete the memory measures. Analyses were computed on available data; therefore, different analyses reflect slightly different sample sizes. Participants volunteered and received $25 compensation, or the equivalent monetary incentive for Japanese and Indian students (not a direct exchange of US $25). Volunteers responded to advertisements for the study posted on or near campus. At the end of the study, participants were fully

Table 1 Participant samples

Culture	n	Female (%)	Age	
			M	*SD*
Japanese[a]	91	63	20.2	2.3
Indian[b]	160	64	21.4	2.6
Asian American[c]	33	67	20.6	1.9
Hispanic[d]	80	79	21.7	5.5
European American[c]	46	83	20.9	4.3
Total	416	68	21.1	3.5

[a] Recruited from International Christian University and Meisei University, both in Tokyo.
[b] From Utkal University in Bhubeneswar, a city in the state of Orissa, Indian Institute of Management, President's College, Jadavpur University, Indian Institute of Social Welfare and Business Management, Calcutta University-Raja Bazaar, St. Xavier's College, and Ramakrishna Mission at Nurendrapur, all in and around Calcutta.
[c] From the University of Illinois.
[d] From California State University at Fresno. Hispanic respondents were recruited only if they spoke Spanish at home.

debriefed. Table 1 describes the samples. Portions of the data that examined other questions are presented elsewhere (on cross-situational consistency across cultures, see Oishi, Diener, Scollon, & Biswas-Diener, 2004; on dialectical emotions, see Scollon, Diener, Oishi, & Biswas-Diener, 2005).

Measures

At the beginning of the study, participants completed global report measures concerning emotions, after which they began the week-long experience sampling portion of the study. At the end of the week, participants recalled their emotions from the experience sampling week. All materials were in English, except for those presented to Japanese respondents. Given India's diversity of languages and the fact that English is one of the country's official languages, translation of materials was not necessary for the Indian college students.[3]

Global measure. Before beginning the experience sampling portion of the study, participants indicated how much of the time they typically felt eight specific emotions (described later) during the past month on a scale ranging from 1 (*never*) to 7 (*always*). As Robinson and Clore (2002b) have shown, when participants are asked to reference a large time frame, they rely on heuristic information to respond to the question, rather than careful retrieval and aggregation of affective memories. Thus, this measure can be considered a general measure of affect that approximates a person's self-concept. Importantly, this measure bears no overlap in time with the experience sampling or recalled measures.

Experience sampling of the week. During their waking hours, participants carried a device that was preset to sound an alarm at random moments throughout a 2- to 3-hour interval 5 times a day for 7 days.[4] When signaled, participants completed mood ratings according to how they were feeling "right before the alarm sounded." We specified the time "right before the alarm" to remove any effects of the alarm itself. Although in most instances respondents could complete the mood form immediately after being signaled, if it were impossible to do so at the moment (e.g., during a test), participants were allowed to complete the form up to 30 minutes after the

---

[3] Kim-Prieto et al. (2004) tested the effect of language on emotional experience using emotion ratings from multiple sites in various countries. At some sites, participants responded in their native language, whereas at other sites, participants responded in English. Using hierarchical clustering, they found that samples did not cluster by language, but instead clustered according to geographical region. Both the Indian sample that completed English measures and the Indian sample that completed Bengali measures were closest in the clustering to each other and China. The Indian sample that used Hindi measures clustered with the United States and Australia—a finding better explained by exposure to Western culture (because that specific sample was drawn from a business school) rather than language, because Americans and Australians completed measures in English.
[4] Participants completed mood ratings directly on a personal digital assistant that also served as the signaling device, with the exception of participants in India who wore alarm watches as the signaling device and completed identical measures in paper-and-pencil form. Watch alarms were programmed to occur roughly once every 2–3 hours, 5 times a day. Participants in the Indian sample turned in their forms each day to guard against any late reporting.

alarm sounded. Participants were explicitly told not to complete the mood ratings beyond the half-hour time frame. The average response rate was 75%. Participants completed additional mood ratings when they first woke up and before going to bed each day. When signaled, participants recorded to what degree they were feeling the specific emotions on a scale ranging from 0 (*not at all*) to 6 (*with maximum intensity*).

Proportion or frequency of emotions. Ratings for each occasion were transformed into dichotomous variables indicating whether the emotion was currently being experienced (i.e., any nonzero response) or not (i.e., any zero response). We then computed the proportion of time each specific emotion was reported over the entire week. These values specifically reflect the amount of time various emotions were experienced and do not take into account the intensity of those emotions.

Intensity of emotions. We computed the (week-long) mean level of intensity for each of the eight emotions by summing a person's ratings on each emotion and dividing by the total number of occasions on which the emotion rating was nonzero. In other words, this score reflects the mean level of intensity for a particular emotion only when that emotion was felt (for a detailed discussion of the rationale for this procedure, see Diener, Larsen, Levine, & Emmons, 1985).

Retrospective measure. On the last day of the experience sampling week, participants recalled the percentage of time they experienced each of the specific emotions during the week in which they carried the signaling device. Responses could range from 0 to 100% of the time for each emotion. Instructions specified that the percentages did not need to sum to 100% because participants may have felt more than one emotion at the same time. Note that this is a measure of the proportion of time a person experienced specific emotions.

Choice of emotions. For each type of assessment (global, online frequency, online intensity, and recall), we sampled four positive emotions (pride, affection, joy, and happiness) and four negative emotions (irritation, guilt, sadness, and worry).[5] These emotions were selected to represent major forms of pleasant and unpleasant emotion (Diener, Smith, & Fujita, 1995) and served as a compromise between an exhaustive list of emotions and the quick, short list required by the experience sampling method (for a practical review of experience sampling methodology, see Kim-Prieto, Fujita, & Diener, 2004). Recognizing that we could not sample all the emotions, these eight emotion terms were selected because they are diverse and appear in many emotion systems such as Ortony, Clore, and Collins (1988); Shaver, Wu, and Schwartz (1992); Plutchik (1980); and Izard (1977). In addition, we avoided extreme emotions

---

[5] Proud, affectionate, joyful, happy, irritated, guilty, sad, and worried were translated into Japanese by Shigehiro Oishi, a native Japanese speaker who is familiar with Japanese translations of emotion words used in previous cross-cultural research (e.g., Kitayama et al., 2000; Suh, Diener, Oishi, & Triandis, 1998). Furthermore, Kengo Takeno, a Japanese Ph.D. student in psychology at International Christian University in Tokyo, checked the Japanese translations and made minor changes to ensure accuracy. The Japanese emotion terms were *hokori, aijo, ureshii, shiawase, iraira, zaiakukan, kanashii,* and *sinpai*, respectively.

such as "rage" and "elation" because they are infrequent, and we were interested in everyday common emotions.

One caveat to this selection of emotions is that these terms are established meaningful terms in Western theories of emotion (although Shaver et al. [1992] found these emotions in the Chinese emotion lexicon). Conceivably, the English emotion lexicons might not adequately represent the emotional lives of non-Western individuals. Therefore, we also performed hierarchical cluster analyses on the frequency of online emotions which included two pleasant indigenous emotions (*shitashimi* and *fureai*) and two unpleasant indigenous emotions (*oime* and *rettokan*) in the Japanese sample, and one pleasant (*sukhi*) and one unpleasant (*aviman*) indigenous emotion in the Indian sample, in addition to the previously mentioned eight emotions. The cluster analyses should reveal whether indigenous emotions form distinct clusters from the traditional clusters of pleasant and unpleasant affect commonly found in studies of Western emotion.

The indigenous emotions are unique in that they do not have English equivalents. Nevertheless, we will try to give the reader a general sense of what it means to feel these emotions, keeping in mind that there is no one-to-one translation of these emotions. For example, the Indian term *aviman* is best described as a feeling of prideful loving anger, and the term *sukhi* is similar to peace and happiness. A Japanese individual might use the term *fureai* when she feels a sense of connectedness to someone else. *Shitashimi* is used to describe a sense of familiarity. *Oime* refers to a feeling of indebtedness, and *rettokan* means to feel inferior. A noted similarity among these indigenous emotions is that they tend to implicate the person's social world. This is consistent with Mesquita's (2001) notion that in collectivist cultures, an emotion reflects the self in relation to others, whereas in individualist cultures, emotions refer to the self as a separate, bounded entity. Unfortunately, indigenous emotion ratings for Japanese and Indians were not available in the global and recall measures.

Results

Do Cultures Differ in Frequency of Specific Emotions?

A one-way multivariate analysis of variance (MANOVA) performed on the frequency of specific emotions revealed significant differences between cultures, Wilks's Lambda $= 0.50$, $F(32, 1, 381) = 8.98$, $p < 0.001$, $\eta^2 = 0.16$. Univariate tests revealed significant cultural differences for all emotions, $Fs(4, 381) > 3$, $ps < 0.02$.[6] Figure 1 shows the mean levels of frequency of specific emotions for each cultural group. Several interesting points are worth noting about this figure. First, there is considerably more cultural variability in the pleasant emotions than in

---

[6] In the cases where the assumption of homogeneity of variance was violated, a Kruskal–Wallis test yielded parallel results.

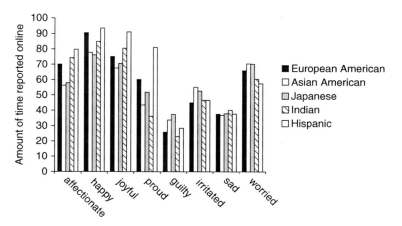

Fig. 1 Amount of specific emotions reported online by cultural group

unpleasant emotions, a finding that replicates Eid and Diener (2001). As expected, the largest difference between cultures was in reports of pride, $F(4, 381) = 25.07$, $p < 0.001$, $\eta^2 = 0.21$. Hispanic Americans felt the most pride ($M = 81.0\%$, $SD = 23.7$), and the three Asian cultures reported the lowest frequency of pride, with Indians reporting the least pride ($M = 36.1\%$, $SD = 32.5$). These findings are consistent with previous formulations about pride in Asian societies (M. Diener et al., 2003; Kitayama et al., 1995, 2000; Menon & Shweder, 1994)—that pride is not highly valued because it separates individuals from others. Interestingly, because Hispanic culture is also purportedly collectivistic (e.g., Triandis et al., 1984), collectivism alone cannot explain cultural differences in mean levels of pride. If it did, we would expect Hispanics to be very low in pride, but instead they are the highest.

Another notable feature of Fig. 1 is that cultural variability for sadness was virtually zero, as indicated by nearly identical means for the different groups but also $F(4, 381) = 0.18$, $p = 0.95$, $\eta^2 = 0.002$, whereas the cultures varied more in terms of guilt, $F(4, 381) = 4.64$, $p < 0.01$, $\eta^2 = 0.05$. Consistent with Kitayama et al. (1995, 2000), Japanese ($M = 37.4\%$, $SD = 28.2$) and Asian Americans ($M = 33.8\%$, $SD = 26.5$) reported more guilt than European Americans ($M = 26.0\%$, $SD = 25.0$) and Hispanics ($M = 28.4\%$, $SD = 27.3$). Unexpectedly, however, Indians reported the least amount of online guilt ($M = 23.0\%$, $SD = 24.8$).

In general, the ordering of the cultural groups remained relatively consistent across the specific emotions, with Hispanic and European Americans feeling the most pleasant and least unpleasant in online reports. The three Asian cultures were consistently lower in pleasant affect and higher in unpleasant affect, although their ordering varied slightly depending on the specific emotion. The pattern of cultural differences resonates with previous studies using global and retrospective reports (e.g., E. Diener, M. Diener, et al., 1995) and echoes the finding that European American and Hispanic cultures tend to place greater emphasis on good feelings (e.g., Diener et al., 2000; Heine et al., 1999; Kitayama et al., 2000; Triandis et al., 1984) and rate pleasant emotions as more desirable and appropriate than individuals in Asian societies (Diener & Suh, 1999; Eid & Diener, 2001).

As expected, cultural differences also emerged in global and recalled reports of pride, $F(4, 406) = 22.97$, $p < 0.001$, $\eta^2 = 0.19$, and $F(4, 373) = 21.72$, $p < 0.001$, $\eta^2 = 0.19$, respectively. Specifically, Hispanic ($M = 4.62$, $SD = 1.7$) and European Americans ($M = 3.69$, $SD = 1.3$) reported the highest levels of pride, whereas Indians ($M = 2.71$, $SD = 1.5$) reported the lowest pride in global measures. Hispanic and European Americans also recalled the most amount of pride ($Ms = 46.8$ and 27.0, $SDs = 32.0$ and 26.2, respectively), and Asian Americans recalled the least amount of pride ($M = 13.2$, $SD = 13.4$), followed by Indians ($M = 16.4$, $SD = 19.4$). Cultural differences emerged in global reports of guilt, $F(4, 406) = 8.80$, $p < 0.001$, $\eta^2 = 0.08$, with Japanese scoring the highest ($M = 3.04$, $SD = 1.5$), followed by Hispanics ($M = 2.48$, $SD = 1.2$) and Asian Americans ($M = 2.45$, $SD = 1.0$). European Americans scored lowest in global reports of guilt ($M = 2.09$, $SD = 0.78$). No significant group differences emerged for recall of guilt, $F(4, 374) = 2.09$, $p = 0.08$, $\eta^2 = 0.02$, although the Japanese again scored the highest ($M = 17.0$, $SD = 22.2$).

Do Indigenous Emotions Add to Conclusions About Average Emotional Well-Being?

To answer this question, we submitted dissimilarity matrices of emotion terms to a hierarchical cluster analysis using complete linkage.[7] As shown in Fig. 2 and 3, for the Japanese and Indians, two clusters of pleasantness and unpleasantness emerged at the highest level. Importantly, the indigenous emotions did not form separate clusters in either sample. Instead, the indigenous emotions simply clustered with the expected pleasant and unpleasant clusters. Interestingly, pride clustered with the negative emotions for Indians, and was closest to the indigenous emotion aviman. The proximity of pride to aviman makes sense, given the definition of aviman ("prideful loving anger"). For the Japanese, however, pride clustered with the positive emotions, although of all the positive emotions, pride was the closest to the negative emotions. For the Japanese sample, the pleasant cluster was bifurcated into happy-joyful versus shitashimi-fureai-affectionate-proud and the unpleasant cluster split into irritated-worried versus sad-rettokan-oime-guilt at the second highest level.

Examination of the amount of time Japanese and Indians reported feeling the indigenous emotions showed that these emotions were either uncommon or ex-

---

[7] To create a dissimilarity matrix, we first created a correlation matrix among the frequency of specific emotions (this number was 12 for the Japanese and 10 for the Indians). We then subtracted each element of the correlation matrix from unity ($1 - r$) to form a dissimilarity matrix of 12×12 for the Japanese sample and 10×10 for the Indian sample. All clustering was performed on these dissimilarity matrices.

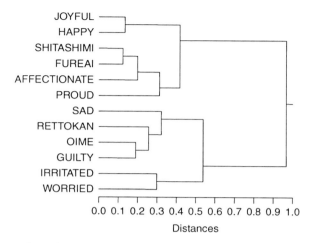

Fig. 2 Dendogram from cluster analysis of Japanese indigenous emotions with translated english emotions
Note. Clustering method was complete linkage. *Shitashimi, fureai, rettokan,* and *oime* are indigenous Japanese terms.

perienced to the same degree as the other eight emotions. For example, the most frequently experienced indigenous emotion among the Japanese was shitashimi ($M = 63\%$, $SD = 27.3$), whereas happiness was reported, on average, 76% of the time ($SD = 22.1$). The negative indigenous emotions (oime and rettokan) were even

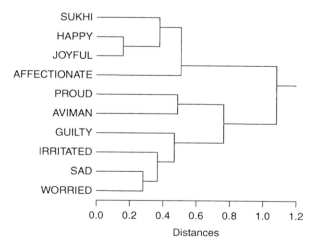

Fig. 3 Dendogram from cluster analysis of Indian indigenous emotions with translated english emotions
Note. Clustering method was complete linkage. *Aviman* and *sukhi* are indigenous Indian emotion terms.

less frequently reported ($Ms = 29\%$ and 31%, $SDs = 27.2$ and 29.3, respectively), whereas the least frequently reported nonindigenous negative emotion for the Japanese was sadness ($M = 38\%$, $SD = 30.4$). Indians reported feeling sukhi 78% ($SD = 27.4$) of the time, whereas they felt happy, on average, 85% of the time ($SD = 16.9$). Aviman was reported only 32% of the time ($SD = 32.4$). Although this was more frequent than guilt (23%, $SD = 24.8$), it was much less frequent than worry, which was reported 61% of the time ($SD = 27.4$). In sum, the present analyses indicate that these specific indigenous emotions are fairly well-represented by Western emotion words.

Cluster analyses were also conducted on the other three cultural groups. Again, the highest level of clusters divided pleasant and unpleasant emotions in each culture, suggesting that there is a tendency for individuals who experience one pleasant emotion to experience the other pleasant emotions as well, over time. Likewise, individuals who frequently felt one unpleasant emotion also felt the other unpleasant emotions. It is important to note that the general clustering of pleasant and unpleasant emotions together in all five cultural groups does not contradict the idea that people in different cultures might classify different emotions as desirable or undesirable (or positive or negative in the narrative sense). Our data do not speak to the perceived normative desirability of the emotions. Instead, our cluster analyses point to a general individual difference tendency such that some individuals are prone to a spectrum of pleasant emotions, and some individuals are predisposed to a variety of unpleasant emotions, and these two dispositions are separable across cultures.

Do Cultures Differ Across Different Types of Measures?[8]

Because the online frequency and recall scores were based on a 100-point scale whereas the other ratings were based on a 7-point scale, it was first necessary to standardize the measures so they would be in the same metric. We then performed a repeated measures MANOVA on the standardized emotion terms (with the four methods of assessment serving as the within-subjects factor). Table 2 shows the results of the MANOVAs, which were conducted separately for each emotion to aid in interpretation. Method $\times$ Culture interactions emerged for all emotions (indicating nonparallel profiles), but effect sizes for these interactions were miniscule—the

---

[8] We were unable to test for any gender by culture interaction effects due to instability in estimates with moderate sample sizes. However, for the samples that were somewhat larger, we conducted within-culture tests of gender effects. Japanese males and females did not differ on any of the measures. Among Indians, significant differences emerged between males and females, $F(1, 150) = 7.46$, $p < 0.01$, such that females ($M = 2.98$, $SD = 0.79$) reported greater intensity of online pleasant emotion than males ($M = 2.65$, $SD = 0.58$), and females reported greater intensity of online unpleasant emotion ($M = 2.35$, $SD = 0.79$) than males ($M = 2.10$, $SD = 0.62$). Marginally significant differences emerged for global and recalled unpleasant emotion that were in the direction of females reporting more unpleasant emotion. A marginally significant difference emerged for frequency of online unpleasant emotion, such that males reported feeling unpleasant a greater proportion of time than females.

Table 2 Multivariate tests and effect sizes

	Method	Culture	Method × Culture
Affectionate	$\Lambda = 1.0$, $F(3, 346) = 0.26$, $\eta^2 = 0.00$	$F(4, 348) = 7.47^{**}$, $\eta^2 = 0.08$	$\Lambda = 0.94$, $F(12, 916) = 1.96^{**}$, $\eta^2 = 0.02$
Happy	$\Lambda = 1.0$, $F(3, 351) = 0.32$, $\eta^2 = 0.00$	$F(4, 353) = 14.90^{**}$, $\eta^2 = 0.14$	$\Lambda = 0.91$, $F(12, 929) = 2.76^{**}$, $\eta^2 = 0.03$
Joyful	$\Lambda = 1.0$, $F(3, 348) = 0.45$, $\eta^2 = 0.00$	$F(4, 350) = 10.15^{**}$, $\eta^2 = 0.10$	$\Lambda = 0.84$, $F(12, 921) = 5.36^{**}$, $\eta^2 = 0.06$
Proud	$\Lambda = 0.97$, $F(3, 327) = 3.27^{**}$, $\eta^2 = 0.03$	$F(4, 329) = 29.86^{**}$, $\eta^2 = 0.27$	$\Lambda = 0.93$, $F(12, 865) = 2.13^{**}$, $\eta^2 = 0.03$
Guilty	$\Lambda = 0.96$, $F(3, 307) = 4.29$, $\eta^2 = 0.04$	$F(4, 309) = 4.52^{**}$, $\eta^2 = 0.06$	$\Lambda = 0.92$, $F(12, 813) = 2.19^{**}$, $\eta^2 = 0.03$
Irritated	$\Lambda = 0.98$, $F(3, 348) = 2.14$, $\eta^2 = 0.02$	$F(4, 350) = 2.62^{**}$, $\eta^2 = 0.03$	$\Lambda = 0.83$, $F(12, 921) = 5.64^{**}$, $\eta^2 = 0.06$
Sad	$\Lambda = 98$, $F(3, 335) = 2.01$, $\eta^2 = 0.02$	$F(4, 337) = 1.55^{**}$, $\eta^2 = 0.02$	$\Lambda = 0.92$, $F(12, 887) = 2.49^{**}$, $\eta^2 = 0.03$
Worried	$\Lambda = 0.99$, $F(3, 350) = 1.68$, $\eta^2 = 0.01$	$F(4, 352) = 5.75^{**}$, $\eta^2 = 0.06$	$\Lambda = 0.92$, $F(12, 926) = 2.49^{**}$, $\eta^2 = 0.03$

Note. Multivariate test statistic was Wilks's Lambda (Λ). The repeated measures factor was Method, and refers to the four types of measures (global self-concept, online frequency, online intensity, and recalled emotion).

$^{**} p < 0.05$.

largest effect size being 0.06 for joyful and irritated. No main effects for method emerged. However, a main effect for culture emerged for every emotion. Most of the effect sizes for culture were small, but in a few instances this culture effect was larger. Specifically, the effect sizes (η^2) for culture were 0.14 for happiness and 0.10 for joy, and the largest effect size for culture was for the emotion pride ($\eta^2 = 0.27$).

Aggregation of emotion terms. In the interest of brevity, we do not present all 160 means for each emotion for each method of assessment for each cultural group (i.e., $8 \times 4 \times 5$). Instead, we created composite scores from the specific emotions, and describe the convergence of measures based on these aggregated terms.

For all measures, happiness and joy were averaged to create a pleasant emotion (PE) score, and guilt, irritation, sadness, and worry formed an unpleasant emotion (UE) score. This choice of aggregation was based on several convergent lines of research. First, the dimensions of pleasantness and unpleasantness have been replicated in multiple studies using cross-cultural samples (e.g., Kim-Prieto et al., 2004; Scollon et al., 2005), even in studies that began with indigenous emotion terms rather than using translations of English emotion words (e.g., Shaver et al., 1992; Watson, Clark, & Tellegen, 1984). Second, Scollon et al. (2005) and Eid and Diener (2001) found less cultural variability in unpleasant emotions, and Scollon et al. (2005) found strong evidence that the negative emotions consistently covaried with one another, regardless of culture. Thus, we elected to aggregate the four unpleasant emotion terms (guilt, irritation, sadness, and worry). See Table 3 for reliability coefficients (Cronbach's alphas).

For pleasant feelings, however, there appears to be greater cultural variability. In particular, pride and affection are sometimes associated with negative emotions, especially in Asian cultures. First and most simply, the mean levels of pride reflect differences in cultural norms regarding this emotion, replicating other cross-cultural investigations of pride (e.g., Stipek, 1998). Second, Kim-Prieto et al. (2004) conducted a cluster analysis of emotion in 46 nations and found that at higher level clusters, pride clustered with the negative emotions in India and other non-Western societies. In the present study, pride also clustered with the unpleasant emotions for the Indian sample. Third, Scollon et al. (2005) found that pride loaded on the

Table 3 Internal consistency (alphas) for pleasant and unpleasant emotion indices by method and culture

Culture	Pleasant emotion[a]				Unpleasant emotion[b]			
	Global	Frequency Online	Intensity Online	Recall	Global	Frequency Online	Intensity Online	Recall
European American	0.84	0.74	0.93	0.77	0.71	0.85	0.70	0.68
Asian American	0.85	0.93	0.94	0.91	0.72	0.86	0.76	0.60
Japanese	0.67	0.92	0.90	0.89	0.54	0.86	0.79	0.77
Indian	0.84	0.92	0.92	0.87	0.61	0.86	0.82	0.80
Hispanic	0.86	0.91	0.93	0.89	0.66	0.86	0.80	0.75

[a] Computed from two items: happy and joyful.

[b] Computed from four items: guilty, irritated, sad, and worried.

pleasant and unpleasant factors for Asians, and affectionate showed some mild associations with unpleasant feelings as well. Similarly, Shaver et al. (1992) noted that among Chinese respondents, love did not emerge as a basic emotion with positive valence. Instead, for the Chinese, love-related concepts clustered near sadness and other negative emotions related to attachment and loss. Lutz's (1982) observation that the Ifaluk have an emotion called *fago* that represents a combination of love, sadness, pity, and compassion also converges with the notion that affection may not be purely positive in non-Western cultures. In contrast, happiness and joy are generally rated as desirable in most cultures (Sommers, 1984). Indeed, Shaver et al. (1992) found that happiness/joy emerged as a basic emotion concept in several cross-cultural samples, including the Chinese. Therefore, in aggregating across the pleasant emotions, we elected to use a 2-item PE scale (formed by averaging happiness and joy). See Table 3 for reliability coefficients (Cronbach's alphas).

Cultural differences emerged on all measures of PE and UE, Wilks's Lambda = 0.62, $F(32, 1,278) = 5.62$, $p < 0.001$. Univariate tests indicated cultural differences on all measures except frequency of online UE and recall of online UE (see Table 4 for means and univariate F tests). Table 4 also shows that, across the board, participants tended to underestimate their emotional experiences in their recall. Whereas the overall mean frequency of online PE was 81%, the overall mean recall of PE was 49%. Similarly, participants reported negative emotion on average 45% of the time online but recalled that figure as only 25%. These underestimates most likely reflect the difficult nature of the task. In particular, participants may have discounted or not remembered instances in which they felt an emotion only slightly.

As shown in Table 4, Hispanic American respondents scored highest on all measures of PE, followed by European Americans. The three Asian groups were consistently lower on the PE measures. In general, the reverse was true for negative emotion—Hispanic and European Americans were very low on these measures, whereas the other three groups (especially the Japanese) were consistently higher. This pattern is most striking in Fig. 4a and b, where we have standardized the measures to the same scale so that comparisons can be made. Although the standardized measures could obscure some of the details due to different variances, an interesting pattern still emerges—the rank ordering of the groups is maintained across the different measures. Again, the groups varied less on the unpleasant emotions (as indicated by less spread of the horizontal lines).

Does Self-Concept Predict Memory for Emotions Across Cultures?

For the memory analyses, we again chose to use indices of PE and UE for the three measures (global, online, and recall) for two reasons. First, we did not have predictions about how the use of self-concept information would vary by specific emotion or by culture. Second, the composite scores form more reliable measures and provide a useful framework for interpreting our findings.

Table 4 Means and standard deviations of measures by culture

Culture	Pleasant emotion (PE)				Unpleasant emotion (UE)			
	Global	Frequency Online	Intensity Online	Recall	Global	Frequency Online	Intensity Online	Recall
European American	4.39 (1.03)	82.87 (18.26)	2.79 (0.72)	49.12 (22.33)	3.18 (0.87)	43.63 (21.98)	1.90 (0.43)	25.90 (15.58)
Asian American	4.35 (1.18)	72.68 (25.15)	2.37 (0.60)	39.77 (23.24)	3.33 (0.81)	49.03 (23.03)	1.96 (0.43)	25.43 (14.54)
Japanese	4.72 (1.13)	73.36 (22.78)	2.53 (0.64)	43.98 (22.02)	3.83 (0.94)	49.57 (23.58)	2.17 (0.60)	28.25 (18.00)
Indian	4.34 (1.26)	82.71 (17.97)	2.87 (0.74)	49.86 (21.60)	2.92 (0.85)	42.57 (22.58)	2.26 (0.74)	24.52 (16.63)
Hispanic American	5.04 (1.16)	92.25 (8.85)	3.21 (0.64)	59.99 (24.64)	3.05 (0.88)	42.56 (23.31)	1.97 (0.55)	20.59 (16.64)
F	5.69*	11.89*	13.10*	7.06*	16.75*	1.77**	5.18*	2.28**
n	411	385	385	377	411	385	384	378

Note. $df = 4$. The theoretical range of scores is as follows: global (1–7), frequency online (0–100%), intensity online (0–6), recall (0–100%). Levene's test for homogeneity of variance was violated for self-concept PE, frequency of online PE, and intensity of online UE. For those cases, a Kruskal–Wallis test indicated significant differences among means for self-concept PE ($\chi^2_{(4)} = 20.40$), frequency of online PE ($\chi^2_{(4)} = 39.45$), and intensity of online UE ($\chi^2_{(4)} = 15.85$).
* $p < 0.01$; ** $p < 0.10$.

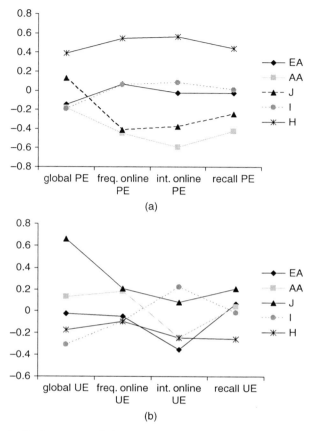

Fig. 4 (a) Standardized measures of pleasant emotion (PE) and (b) unpleasant emotion (UE) by cultural group
Note. EA = European American; AA = Asian American; J = Japanese; I = Indian; H = Hispanic; freq. = frequency; int. = intensity.

We should note, also, that the analyses concerning memory for emotions do not include indigenous emotions because we were interested in making comparisons across groups and across measures, and therefore needed assessments that would be isomorphic. We recognize that our findings must be interpreted with this limitation in mind.

To determine whether self-concept predicts memory for emotions after controlling for online reports, we regressed the retrospective measure of emotion (taken at the end of the experience sampling week) onto both the online and global measures. We performed this analysis separately for each cultural group, and for PE and UE separately, resulting in 10 separate equations. Table 5 presents the standardized betas for each regression. These betas indicate the unique contribution of online emotion and the unique contribution of global self-beliefs to the recall of that emotion,

Table 5 Standardized beta weights from regressions predicting recalled emotion from online and global measures

	Standardized betas			
	Pleasant emotion		Unpleasant emotion	
	Online	Global	Online	Global
European American	0.61***	0.27**	0.56***	0.31**
Asian American	0.37***	0.47***	0.41**	0.39**
Japanese	0.44***	0.26***	0.22**	0.34***
Indian	0.36***	0.33***	0.32***	0.37***
Hispanic	0.18*	0.52***	0.17*	0.52***

$^*p<0.10$; $^{**}p<0.05$; $^{***}p<0.01$.

while controlling for the other predictor. As one might expect, the significant and large betas for online emotion indicate that people are fairly accurate in their recall. Clearly, people have a relatively accurate sense of their own emotional lives—if they did not, this would be alarming. Nevertheless, the global measure still contributes to recall even after controlling for online emotion, as evidenced by the significant betas for the global measure for all groups. In some cases, global self-concept was as strong or stronger of a predictor of memory than online experiences. Furthermore, global self-concept influenced memory in all five cultural groups, and in predicting memory for pleasant and unpleasant emotion.

Interestingly, there were group differences in the degree to which global self-concept influenced memory for emotions. For instance, online emotion was less important to the recall of pleasant and unpleasant emotion in the Hispanic group, and online emotion was a relatively stronger predictor of recall for European Americans than was global self-concept. Although these differences are interesting, we do not have a strong theoretical explanation for why some cultures would use self-concept more. We elaborate on this issue in the discussion section.

Is Memory for Amount of Emotion Experienced (i.e., Frequency) Influenced by Intensity of Online Experience?

To test this question, we regressed recalled emotion onto intensity of online emotion and frequency of online emotion. Because the recall measure was, by definition, a frequency measure, we would expect there to be a high degree of association between the two. However, if intensity of online emotions is also implicated in people's memories, then we would expect intensity of emotion to add to the prediction of recall even after controlling for online frequency. Table 6 shows the standardized betas for frequency and intensity by cultural group for PE and UE separately. Interesting cultural differences emerged in the degree to which intensity predicted recalled reports of frequency. Notably, intensity of PE was related to recalled frequency of PE among European American, Indian, and Hispanic American participants, suggesting that their memory for the frequency of positive emotions was

Table 6 Standardized beta weights from regressions predicting recalled (frequency) of emotion from online frequency and online intensity measures

	Standardized betas			
	Pleasant emotion		Unpleasant emotion	
	Online frequency	Online intensity	Online frequency	Online intensity
European American	0.51**	0.43**	0.82**	0.13
Asian American	0.47**	0.39**	0.57**	0.19
Japanese	0.47**	0.15	0.58**	0.21*
Indian	0.34**	0.34**	0.50**	0.40**
Hispanic	0.09	0.45**	0.52**	0.00

$*p<0.05; **p<0.01.$

colored by the intensity of their positive emotions. Among Japanese respondents, intensity of PE did not contribute to recalled PE ($\beta = 0.15, t = 1.40, p = 0.17$), but intensity of UE predicted recalled UE ($\beta = 0.21, t = 2.34, p = 0.02$). Intensity of online UE also strongly predicted recalled UE for Indian participants ($\beta = 0.40, t = 6.28, p<0.001$). Interestingly, for the Hispanic American group, intensity of PE entirely predicted recall of PE ($\beta = 0.45, t = 3.75, p<0.001$), whereas frequency of PE did not predict recall. In addition, intensity of UE was completely unrelated to recalled UE ($\beta = 0.00, t = 0.02, p = 0.99$) for Hispanics.

These results suggest that retrospective reports of emotions are contaminated by intensity, but the degree to which intensity of online experience is implicated in memory varies by culture and the valence of emotion. Hispanic Americans tended to place greater weight on intense pleasant experiences but no weight at all on intense negative emotions. Indian respondents weighted intensity quite heavily, regardless of valence.

Discussion

Cultural Differences in Specific, Aggregated, and Indigenous Emotions

The present study found cultural differences in pleasant and unpleasant emotion on virtually all types of assessment (global, online, and recall). Consistent with cultural norms regarding the value of pleasant and unpleasant feelings, European Americans and Hispanics displayed the highest levels of pleasant emotion and the lowest levels of unpleasant emotion, whereas Asian Americans, Japanese, and Indians were generally lower in pleasant feelings and higher in unpleasant feelings. In general, the different measures resulted in similar conclusions in that the rank order of the groups was preserved across the methods of assessment.

With regard to specific emotions, we observed the greatest cultural differences in measures of pride. In particular, the three Asian groups, especially the Indians, reported considerably lower levels of pride than European Americans and Hispanics, regardless of type of assessment. Guilt also exhibited large cultural variability, with Japanese and Asian Americans generally reporting the most guilt. These cultural differences are consistent with theories suggesting that European American and Hispanic culture, in general, emphasize pleasant feelings regardless of whether such emotions are engaging or disengaging. In contrast, Asian cultures typically emphasize engaging emotions and de-emphasize disengaging emotions, regardless of the valence of such emotions (Kitayama et al., 1995, 2000). Thus, it is not surprising that European Americans and Hispanics would display the highest levels of pride (pleasant, disengaging) and relatively low levels of guilt (unpleasant, engaging), whereas Asians would display less pride and more guilt.

The present study also included indigenous emotions and found that these specific emotions did not form separate clusters from the dimensions of pleasant and unpleasant affect that are common to Western theories of emotion. It is possible that the sampling of other indigenous emotions might reveal a different structure, but this remains to be explored in future research. Naturally, the indigenous emotions do include specific content that is not included in other emotions. However, the indigenous emotions that were studied would not alter general conclusions at the level of pleasant and unpleasant affect.

Positive and negative emotions. Characterizing emotions simply as positive or negative has come under attack in recent years because these global assignments can oversimplify the emotion domain, especially in the cross-cultural context where what is considered positive or negative may vary. It should be noted that a positive cluster and a negative cluster emerged in each culture, although pride clustered with the negative emotions in India. Presumably, in each culture people view events as either desirable or undesirable, and react with either pleasant or unpleasant emotions, respectively. Pleasant and unpleasant emotions may be universal reactions to events that are seen as either beneficial or detrimental to a person's goals and well-being. At the same time, the present findings confirm earlier speculations that certain specific emotions such as pride may be considered pleasant or unpleasant in particular cultures. Thus, the positive and negative emotion categories may be useful in a cross-cultural context, but care must be taken as to which emotions belong to these categories.

Memory for Emotions Across Cultures

The present study demonstrated that global ratings of affect figure prominently in people's memories of their emotions. For pleasant and unpleasant emotion, there was a sizeable association between global and recalled affect across the cultural groups, even after controlling for online affect. These results are even more remarkable considering that the global and retrospective measures have no overlap in time frame. Furthermore, the present study was a conservative test of the influence of self-concept on memory because participants in experience sampling studies are more likely to attend to their own emotion states and thus should be unusually accurate in remembering them.

The present findings also underscore the need for experience sampling measures in cross-cultural studies of emotion, particularly in studies of clinical phenomena. Whereas cultures did not differ significantly in online reports of unpleasant emotion (particularly sadness), they differed in global reports of unpleasant emotion. Over-reliance on retrospective measures could indicate cultural differences that are not apparent in daily experience.

Although global affect serves as a source of information when recalling emotion, regardless of culture, interesting cultural differences emerged in the degree to which intensity predicted recall (of frequency). Hispanic Americans weighted intensity of pleasant emotion quite heavily, giving no weight at all to the intensity of unpleasant emotions. Indians placed relatively greater impact on intensity of pleasant emotion but equally weighted the frequency and intensity of unpleasant emotions. We speculate that the differential influence of intensity on emotion recall is one mechanism through which cultural and individual differences in subjective well-being reports might emerge, but clearly more research is needed. Unfortunately, emotion scales often ask respondents to report the amount of emotion experienced, without differentiating between frequency and intensity of emotions. In future research, it would also be informative to ask respondents to recall the intensity of their emotions.

Unexpected differences. An unexpected finding was that cultures differed in on-line reports of pleasant emotion. This finding was inconsistent with Oishi's (2002) study. However, in a study by Mesquita and Karasawa (2002), Japanese students rated everyday emotional events as less pleasant than American students. Nevertheless, because we did not have any theoretical predictions for online differences, this finding needs to be interpreted with caution. Furthermore, given the dearth of cross-cultural investigations of online emotions, we cannot make any definitive conclusions about online differences until the finding has been replicated. One possibility is that online differences are sample-specific; therefore, obtaining several diverse samples in each culture should be a goal for future research.

Conceptual overlap. Do global self-beliefs of emotion predict memory for emotions simply because the constructs are conceptually related? Global, online, and recalled assessments of emotion bear some conceptual overlap. After all, a person who was very happy during the experience sampling week probably typically feels happy and therefore has global beliefs about the self that include a lot of positive emotion. And naturally, people's memory and global self-beliefs are grounded in reality to some extent. However, the present study demonstrated that there are systematic biases in memory, and these biases can be accounted for by a person's global self-concept. Future research should try to separate these constructs through experimental mood manipulation to determine whether recall can still be predicted from global affect.

Identifying the processes of emotion recall. Based on Robinson and Clore's (2002a) theory, heuristic information may "fill in" when individuals lack concrete, episodic knowledge (see also Roediger & McDermott, 2000). However, another possibility is that strong norms for particular emotions in some cultures may also increase the use of heuristic information. The present data do not speak to the distinction between these two processes, although this question deserves some attention in future research. One way to examine this in future research is to have participants recall their emotions under different conditions of cognitive load or following cultural priming manipulations. If use of heuristics is driven by memory decay, we would expect a greater correspondence between the global self-beliefs and recall when recall takes place under cognitive load. If use of heuristic information is driven by cultural norms, then we might observe stronger associations between global self-beliefs and recall after priming cultural norms.

Choice of emotions. Our findings are limited to the extent that our grouping of emotions into the dimensions of pleasantness versus unpleasantness is a meaningful way of organizing the data. However, based on structural analyses of emotions (e.g., Kim-Prieto et al., 2004; Scollon et al., 2005; Watson et al., 1984), we believe there was sufficient justification to make the pleasantness-unpleasantness distinction in all five cultural groups. Furthermore, we took care to include in our PE and UE indices only those emotions that exhibited common structure across the five groups. Although alternative ways of organizing the data do exist, the current dimensions of pleasantness and unpleasantness, nevertheless, lend a useful framework for interpreting the present set of findings. In addition, our findings are limited to the extent that our selection of emotion terms was representative of the emotional lives of the different individuals from different cultural backgrounds in our study. It is possible that the inclusion of additional indigenous emotions terms would alter our findings. However, because our goal was to examine whether self-concept influences memory for emotions, we found it necessary to use the same emotion terms across cultures.

Sample characteristics. This study was a first effort to use multiple methods of assessment, including experience sampling, to study multiple cultural groups. However, some caveats about our samples are worth noting. First, we elected to treat the three within-U.S. groups separately, given past research on ethnic differences in emotion and well-being (e.g., Matsumoto, 1993; Okazaki, 1997, 2000) as well as strong ethnic differences in mean levels of emotions in the present study (see Fig. 1 and Table 4). One weakness was that ethnicity was also confounded by geographical differences, leaving open the possibility that group differences were due to geography rather than ethnicity per se. To our defense, however, Schkade and Kahneman (1998) did not find any differences in self-reported life satisfaction between Midwesterners and Californians. Furthermore, our own findings converge with the conclusions of these cultural groups based on global reports of emotion (e.g., E. Diener, M. Diener, et al., 1995). Second, males were somewhat underrepresented in all our samples. However, for all groups, there were more males than females, so any cultural differences that emerged are unlikely due to gender differences. Finally, we did not have even sample sizes for our five groups. These uneven sample sizes present a problem only for the multivariate hypothesis testing, and even so, a simple observation of the means for each culture on the specific emotions suggests clear differences. The uneven sample sizes do not present a problem for regression analyses or for cluster analyses because these analyses were conducted within each culture separately. In these analyses, the sample size only affects the stability of the coefficients and the dissimilarity matrices (on which the clustering was performed) in the same way that sample size influences the stability of a correlation coefficient.

General Conclusion

Despite the inevitable limitations of a single study, the present research is the first to assess emotional experiences in five cultures using the experience sampling method and sampling indigenous emotions. Several important conclusions emerged and point the way toward intriguing lines of inquiry for future research. First, pleasant and unpleasant emotions emerged in all five cultures, although pride grouped with the unpleasant emotions in India. Second, indigenous emotions in India and Japan clustered with Western emotions and did not form separate clusters. Third, the different methods gave some approximate ordering of the groups, but online methods (especially for negative emotion) showed smaller cultural differences than recall methods. The greatest cultural differences emerged in measures of pride. Fourth, there were interesting recall biases for emotions, suggesting that although global self-beliefs influenced recall in each of the cultures, different groups used different types of self-belief information in recalling emotion.

Acknowledgments We would like to thank Dr. Lawrence Hubert for his assistance with the cluster analyses. We would also like to thank Drs. Hideki Okabayashi of Meisei University and Kaoru Nishimura of International Christian University for their help in data collection in Japan. Portions of these data that examine the relation between pleasant and unpleasant affect (Scollon et al., 2005) and situational consistency across cultures (Oishi et al., 2004) are reported elsewhere. However, these articles are concerned with conceptually distinct issues from the one discussed in the present article; therefore, there is no conceptual overlap with the current article.

References

Biswas-Diener, R., & Diener, E. (2001). Making the best of a bad situation: Satisfaction in the slums of Calcutta. *Social Indicators Research, 55,* 329–352.

Christensen, T. C., Wood, J. V., & Feldman Barrett, L. (2003). Remembering everyday experience through the prism of self-esteem. *Personality and Social Psychology Bulletin, 29,* 51–62.

Diener, E., Diener, M., & Diener, C. (1995). Factors predicting the subjective well-being of nations. *Journal of Personality and Social Psychology, 69,* 851–864.

Diener, E., Larsen, R. J., & Emmons, R. A. (1984, August). *Bias in mood recall in happy and unhappy persons.* Paper presented at the 92nd annual meeting of the American Psychological Association, Toronto, Canada.

Diener, E., Larsen, R. J., Levine, S., & Emmons, R. A. (1985). Intensity and frequency: Dimensions underlying positive and negative affect. *Journal of Personality and Social Psychology, 48,* 1253–1265.

Diener, E., Scollon, C. K. N., Oishi, S., Dzokoto, V., & Suh, E. M. (2000). Positivity and the construction of life satisfaction judgments: Global happiness is not the sum of its parts. *Journal of Happiness Studies, 1,* 159–176.

Diener, E., Smith, H., & Fujita, F. (1995). The personality structure of affect. *Journal of Personality and Social Psychology, 69,* 130–141.

Diener, E., & Suh, E. M. (1999). National differences in subjective well-being. In D. Kahneman, E. Diener, & N. Schwarz (Eds.), *Well-being: The foundations of a hedonic psychology* (pp. 434–450). New York: Russell Sage Foundation.

Eid, M., & Diener, E. (2001). Norms for experiencing emotions in different cultures: Inter- and intranational differences. *Journal of Personality and Social Psychology, 81*, 869–885.

Feldman Barrett, L. (1997). The relationships among momentary emotion experiences, personality descriptions, and retrospective ratings of emotion. *Personality and Social Psychology Bulletin, 23*, 1100–1110.

Flannery, W. P. (1999). *The effect of culture on emotion: A critical review and proposed desiderata.* Unpublished manuscript, University of California, Berkeley.

Heine, S. J., Lehman, D. R., Markus, H. R., & Kitayama, S. (1999). Is there a universal need for positive self-regard? *Psychological Review, 106*, 766–794.

Izard, C. E. (1977). *Human emotions.* New York: Plenum.

Kahneman, D. (1999). Objective happiness. In D. Kahneman, E. Diener, & N. Schwarz (Eds.), *Well-being: The foundations of a hedonic psychology* (pp. 3–25). New York: Russell Sage Foundation.

Kim-Prieto, C., Fujita, F., & Diener, E. (2004). *Culture and structure of emotional experience.* Unpublished manuscript, University of Illinois, Urbana-Champaign.

Kitayama, S., Markus, H. R., & Kurokawa, M. (2000). Culture, emotion, and well-being: Good feelings in Japan and the United States. *Cognition and Emotion, 14*, 93–124.

Kitayama, S., Markus, H. R., & Matsumoto, H. (1995). Culture, self, and emotion: A cultural perspective on "self-conscious" emotions. In J. P. Tangney & K. W. Fischer (Eds.), *Self-conscious emotions: The psychology of shame, guilt, embarrassment, and pride* (pp. 439–464). New York: Guilford.

Levine, L. J. (1997). Reconstructing memory for emotions. *Journal of Experimental Psychology, 126*, 165–177.

Lutz, C. (1982). The domain of emotion words on Ifaluk. *American Ethnologist, 8*, 113–128.

Matsumoto, D. (1993). Ethnic differences in affect intensity, emotion judgments, display rule attitudes, and self-reported emotional expression in an American sample. *Motivation and Emotion, 17*, 107–123.

Menon, U., & Shweder, R. A. (1994). Kali's tongue: Cultural psychology and the power of shame in Orissa, India. In S. Kitayama & H. R. Markus (Eds.), *Emotion and culture: Empirical studies of mutual influence* (pp. 241–284). Washington, DC: American Psychological Association.

Mesquita, B. (2001). Emotions in collectivist and individualist contexts. *Journal of Personality and Social Psychology, 80*, 68–74.

Mesquita, B., & Frijda, N. H. (1992). Cultural variations in emotions: A review. *Psychological Bulletin, 112*, 179–204.

Mesquita, B., & Karasawa, M. (2002). Different emotional lives. *Cognition and Emotion, 16*, 127–141.

Oishi, S. (2002). Experiencing and remembering of well-being: A cross-cultural analysis. *Personality and Social Psychology Bulletin, 28*, 1398–1406.

Oishi, S., Diener, E., Scollon, C. N., & Biswas-Diener, R. (2004). Cross-situational consistency of affective experiences across cultures. *Journal of Personality and Social Psychology, 86*, 460–472.

Okazaki, S. (1997). Sources of ethnic differences between Asian American and White American college students on measures of depression and social anxiety. *Journal of Abnormal Psychology, 106*, 52–60.

Okazaki, S. (2000). Asian American and White American differences on affective distress symptoms: Do symptom reports differ across reporting methods? *Journal of Cross-Cultural Psychology, 31*, 603–625.

Ortony, A., Clore, G. L., & Collins, A. (1988). *The cognitive structure of emotions.* New York: Cambridge University Press.

Plutchik, R. (1980). *Emotion: A psychoevolutionary synthesis*. New York: Harper & Row.

Robinson, M. D., & Clore, G. L. (2002a). Belief and feeling: Evidence for an accessibility model of emotional self-report. *Psychological Bulletin, 128*, 934–960.

Robinson, M. D., & Clore, G. L. (2002b). Episodic and semantic knowledge in emotional self-report: Evidence for two judgment processes. *Journal of Personality and Social Psychology, 83*, 198–215.

Robinson, M. D., Johnson, J. T., & Shields, S. A. (1998). The gender heuristic and the database: Factors affecting the perception of gender-related differences in the experience and display of emotions. *Basic and Applied Social Psychology, 20*, 206–219.

Roediger, H. L., III., & McDermott, K. B. (2000). Tricks of memory. *Current Directions in Psychological Science, 9*, 123–127.

Ross, M. (1989). Relation of implicit theories to the construction of personal histories. *Psychological Review, 96*, 341–357.

Schkade, D. A., & Kahneman, D. (1998). Does living in California make people happy? A focusing illusion in judgments of life satisfaction. *Psychological Science, 9*, 340–346.

Scollon, C. N., Diener, E., Oishi, S., & Biswas-Diener, R. (2005). An experience sampling and cross-cultural investigation of the relation between pleasant and unpleasant affect. *Cognition and Emotion, 19*, 27–52.

Shaver, P. R., Wu, S., & Schwartz, J. C. (1992). Cross-cultural similarities and differences in emotion and its representation. In M. S. Clark (Ed.), *Emotion: Review of personality and social psychology* (pp. 175–212). Newbury Park, CA: Sage.

Sommers, S. (1984). Adults evaluating their emotions: A cross-cultural perspective. In C. Z. Malatesta & C. Izard (Eds.), *Emotions in adult development* (pp. 319–338). Beverley Hills, CA: Sage.

Stipek, D. (1998). Differences between Americans and Chinese in circumstances evoking pride, shame, and guilt. *Journal of Cross-Cultural Psychology, 29*, 616–629.

Suh, E., Diener, E., Oishi, S., & Triandis, H. C. (1998). The shifting basis of life satisfaction judgments across cultures: Emotions versus norms. *Journal of Personality and Social Psychology, 74*, 482–493.

Triandis, H. C., Marin, G., Lisansky, J., & Betancourt, H. (1984). Simpatia as cultural script of Hispanics. *Journal of Personality and Social Psychology, 47*, 1364–1375.

Watson, D., Clark, L. A., & Tellegen, A. (1984). Cross-cultural convergence in the structure of mood: A Japanese replication and a comparison with U.S. findings. *Journal of Personality and Social Psychology, 47*, 127–144.

Positivity and the Construction of Life Satisfaction Judgments: Global Happiness is Not the Sum of its Parts

Ed Diener, Christie Napa Scollon, Shigehiro Oishi, Vivian Dzokoto and Eunkook M. Suh

Abstract The present study investigated how reports of satisfaction with specific versus global domains can be used to assess a disposition towards positivity in subjective well-being reports. College students from 41 societies ($N = 7167$) completed measures of life satisfaction and ratings of global and specific aspects of their lives. For example, participants rated satisfaction with their education (global) and satisfaction with their professors, textbooks, and lectures (specific). It was hypothesized that global measures would more strongly reflect individual differences in dispositional positivity, that is, a propensity to evaluate aspects of life in general as good. At both the individual and national levels, positivity predicted life satisfaction beyond objective measures. Also, positivity was associated with norms about ideal life satisfaction such that countries and individuals who highly valued positive emotions were more likely to display positivity. The difference between more global versus more concrete measures of satisfaction can be used as an indirect and subtle measure of positivity.

Previous studies examining subjective well-being (SWB) at the national level showed notable differences among countries. Thus far, differences in living conditions, income, and cultural values have been offered as explanations for these nation differences in happiness. However, such variables have not been able to consistently account for why some countries are not as happy as national economic indicators or cultural variables would predict—and likewise, why other countries are happier than we might expect. For instance, despite their finding that the wealth of nations is a strong predictor of SWB, E. Diener, M. Diener, and C. Diener (1995) found that Japan was considerably less happy than its economic prosperity would predict. And, although Colombia ranked among the poorest of countries, and has high levels of violence, it was the 8th happiest of 55 nations in that study. Similarly, other Pacific Rim nations besides Japan have also been found to score unexpectedly

E. Diener (✉)

Department of Psychology, University of Illinois, Champaign, IL 61820, USA
e-mail: ediener@uiuc.edu

E. Diener (ed.), *Culture and Well-Being: The Collected Works of Ed Diener*, Social
Indicators Research Series 38, DOI 10.1007/978-90-481-2352-0_11,
© Springer Science+Business Media B.V. 2009

low on SWB, while other Latin nations score higher than expected based on economic conditions (E. Diener, M. Diener, et al., 1995; Veenhoven, 1993). Attempts to understand this apparent inconsistency have turned toward cultural explanations of SWB. In particular, individualism–collectivism (I–C; Hofstede, 1980; Triandis, 1989), also referred to as independence-interdependence (Markus & Kitayama, 1991), was suggested as one possible influence on SWB. And yet, even though individualism correlates positively with SWB measures, the I–C dimension does not fully account for Japan's low levels of SWB and Colombia's high levels of SWB because the two countries are nearly equal in collectivism (E. Diener, M. Diener, et al., 1995).

Thus, the question remains of what accounts for the relatively unhappy Japanese and the relatively happy Colombians? Are differences in SWB across nations embedded in culture in the differing ways in which people respond to the question of life satisfaction? We propose that a positive disposition, influenced by cultural norms and practices, can explain why some nations are higher in SWB than we might expect based on wealth. The present study sought to explore this hypothesis in two ways. First, we analyzed how a positivity set, or propensity to make positive evaluations in general, might influence responses across cultures. Secondly, we examined how dispositional positivity relates to cultural norms.

A Propensity View of SWB

Kozma, Stone, and Stones (2000) found that the best explanation for the stability in SWB is a "propensity model." According to this formulation, there is a dispositional component to SWB that operates much like a trait and accounts for the stability in SWB despite environmental change. In support of their propensity model, Kozma et al. found that the best predictor of SWB—an even better predictor than environmental factors, personality variables, and satisfaction with important life domains—was past SWB. Furthermore, environmental and personality variables could not fully explain the stability in SWB. In other words, the propensity component of SWB may be related to but not entirely explained by personality.

Although Kozma et al. (2000) provide support for a propensity or disposition component to SWB, they did not examine how cultural variables may influence the level of positivity. Thus, a major aim of the present study was to examine how individual differences in positivity may be driven by cultural norms that determine the degree to which happiness is valued and considered desirable. If level of positivity is influenced by cultural factors, this might explain some of the national differences in SWB. Thus, in attempting to resolve the Japan–Colombia paradox, we explain Latin American countries' high levels of SWB as a propensity to view life experiences in a rosy light because they value positive affect and a positive view of life. By the same token, Japan's relatively low SWB suggests a relative absence of the propensity to evaluate aspects of life positively.

In order to examine how dispositional positivity may influence constructions of life satisfaction judgments, we first had to consider how to measure positivity. In what ways would individuals who have a propensity towards the positive display such evaluative tendencies? And more importantly, how could we separate positivity from objective conditions in evaluations? These questions led us to examine more closely how individuals construct different types of evaluations in general—in particular, the differing ways in which individuals form global and specific judgments.

Global Versus Specific Judgments

Most of the research on life satisfaction has relied on brief, global self-report instruments. Because SWB is by definition *subjective*, self-reports are desirable in that they emphasize subjective experience rather than relying on "experts" to judge another's happiness. These measures often ask about a person's lifetime, or large periods of time such as the last year, and they tend to focus on broad domains such as one's life, job, or marriage. For example, respondents may be asked to evaluate statements such as "In most ways my life is close to my ideal" (Satisfaction With Life Scale; Diener, Emmons, Larsen, & Griffin, 1985), or they may be asked to respond to the question "How do you feel about your life as a whole?" on a scale ranging from "Delighted" to "Terrible" (Andrews & Withey, 1976). Asking participants to rate such broad categories as one's "life as a whole," or one's job as a whole, raises a number of issues. Schwarz and Strack (1991) noted that such questions may, in fact, "request something impossible from the respondent" (p. 29). Asking people to evaluate their happiness invites a host of potential heuristic strategies because individuals do not carry out careful calculations of summing weighted positive and negative experiences to arrive at a general happiness value. One would expect such computations to be time consuming, and the average person is able to provide an evaluation of his or her life in an astonishingly short amount of time—usually less than a minute (Schwarz & Strack, 1991). Recently it has been suggested that when asked to evaluate their life satisfaction, people rely on heuristic strategies, current affect, and other information that is readily available (Strack, Martin, & Schwarz, 1988; Schwartz & Clore, 1983). When primed with certain information, people may use that information (or perhaps weight it more heavily) in judgments about their overall happiness.

In short, asking people to generate a composite judgment about their lives is a complex task that may not reflect a systematic, bottom–up computational assessment (Schwarz & Strack, 1991, 1999). Until now, most researchers considered this to be an artifact and shortcoming of global assessment measures. However, we suggest that *because* global evaluations may reflect dispositional tendencies, such measures can provide valuable information about the nature of SWB. It is important to note that dispositional tendencies are likely to have their greatest influence on global judgments, and this tendency is maximized for life satisfaction measures. Because global evaluations are often vague, they allow greater freedom for individuals to project their norms, view of life, and self-beliefs onto the assessment item. When asked to evaluate specific or more concrete domains, however, individuals are more constrained by how they feel and think about the actual domains, inherently leaving less room for possible top–down influences. Although a positive disposition might influence one's reactions to concrete and specific aspects of life, in the case of broader domains this disposition can influence not only actual experience, but also one's memory and judgment of specific aspects as well. Thus, a positive disposition is likely to have stronger effects on global reports.

To some extent the two types of measures, global/abstract and specific/concrete, may reflect different types of SWB—global measures may be more reflective of a person's disposition while specific measures may reflect actual experiences. Thus, we would expect the two measures to yield different conclusions about the SWB of a nation or an individual. With this in mind, we may be able to capitalize on the different evaluations people make at the distinct levels of judgment. In fact, disparities between the two types of evaluations would suggest that overall happiness is not the sum of its parts. Furthermore, although global measures may be less tied to actual experience, knowing which individuals and societies possess a propensity to respond to global measures in a positive way may provide us with valuable information about the nature of SWB.

In the following study, we suggest one way of capturing the positivity disposition: by assessing the degree to which individuals evaluate global domains more positively than specific domains. To the degree that individuals weight specific aspects of their lives to arrive at global judgments, we would expect the mean evaluation of specific domains to equal the evaluation of the broader domain. However, for individuals who might be likely to display positivity, global judgments should reflect inflation over the specific judgments. We elected to index positivity by comparison between satisfaction with various levels of abstraction for several reasons. First, this method does not rely directly on the use of numbers (because it is the difference between two sets of numbers), and therefore is not contaminated by the artifact of preference for high or low measures that might contaminate other measures. Second, our index is indirect or implicit—relying on a calculation we make rather than on direct self-report—and therefore should minimize self-presentation artifacts. Finally, our indirect measure of positivity is not a direct report of self-concept, and therefore should not be influence by artificial response tendencies that might also influence reports of SWB.

Overview and Predictions

In summary, the present study sought to explore how life satisfaction is constructed, with the hypothesis that part of the construction relies more heavily on positivity in some nations than in other nations. Rather than dismissing differences in responding style as artifacts of global measures of life satisfaction, we suggest that these differences offer valuable insight into how satisfaction judgments are formed. Our three hypotheses are:

Hypothesis 1: Individuals and nations will differ in positivity as measured by the degree to which they evaluate global life aspects more positively than specific aspects.

Hypothesis 2: Positivity will predict overall life satisfaction at both the individual and national level beyond objective measures such as income.

Hypothesis 3: Positivity will correlate with how much people at both the individual and national levels believe it is desirable to feel satisfied (i.e., ideal life satisfaction).

Method

Sample

Participants included 7,167 college students (2,780 males, 4,301 females, and 86 not reporting gender) from 41 societies sampled as part of the International College Student Data (ICSD), collected in collaboration with international colleagues during 1995–1996. The ICSD project was undertaken in an effort to understand various issues relating to societal and cultural differences in subjective well-being. Eighty-five percent of the respondents were 18–25 years old. The 41 societies and their respective sample sizes are summarized in Table 1.

Measures

In many nations our respondents were fluent in English and responded to the English version of our survey, but in some countries the questions were presented in the native language (e.g., Egypt). In the cases where translation was necessary, questionnaires were translated from English to native languages by bilingual collaborators who were all professional psychologists associated with major universities in each country. Shao (1993) reported a high correspondence between the translated versions and the English version for the four languages in which systematic back-translation was conducted.

Life Satisfaction

Life satisfaction was assessed by the Satisfaction With Life Scale (SWLS; Diener, Suh, Smith, Shao, 1985). The SWLS is a five-item measure that asks respondents to rate their global life satisfaction from their subjective perspective. Sample items include"I am satisfied with my life" and "The conditions of my life are excellent." The response ranges from 1 (strongly disagree) to 7 (strongly agree) and are summed to yield a possible total score ranging from 5 to 35. The SWLS possesses adequate psychometric properties (see Pavot & Diener, 1993) and has demonstrated its validity among Korean (Suh, 1994), mainland Chinese (Shao, 1993), and Russian

Table 1 Means for satisfaction with life and positivity by nation

Nation	N	SWLS (5–35)	Positivity	Ideal SWLS
Puerto Rico	87	25.26	0.48	30.70
Colombia	99	26.40	0.39	31.02
Spain	323	22.37	0.30	31.02
Taiwan	532	20.12	0.25	29.18
Indonesia	90	21.89	0.23	26.44
Peru	129	23.31	0.23	28.98
Portugal	139	22.98	0.22	29.53
Slovenia	50	24.42	0.20	28.80
USA	442	23.64	0.20	28.92
Argentina	90	22.44	0.19	27.72
Ghana	118	20.12	0.17	25.63
Bahrain	124	19.85	0.15	23.64
Thailand	92	23.62	0.13	24.56
Denmark	88	25.00	0.11	29.12
S. Africa	370	20.97	0.11	28.44
Italy	288	21.52	0.10	29.38
Australia	289	23.05	0.09	31.14
Kuwait	252	22.57	0.09	26.08
Germany	107	23.27	0.06	29.07
Singapore	131	22.40	0.06	28.65
Zimbabwe	109	18.05	0.06	23.91
Nigeria	243	21.42	0.05	25.56
Guam	183	21.40	0.03	26.31
Austria	164	24.28	0.01	29.73
Nepal	98	20.93	0.00	23.77
Estonia	117	20.91	−0.01	27.94
India	93	22.12	−0.03	25.73
Brazil	112	21.61	−0.04	29.07
Greece	129	20.73	−0.06	29.09
Hungary	74	22.54	−0.13	29.85
Tanzania	134	20.88	−0.13	22.09
Norway	99	25.24	−0.14	30.54
Finland	91	23.46	−0.15	29.62
Hong Kong	142	19.31	−0.25	25.38
Pakistan	153	22.83	−0.25	27.36
Egypt	119	22.01	−0.28	30.65
Turkey	100	18.87	−0.34	26.44
Japan	200	20.20	−0.42	25.75
China	544	16.43	−0.43	19.80
Korea	277	18.72	−0.44	25.01
Lithuania	99	18.71	−0.44	27.68

Nations are ordered by their score on measures of positivity. SWLS = Satisfaction With Life Scale.

(Balatsky & Diener, 1993) samples. The overall alpha for the SWLS (N = 7014) was 0.81, and the mean alpha coefficient across the 41 nations was 0.78; more than half of the nations had alphas greater than 0.80.

Life Satisfaction Norms

In addition to having participants rate their own life satisfaction using the SWLS, we also asked participants rate the ideal level of SWLS—how they thought the ideal person would complete such items.

Positivity Disposition

In order to examine the positivity disposition that may be inherent in rating broad versus specific domains, we examined the following ratings: (1) Satisfaction with one's education (broad) versus satisfaction with one's professors, textbooks, and lectures (specific). The latter three ratings were averaged to form the specific measure of satisfaction with education. (2) Satisfaction with one's recreation (broad) versus satisfaction with sports and television (specific). Again, the two specific ratings were averaged. (3) Satisfaction with oneself (broad) versus satisfaction with one's grades and health (specific aspects of the self). The narrow subdomains were selected because they appeared to be variables that would be relevant to students' satisfaction with the global domains in all the societies we sampled. A composite broad satisfaction value was computed at the individual level by averaging the three broad ratings, and a specific satisfaction value was computed by averaging the mean of the three specific ratings. Given adequate sampling of domains, the broad and specific domains ought to be isomorphic, and therefore satisfaction at the two levels ought to be identical unless there are dispositions that influence one level that do not influence the other level. The major SWB dependent variable was the Satisfaction With Life Scale (Diener et al., 1985).

Results

The first column of Table 1 summarizes the life satisfaction means for each society. The mean satisfaction score for the 41 societies was 21.85 (SD = 2.13). China was the least satisfied, while Colombia reported the greatest levels of life satisfaction. Consistent with previous studies (E. Diener, M. Diener, et al., 1995; Veenhoven, 1993), the mean SWLS score for Japan was lower than we might expect based on economic development. Additionally, other studies have also demonstrated that China and other Asian societies tend to report relatively low satisfaction (E. Diener, M. Diener, et al., 1995; Diener, Suh, Smith, & Shao, 1995).

Overview of Analyses

We first analyzed the data at the individual level and later at the national level. At the individual level, all independent and dependent measures were standardized within countries in order to control for nation differences. The resulting scores rely on a person's relative standing within nations. In contrast, the nation-level analyses are based on analyzing means of countries. Thus, the two levels of analyses are independent of each other.

Analyses at the Individual Level

Table 2 summarizes the zero-order correlations between SWLS scores, global domain satisfaction scores, and specific domain satisfaction scores. Correlations above the diagonal represent analyses at the individual level. Correlations on the diagonal that are not in parentheses indicate the reliability coefficients for each measure at the individual level. As shown, the global score was a significantly better zero-order predictor of life satisfaction than the specific score, $t = 11.06$, $p < 0.001$ (J. Cohen & P. Cohen, 1983; Steiger, 1980). This relation is particularly robust considering the reliability for the specific score was greater than the reliability for the global score. Furthermore (not shown), positivity (the residual of global domains mediated by the specific domains) significantly correlated with the standardized SWLS scores, $r_{(6974)} = 0.32$, $p < 0.001$.

Our next set of analyses involved computing a "positivity score" for each participant by regressing the global score onto the specific score. The resulting standardized regression residual was then used as a measure of positivity for each individual (after Kurman & Sriram, 1997). To simplify a bit, this residual score captured the degree to which people were more likely to judge broader and vaguer categories as better (i.e., more positive). For the positivity score, positive values indicated that the person judged global categories more positively than specific categories, and negative values indicated the opposite. We entered income and the residual positivity score simultaneously into a regression equation predicting life satisfaction (SWLS). The top portion of Table 3 summarizes the results of the regression analyses at the individual level. Although both income and positivity significantly predicted life satisfaction, the beta for the residual positivity score was much stronger than

Table 2 Zero-order correlations between global and specific scores and life satisfaction

	Global	Specific	SWLS
Global	**0.61 (0.72)**	0.70	0.49
Specific	0.79	**0.67 (0.79)**	0.38
SWLS	0.72	0.56	**0.81 (0.78)**

Correlation above the diagonal are for analyses at the individual level. Correlations below the diagonal are for analyses at the nation level—calculated from the nation's mean level of scores on each measure. The diagonal shows the reliability coefficient (alphas in parentheses represent reliability calculated at the national level). Sample sizes at the individual level range from $N = 6976$ to $N = 7124$ due to missing data. At the national level, all correlations reflect an N of 41. All correlations are significant at $p < 0.001$ level.

Table 3 Regression analyses predicting life satisfaction from income and positivity

Variable	Standardized coefficient	Standard error	Total R^2
Individual level			
Income	0.11**	0.01	0.11
Positivity	0.31**	0.01	
National level			
Income	0.38*	0.17	0.34
Positivity	0.36*	1.30	

* $p < 0.05$; ** $p < 0.001$.

that for income, suggesting that our measure of positivity captures an aspect of life satisfaction beyond objective measures.

Analyses at the Nation Level

The right two columns of Table 1 summarize the nation aggregated data, from the society scoring the highest in mean positivity disposition (Puerto Rico, +0.48) to the society scoring the lowest in mean positivity disposition (Lithuania and Korea tied, −0.44). The United States tied with Slovenia for the 8th highest score in positivity, with a residual score of 0.20. The United States' standing among our 41 nations is consistent with Matlin and Stang's (1978) research on the "Pollyanna Principle," which showed that Americans preferred the positive over the negative in several cases—in choosing between positive and negative words, memories, faces, and reporting of news. Thus, it is not surprising that most Americans also rate their lives as happy (E. Diener & C. Diener, 1996). Notably, both Japan and China were among the lowest in positivity, with residual scores of −0.42 and −0.43, respectively. Meanwhile, Colombia, the nation with the highest SWLS score in our sample, had the second highest score for positivity (+0.39).

The correlations below the diagonal presented in Table 2 summarize the zero-order correlations between mean SWLS, global domain satisfaction, and specific domain satisfaction scores at the nation level. Correlations on the diagonal that are in parentheses indicate the reliability coefficients for each measure at the national level. Although global and specific scores were highly correlated between nations, the mean global score correlated more highly with life satisfaction than the specific scores. Furthermore, the residual positivity scores (not shown) correlated as strongly with life satisfaction as the specific scores themselves ($r_{(39)} = 0.57$, $p < 0.001$), thus verifying the importance of positivity to life satisfaction judgments.

Regression analyses also supported the strength of our measure of positivity as a better predictor of life satisfaction among nations than objective measures, as shown in the bottom portion of Table 3. When per capita national wealth and the average positivity score were simultaneously entered into a regression equation predicting national levels of life satisfaction (mean SWLS score), positivity was as good a predictor as national wealth.

Top–Down Versus Bottom–Up Theories

The residual positivity score can also be compared to satisfaction with important life domains as a test of top–down versus bottom–up theories. After all, if global measures of satisfaction are simply the sum of happiness across narrower domains, it follows that satisfaction with the most important domains should strongly predict overall life satisfaction. Returning to analyses at the individual level, we examined five important life domains that did not include the three global domains that we have already mentioned. These five important domains were health, finances, friends, family, and religion. Results of the regression analyses at the individual level are summarized in the top half of Table 4. At the individual level, the residual positivity scores predicted overall life satisfaction beyond the important domains scores. Thus, overall life satisfaction appears to be more than a cognitive computation or summing up of satisfaction in the important areas of one's life. Our measure of positivity added substantially to the prediction of life satisfaction. Interestingly, similar analyses at the nation level (shown in the bottom half of Table 4) revealed that the important domains did not emerge as a significant predictor of overall life satisfaction, but the residual positivity score significantly predicted SWLS scores. The robust findings at the nation level suggest that mean levels of national well-being are especially influenced by the positivity tendency. Alternatively, satisfaction with important domains may demonstrate low predictive power at the national level because people's satisfaction with these domains depends largely on their relative standing within their nation.

Bottom–up versus top–down processes can also be tested by examining the predictive power of objective variables such as income on financial satisfaction compared with the predictive power of our measure of positivity. If bottom–up processes are at work, an individual's satisfaction level should be a function of objective life events (Diener, 1984). In a regression equation predicting financial satisfaction from objective income (a bottom–up variable) and the residual positivity score (a dispositional variable), both income and positivity significantly predicted financial satisfaction at the individual level (as shown in the top portion of Table 5). Similarly, at the national level, we predicted average financial satisfaction from the

Table 4 Regression analyses predicting life satisfaction from important domains and positivity

Variable	Standardized coefficient	Standard error	Total R^2
Individual level analyses			
Important domains	0.42**	0.01	0.27
Positivity	0.23**	0.01	
National level analyses			
Important domains	0.24	1.37	0.36
Positivity	0.43*	1.50	

Satisfaction with important domains includes one's health, finances, friends, family, and religion.
* $p < 0.02$; ** $p < 0.001$.

Table 5 Regression analyses predicting financial satisfaction from income and positivity

Variable	Standardized coefficient	Standard error	Total R^2
Individual level analyses			
Income	0.18**	0.01	0.06
Positivity	0.15**	0.01	
National level analyses			
Income	0.05	0.04	0.13
Positivity	0.34*	0.27	

* $p < 0.05$; ** $p < 0.001$.

average income and the average positivity score by nation. The bottom portion of Table 5 summarizes the results at the national level. A similar pattern emerged in that the beta for positivity was greater than the beta for objective income. However, positivity only approached significance here, while objective income was not significant.

Cultural Norms and Dispositional Positivity

In order to examine the cultural influences on dispositional positivity we correlated our measure of positivity with the ideal SWLS scores—that is, how satisfied participants thought people should ideally be. The far right column of Table 1 summarizes the mean ideal SWLS scores for each nation. At both the individual and national level, positivity significantly correlated with ideal life satisfaction ($r_{(6845)} = 0.09$, $p < 0.001$ and $r_{(39)} = 0.39$, $p < 0.02$, respectively) suggesting that norms for satisfaction might have some influence on positivity.

Discussion

The thrust of the present study is that different influences operate on the two levels of satisfaction judgments (global versus specific). Our measure of positivity, which reflected the degree to which people judge broad categories more positively than narrow categories, provides one systematic way of assessing individual and cross-cultural differences in SWB. Additionally, we demonstrated that this measure of positivity is a good predictor of life satisfaction above and beyond other variables that in past studies have been shown to correlate with SWB, namely income and satisfaction with important domains (Campbell, Converse, & Rodgers, 1976; Diener, Suh, Smith, Shao, 1995). At the individual level both positivity and bottom–up influences were significant predictors of SWB—that is, life satisfaction depends on how good the various objective life domains are perceived to be in a person's life, but it is additionally influenced by the degree to which the person judges global domains more positively than specific domains. At the national level, positivity showed strong influences on national levels of SWB. Income only moderately predicted national SWB, and satisfaction with important domains was much less important. The contrast in findings among the two levels of analyses suggests that bottom–up influences may account for more individual variation in well-being whereas positivity may account for more cultural variability in life satisfaction. Additionally, these results are consistent with Kozma et al.' study (2000) that supported a "propensity" approach to SWB and that also showed that top–down processes were more important in SWB than bottom–up processes.

What, then, *is* the global positivity disposition? One explanation is that positivity is related to cultural norms regarding the value of happiness and positive emotion— that is, how satisfied people think it is desirable to be. Correlations between ideal SWLS and positivity revealed some support for this explanation. In returning to the question we began with, why Japan reports relatively low SWB and Latin American countries report high SWB, a propensity explanation suggests that the Pacific Rim societies do not have a strong tendency to evaluate abstract domains in a positive way, whereas Latin American countries have a propensity to evaluate most global domains positively. The concordance between average life satisfaction in nations and the residual positivity score shown in Table 1 is striking. Part of the positivity propensity may be rooted in cultural norms regarding the value of believing aspects of life, in general, to be good. The Confucian countries in our sample did not hold strong norms of positivity compared to the other nations. The Latin American countries, on the other hand, showed strong normative beliefs about the value of positivity. Because the correlations between ideal SWLS and positivity were not corrected for measurement error, they are likely to be stronger at the latent level. Clearly future research should turn to investigations of the origins of the positivity disposition both at the individual and cross-cultural level.

Is positivity a fact or artifact? The answer might depend on the phenomenon the researcher is trying to understand. Positivity might color the way people perceive the world and recall information, and is not necessarily merely a bothersome response artifact. Positivity might result from cultural norms that influence responding to surveys, but might also influence how people recall their experiences and make decisions about the future. On the other hand, positivity might play a smaller role in people's on-line experiences in specific situations. This is certainly an area in need of more in-depth research.

Because global measures are less tied to actual experience than specific measures, a question that arises is why use global measures at all. Perhaps in order to get accurate evaluations of a broad experience, researchers should sum evaluations at the specific or concrete level to gain a more accurate evaluation of the experience as a whole. With regard to the question of life satisfaction, how a person responds to the question "How do you feel about your life as a whole?" may be inseparable from the way he or she answers global evaluations. Kahneman (1999) suggested that answers to such questions are "fallible estimates" (p. 5) of true experience. In fact, Kahneman (1999) argues that in order to achieve measures of "objective happiness," researchers should rely on the experience sampling method rather than global questions of life satisfaction. Experience sampling or measures of "on-line" affective experience can be taken to be the most specific level of measurement possible, and therefore less vulnerable to biases in memory or responding.

What then is the "real" happiness? Is it how a person answers the question "How satisfied are you with your life in general?" or is it the sum of an individual's moment-to-moment emotional experiences? The answer is both—global and specific domain satisfactions and experience sampling likely tap two different types of SWB. Furthermore, we caution against altogether abandoning global assessment instruments for the more "objective" on-line measures for a number of reasons. First, experience sampling can be expensive because it requires equipment such as beepers or palm top computers for each respondent. Second, because human beings do not form their global satisfaction judgments based on the sum of long-term emotions, would it be entirely accurate for psychologists to rely solely on the sum of specific evaluations? After all, positivity is part of the way people perceive the world. A complete understanding of any human experience "as a whole" requires both types of measurement. Finally, global measures provide useful information about the individual's view of the world, regardless of the degree to which the person's judgment is based on specific experience.

Additionally, global evaluations might have important implications for decision making. To illustrate this point, we use the example of vacations. In reality, a vacation can be quite stressful (flights are delayed, reservations lost, and one can never be completely certain that the luggage will arrive), conflictual (trying to meet each family member's needs), or even boring at times. However, ask people how they felt about their vacations overall, and the answer most likely will be positive—a vacation is remembered as relaxing and fun (Mitchell, Thompson, Peterson, & Cronk, 1997). Furthermore, in deciding on whether or not to go on vacation next year, the moment-to-moment emotional experiences are most likely forgotten, leaving people to rely on their pleasant memories and global evaluations of the vacation in planning for the next one. Thus, global evaluations might predict future behavior even after controlling for on-line experience.

Although the present study offers new insight into the construction of life satisfaction judgments, additional research is necessary in order to understand the causes and consequences of global and specific judgments. Future research should investigate the mechanisms through which culture exerts its influence on positivity in addition to other factors that might operate on positivity.

There were a number of limitations in the present study that should be corrected in future research. For example, broader and more representative samples of nations would be beneficial. A necessary step is to sample a greater number of narrow and broad domains, and insure that the narrow domains represent an equally representative set of components for each culture. The indirect measure of positivity we constructed should be compared to other more direct measures of positivity. Finally, other methodologies such as ecological experience sampling would also help us disentangle the influence of positivity on immediate affective experience versus global recall of this experience.

References

Andrews, F. M. & Withey, S. B. (1976). *Social indicators of well-being: America's perception of life quality*. New York: Plenum Press.

Balatsky, G., & Diener, E. (1993). Subjective well-being among Russian students. *Social Indicators Research, 28*, 225–243.

Campbell, A., Converse, P. E. & Rodgers, W. L. (1976). *The quality of American life*. New York: Russell Sage.

Cohen, J. & Cohen, P. (1983). Applied multiple regression/correlation analysis for the behavioral sciences. Hillsdale, NJ: Lawrence Erlbaum.

Diener, E. (1984). Subjective well-being. *Psychological Bulletin, 95*, 542–575.

Diener, E., & Diener, C. (1996). Most people are happy. *Psychological Science, 7*, 181–185.

Diener, E., Emmons, R. A., Larsen, R. J. & Griffin, S. (1985). The satisfaction with life scale. *Journal of Personality Assessment, 49*, 71–75.

Diener, E., Diener, M. & Diener, C. (1995). Factors prediction the subjective well-being of nations. *Journal of Personality and Social Psychology, 49*, 851–864.

Diener, E., Suh, E., Smith, H. & Shao, L. (1995). National differences in reported subjective well-being: Why do they occur?. *Social Indicators Research, 34*, 7–32.

Hofstede, G. (1980). Culture's consequences: International differences in work-related values. Beverly Hills, CA: Sage.

Kahneman, D. (1999). Objective happiness. In D. Kahneman, E. Diener, & N. Schwarz (Eds.), *Well-being: The foundations of a hedonic psychology* (pp. 3–25). New York: Russell Sage Foundation.

Kozma, A., Stone, S. & Stones, M. J. (2000). Stability in components and predictors of subjective well-being (SWB): Implications for SWB structure. In E. Diener & D. R. Rahtz (Eds.), *Advances in quality of life theory and research* (Vol. I, pp. 13–30). London: Kluwer Academic Publishers.

Kurman, J., & Sriram, N. (1997). Self-enhancement, generality of self-evaluation, and affectivity in Israel and Singapore. *Journal of Cross-Cultural Psychology, 28*, 421–441.

Markus, H. R., & Kitayama, S. (1991). Culture and the self: Implications for cognition, emotion, and motivation. *Psychological Review, 98*, 224–253.

Matlin, M. W., & Stang, D. J. (1978). *The Pollyanna Principle: Selectivity in language, memory, and thought*. Cambridge, MA: Schenkman.

Mitchell, T. R., Thompson, L., Peterson, E. & Cronk, R. (1997). Temporal adjustment in the evaluation of events: The "rosy view". *Journal of Experimental Social Psychology, 33*, 421–448.

Pavot, W., & Diener, E. (1993). Review of the satisfaction with life scale. *Psychological Assessment, 5*, 164–172.

Schwarz, N., & Clore, G. L. (1983). Mood, misattribution, and judgments of well-being: Informative and directive functions of affective states. *Journal of Personality and Social Psychology, 45*, 513–523.

Schwarz, N., & Strack, F. (1991). Evaluating one's life: A judgment model of subjective well-being'. In F. Strack, M. Argyle, & N. Schwarz (Eds.), *Subjective well-being: An interdisciplinary perspective* (pp. 27–47). Oxford: Pergamon Press.

Schwarz, N., & Strack, F. (1999). Reports of subjective well-being: Judgmental processes and their methodological implications. In D. Kahneman, E. Diener, & N. Schwarz (Eds.), *Well-being: The foundations of hedonic psychology* (pp. 61–84). New York: Russell Sage Foundation.

Shao, L. (1993). *Multilanguage comparability of life satisfaction and happiness measures in mainland China and American students*. Unpublished master's thesis University of Illinois, Urbana-Champaign.

Steiger, J. H. (1980). Tests for comparing elements of a correlation matrix. *Psychological Bulletin, 87*, 245–251.

Strack, F., Martin, L. L. & Schwarz, N. (1988). Priming and communications: Social determinants of information use in judgments of life satisfaction. *European Journal of Social Psychology, 18*, 429–442.

Suh, E. (1994). Emotion norms, values, familiarity, and subjective well-being: A cross-cultural examination. Unpublished master's thesis, University of Illinois, Urbana-Champaign.

Triandis, H. C. (1989). The self and social behavior in differing cultural contexts. *Psychological Review, 96*, 506–520.

Veenhoven, R. (1993). *Happiness in nations*. The Netherlands: Risbo.

Most People Are Pretty Happy, but There Is Cultural Variation: The Inughuit, the Amish, and the Maasai

Robert Biswas-Diener, Joar Vittersø and Ed Diener

Abstract E. Diener and C. Diener (1996; Psychological Science 7: 181–185) suggested that most people are happy, and offered support for this claim from surveys in industrialized societies. We extend their findings to include people who lead materially simple lives and live in cultures far removed from those of typical survey respondents. We found that the Kenyan Maasai, the United States Amish, and the Greenlandic Inughuit, all reported positive levels of life satisfaction, domain satisfaction, and affect balance (more frequent positive emotions than negative ones). Across satisfaction and affect measures, including methods in addition to global self-reports, our 358 respondents from these cultures were one average, positive on all 54 scales, and significantly above neutral on 53 of them. Across all measures and samples 84% of participants scored above neutral. However, nobody was perfectly happy and satisfied, and the groups reported unique configurations of satisfaction and affect. Although all three groups were high in satisfaction with social domains, the Amish reported lower satisfaction with self-related domains, and the Maasai and Inughuit were relatively lower in satisfaction with material domains. All three groups reported frequent positive emotions, but only the Maasai reported frequent feelings of pride. Thus, the fact that most people tend to be moderately happy does not mean that they are ecstatic, or that there is no variation across cultures in happiness.

In 1996, E. Diener and C. Diener claimed that most people are happy, and implied that this is a natural state gifted to us by evolution. They reviewed evidence showing that a wide range of people, on average, report positive (above neutral) levels of well-being. From an evolutionary perspective these results make sense: the predominance of pleasant emotions would facilitate approach behaviors, because these emotions lead to the broadening and building of resources (Fredrickson, 2001), and high activation pleasant emotions include facets such as activity and energy that are almost synonymous with approach behavior. The importance of these approach-oriented behaviors might be particularly beneficial for an intelligent

E. Diener (✉)
Department of Psychology, University of Illinois, Champaign, IL 61820, USA
e-mail: ediener@uiuc.edu

E. Diener (ed.), *Culture and Well-Being: The Collected Works of Ed Diener*, Social Indicators Research Series 38, DOI 10.1007/978-90-481-2352-0_12,
© Springer Science+Business Media B.V. 2009

species that can move between new and different environments. This is congruent with Ito, Cacioppo, and Lang (1998) positivity-offset theory, the idea that people have a slightly positive hedonic tone that stimulates approach behaviors when no hedonic stimuli are active.

But, because the data reviewed by E. Diener and C. Diener came almost entirely from people in industrialized societies, another explanation is possible: that some factor related to life in industrialized culture contributed to the reports of positive well-being. For example, there could be emotion norms for positivity common to industrial cultures, which tend toward individualistic definitions of self (Triandis, 1995). Another possibility is that people reported happiness because industrial society largely meets human needs. Industrialized countries tend, for example, to have better infrastructure, better health care systems, better human rights records, more formalized social welfare programs, lower unemployment, and higher rates of education for both sexes than their "third world" counterparts. These advantages could lead to an increase in subjective well-being (SWB). In the present article, we extend the analysis of E. Diener and C. Diener to cultures that are substantially different from industrialized culture, including collectivisit culture and materially simple culture. We examine the Maasai of Kenya, traditional pastoralists who have few modern amenities and little exposure to western media, the Amish, who consciously reject modern values and technologies, and the Inughuit of Greenland, who live in a harsh environment and retain many elements of a hunting lifestyle.

In addition to sampling culturally distinct groups, we have included several types of measures in our studies to more strongly test the generality of E. Diener and C. Diener's conclusions. In terms of content, we examined both cognitive and affective components of SWB including life satisfaction, reports of satisfaction with specific domains (e.g., food, friendships, and physical appearance), and affect balance (positive minus negative emotions). We also employed several different methodologies to assess SWB. In addition to the global self-reports scales that are frequently used in this field, we also measured happiness by the reports of friends and family members of the respondents.

Another measure used with the Maasai (Study 1) and the Amish (Study 2) was based on memory—the degree to which the respondent could remember more positive than negative life events in two separate timed periods. Finally, with the Inughuit (Study 3), we also used the Experience Sampling Method (ESM), in which respondents' moods were recorded at periodic times during the day while the respondents were engaged in various activities. This measure has advantages over global reports in that it records moods in the moment rather than remembered mood states that can be subject to recall (Thomas & Diener, 1990).

The question of whether people are mostly happy is of theoretical importance to several different fields. In the area of emotion scholarship, it is essential to know whether certain moods predominate in people's experience, and whether certain moods tend to occur in the absence of significant events. If positive moods predominate, they certainly deserve more attention from emotion theorists, and exploring the reasons for dominance of pleasant emotions becomes a research priority. For the field of SWB, if most people tend to be above neutral in the absence of significant emotional stimuli, a reframing of issues in this field is in order. The search would be focused not on what makes people happy, but instead on what makes people unhappy, and what moves them up or down within the positive zone. Finally, if people have a tendency to be happy in the absence of hedonic stimuli, this has potential implications for our understanding of human nature in terms of the influence of approach tendencies on human history.

For overviews of SWB, the reader is referred to Diener, Suh, Lucas, and Smith (1999), and Myers (1992).

Methods

Respondent Samples

Research participants in our three studies responded to questions related to subjective well-being. Respondents answered questions relating to cognitive self-appraisals of psychological well-being, including general life satisfaction and specific life domain satisfaction. In addition, they reported their frequency of experience of positive and negative affect. The respondents also provided general demographic information (e.g., age, education, and income) and information related to their life circumstances (e.g., number of people sharing their home, exposure to western media, and a short biography). In two of our studies (Studies 1 and 3) peer reports were obtained for general life satisfaction and affect. We were able to obtain a limited amount of experience sampling data from the Inughuit (Study 3).

Study 1: The Maasai

Our sample of 127 Maasai came from 10 villages in four locations in Southwestern Kenya. The Maasai are traditional pastoralists, who have been living in Northern Tanzania and Southern Kenya since around A.D. 500 (Galaty, 1986). The Maasai resisted colonial incursions into their culture and retain most of their pre-colonial language, values, and practices. They commonly practice circumcision on young adults, engage in polygamy, arrange marriages, conduct child marriages, and require a period of warriorhood for young men. They maintain a form of political-religious leadership, embodied in the "Laibon" (medicine man). Maasai society is structured around age groups, or generations, that advance together across common developmental milestones (e.g., warriorhood, young elders, senior elders). Most traditional Maasai do not have paying jobs, but instead do gender-specific tasks related to cooking, child rearing, and herding. The Maasai have no running water or electricity, live in simple houses made from sticks, mud, and dung, and exist largely outside the cash economy of Kenya. The "morani," or warriors, still use traditional weapons such as bow and arrows, spears, and clubs. The Maasai diet consists largely of milk, tea, cornmeal, and limited amounts of meat. Few of the respondents in the current study spoke English or Swahili, had attended school, or had been exposed to modern media such as magazines or television. Past research suggests that despite obvious cultural differences, there are also certain similarities between Maasai and other cultures such as male-biased attitudes and the perception of time (Cronk, 1999).

The Maasai were recruited through word of mouth, and villages were given a small monetary contribution for participation in the research. After obtaining consent to conduct research from village leaders, the researchers requested and were granted access to a demographically diverse sample including men and women, as well as adults of varying ages. Because, we interviewed between 10 and 22 people in each village (where total populations, including children, averaged about 30) we were able to guard against selection biases. No one refused to participate in the study. Because, the Maasai are largely illiterate, questions were administered orally, in interview format by translators trained in psychological interviewing. For questions requiring a scale response, scales were presented graphically as segmented bars on a sheet of Paper. The use of scales was explained and interviews did not begin until each respondent understood their use. Previous research has been conducted with the Maasai (e.g., Kirk, 1977; Ma & Schoenemann, 1997), including a pilot study by the current authors in 1997, that suggests the Maasai are capable of understanding psychological concepts and can effectively participate in structured research. In an effort to make the respondents more comfortable with the research setting we included general, qualitative questions at the beginning of the interview. To alleviate possible concerns related to confidentiality, the interviewers were Maasai from a nearby region who had no social connections to the respondents or their friends and family members. All materials were translated from English to Maa by a native Maa speaker and key words and terms were back-translated by an independent native Maa speaker. In the infrequent case of translation disagreement a suitable word was arrived at after discussion between the principle investigator and both translators. Discussions included equivalency of concepts as well as local lexical norms.

Study 2: The Amish

We studied 52 people from an Old Order Amish community in central Illinois and a New Order Amish settlement in southern Illinois. The Amish are a conservative religious order tracing their spiritual roots to the Anabaptist movement in Reformation-era Europe (Hostetler, 1993). The earliest Amish immigrants to the United States came from Switzerland, and members of Amish society continue at home to speak "Pennsylvania Dutch," a German dialect, in addition to English. The Amish focus on "gelassenheit," or submission to God, guides their rituals, values, and behaviors (Kraybill, 1989). Food, health, and family unity are viewed as gifts from God. Although the Amish can be friendly to outsiders, their basic view is one of detachment from the outside secular world. In an effort to avoid the "perils of worldliness" the Amish widely shun automobiles, tractors, telecommunications, electricity, and other modern technologies. Although the New Order Amish take a more liberal view of the use of electricity and telephones, they retain the same strict moral, social, and spiritual values as their Old Order counterparts. Both communities are particularly suspicious of the potential negative social impact of mass media technologies such as television and the Internet. Most Amish children are educated no further than the eighth grade in Amish-only schools with a Christian curriculum.

Old Order Amish research participants were recruited by word of mouth and through classroom presentations. To gain the trust of this relatively closed community the principle investigator spent time visiting with Amish families, and obtaining the consent of community leaders to conduct the research. In the New Order Amish community, the principle investigator stayed with the local bishop and was introduced to potential research participants. Because, social introductions were necessary for recruitment purposes, the sample was largely one of convenience. However, the principle investigator actively requested introductions to Amish participants representing distinct demographic variables such as marital status, occupation, and age. Only three people refused to participate in the study. In an effort to introduce the research in an ecologically valid way, the principle investigator ate meals with many research participants and spent time answering questions after the research was concluded. Some respondents were recruited through school presentations, where the principle investigator discussed world cultures with the schoolchildren and their parents. The research materials were presented in English, in written form, and were completed at home, with the principle investigator available to answer questions. In some cases, respondents were allowed to complete surveys on their own and mail them back to the researchers after promising to complete them alone, and in a single sitting. The Amish are educated through grade school and are familiar with modern testing procedures.

Study 3: The Inughuit

Our sample of 179 Inughuit were contacted in the Greenlandic villages of Qaanaaq, Qeqertaq, and Siorapaluk, as well as in nearby hunting and fishing camps. The Inughuit, the name of the local Inuit tribe, live at 79° latitude, the most extreme latitudes of any traditional human society. The surrounding landscape is largely rock, sea, and glacier, with few large plants and no possibility for sustainable agriculture. The sun remains above the horizon 24 h a day during the summer months and never rises during the winter months. Many Inughuit are predominantly hunting-minded and their basic values are still anchored in the cultural traditions of a sharing ideology commonly found in hunting societies (Ingold, 1986). Historically, the Inughuit lived in virtually complete isolation, but today are increasingly exposed to western life, with modern jobs and a cash economy. Although many Inughuit homes have recently been modernized to include electricity, running water, and central heating, people typically live in crowded conditions and without flush toilets. It is common to see a hunter carving a seal or caribou on the kitchen floor, as children watch television. We have some indications that recent technological changes have not dramatically altered Inughuit life satisfaction. One of us (JV) conducted field-work in Siorapaluk in 1989–1990, when neither electricity nor television were available. In 1989, a single life satisfaction item, using a 1–7 scale, was used yielding a sample mean of 5.0 ($n = 19$). Thus, it seems unlikely that the level of satisfaction obtained from our current study is due the transformation to a more modern life style, because the life satisfaction reported in the current study is identical.

Most participants in this study were recruited in Qaanaaq, the administrative center for the municipality (population 620; Statistical Yearbook, 2000). In Qaanaaq, participants were recruited from bulletin board advertisements, announcements in the local radio, and by word of mouth (in the settlements we conducted a door-to-door invitation procedure). In addition, we travelled to the most popular whale hunting and fishing camps to recruit individuals who were actively engaged in these endeavors. Our response rate in the settlements was close to 100% and about 80% in the hunting and fishing camps. Respondents were offered small monetary compensation for participation in the study. All materials were presented in written form, in Greenlandic (two surveys were presented in English and Danish), and completed in a quiet setting where the researchers were available to answer questions. In Qaanaaq, participants were asked to return to the research cite the following day to complete additional surveys (peer report forms). The surveys were originally translated by a professional translator and key words and phrases were back-translated by an independent professional translator. The two translations were found to be equivalent. In addition, a small number of Experience Sampling Method data were collected through random visits to participants (see below).

Measures

Respondents from all three cultures answered the five-item Satisfaction with Life Scale (SWLS; Diener, Emmons, Larsen, & Griffin, 1985). The SWLS has been shown to have good psychometric properties (Pavot & Diener, 1993) and has been used widely across cultures (e.g., Diener, Scollon, Oishi, Dzokoto, & Suh, 2000). Participants from all three cultures also rated satisfaction with 14 life domains (e.g., family, food, and intelligence) using a 7-point satisfaction scale on which 7 was "Totally Satisfied," 4 was "Neutral," and 1 was "Totally Dissatisfied." Identical domain satisfaction questions have been used cross-culturally in previous research (Napa-Scollon et al., 2005). Domain satisfaction measures augment general life satisfaction measures, because they can be more closely tied to concrete experiences, and are less global than life satisfaction (Schwarz & Strack, 1999). Participants in all three cultures also indicated how frequently they felt various emotions during the past month, and for this report we analyzed four positive (joy, affection, pride, and contentment) and four negative emotions (guilt, sadness, anger, and worry) that were common to all three sample surveys, The emotion frequency scale varied from 1, "Never," to 7, "Always." All respondents also provided basic demographic information.

For the Maasai (Study 1) and Amish (Study 2), we employed a memory-based method to assess saliency of positive memories and the predominance of positive over negative memories. In this method, respondents were asked to list as many positive and negative memories as they could remember in separate, timed one minute sessions. The order of positive and negative memory tasks was alternated for every-other participant to control for order effects. The Maasai were asked to list memories aloud, while the Amish were asked to write them down. Later, we computed a memory balance score, subtracting the total number of negative memories from the total number of positive memories. These types of memory measures have been used previously in cross-cultural research (e.g., Balatsky & Diener, 1993) and have been found to show convergent validity with other measures of SWB (Sandvik, Diener, & Seidlitz, 1993).

Finally, with the Inughuit (Study 3), we collected ESM data from 22 respondents. We did this by approaching research participants at random times throughout the day, as they were engaged in various tasks, and asked them to report how much they were currently feeling on the eight emotions on a scale ranging from not at all to extremely intensely. Although a zero to six scale was used, we transformed it to a 1–7 scale for presentation purposes in this paper, so that it would be equivalent to other measures. Although 55 respondents originally agreed to participate in this phase of the study, we could not find many participants on the 12 occasions we searched for them, and some participants decided to withdraw from this part of the study. We elected to retain the 22 respondents who had 8 or more reports, because this number seemed adequate to obtain a somewhat stable and representative affect balance score for them. Participants were paid 50 Danish Kroner (approximately US $7.00) for a full set of 12 responses. ESM data has the advantage of assessing "in the moment" mood states and computing average moods based on these reports rather than on recall. Robinson and Clore (2002) have shown that people use heuristic shortcuts, not memory, to report their moods when longer periods of time such as a month or more are reported.

Results

The basic demographic composition of the samples in the three studies can be seen in Table 1. The table also shows life satisfaction and domain satisfactions for the three groups.

The Maasai, Amish, and Inughuit were significantly higher than the neutral point on all measures ($p < 0.001$—for all), with the exception of the Amish ratings of the "Self" domain (NS). In all groups, the vast majority of respondents scored above neutral on the global SWB measures. Similarly, the affect balance score, the difference between positive and negative emotions (shown in Table 2), was significantly above zero ($p < 0.001$—for all) in all three groups, indicating greater experience of pleasant than unpleasant emotions. Using informant reports also shown in Table 2, we found that an overwhelming majority believed their peers have more frequent positive than negative emotions, and the informant affect balance scores were all significantly greater than zero ($p < 0.00.1$). The memory balance score, the difference between positive and negative memories (Table 2), used in Studies 1 and 2, was significantly above zero ($p < 0.001$—for all). Last, the ESM scores (Table 2) collected from the Inughuit (Study 3) were all significantly above zero ($p < 0.001$—for all). Besides analyses at the group level, we also computed the percent of individuals in each group who were above neutral, with neutral and negative being the complementary category. Only for the Amish satisfaction with "Self" was the percent below half (40%), and the average across all 54 groups and

Table 1 Demographics and satisfaction with life and domains

	Maasai		Amish		Inughuit	
N	127		52		179	
Percent females	52		44		59	
Mean age	32.7		42.2		39.3	
Satisfaction scores	Mean	SD	Mean	SD	Mean	SD
Life satisfaction	5.4	0.6	4.4	1.0	5.0	1.0
Percent of sample above neutral	98%		61%		83%	
Domain satisfaction						
Self	6.6	0.6	4.2	1.3	5.7	1.1
Romantic life	6.4	0.9	6.1	0.7	5.4	1.8
Health	6.4	0.9	5.7	1.0	5.7	1.3
Attractiveness	6.4	0.8	5.1	1.3	5.2	1.4
Intelligence	6.3	0.8	4.7	1.3	5.1	1.4
Family	6.3	0.8	5.9	1.1	6.1	1.1
Friends	6.1	0.8	6.1	0.9	5.5	1.6
Morality	6.0	1.0	5.3	1.1	5.0	1.6
Social life	5.9	1.0	5.7	1.0	5.9	1.1
Housing	5.9	1.1	5.7	1.0	5.3	1.7
Material goods	5.9	1.0	5.6	1.1	4.9	1.6
Privacy	5.8	1.0	5.6	1.3	4.7	2.0
Food	5.4	1.0	6.4	0.7	5.8	1.2
Income	5.2	1.3	5.5	1.3	4.1	2.0

Table 2 Measures of effect

	Maasai		Amish		Inughuit	
Emotions	Mean	SD	Mean	SD	Mean	SD
Affection	6.3	0.9	4.9	1.1	5.2	2.0
Joy	6.4	0.8	4.8	0.9	5.1	1.8
pride	5.4	1.4	2.3	0.8	2.9	1.7
Contentment	6.4	1.0	5.1	1.0	4.8	1.9
Anger	2.1	1.0	2.4	0.6	2.7	1.4
Sadness	1.7	0.9	2.7	0.7	2.9	1.6
Guilt	1.7	1.0	2.4	0.7	2.9	1.7
Worry	2.2	1.2	2.8	0.9	2.8	1.5
Affect balance	4.2	1.0	1.6	0.7	1.7	1.9
Percent above neutral	100%		100%		79%	
Peer reported affect balance	3.8	1.0	1.8	0.7	2.1	1.8
Percent above neutral according to peers	100%		89%		85%	
Memory balance percent	1.74		2.75			
above neutral	87%		95%			
Experience sampling percent					2.60	
above neutral					95%	

measures was 84%. Thus, not only do groups on average score above neutral, but most individuals do so as well.

The results from all measures suggest that people are happy; but how happy? We examined the number of individuals in each sample who was at the top of each scale. One Amish respondent reported perfect life satisfaction, but nobody in this sample reported feeling only positive affect and no negative affect. In the Maasai sample two individuals reported always feeling positive emotions and never feeling negative emotions, but no respondent reported perfect life satisfaction. Among the Inughuit, two individuals reported always feeling positive and never feeling negative, and an additional three reported perfect life satisfaction, but no respondent reported both perfect life satisfaction, and perfect affect balance. Thus, respondents were happy, but nobody was perfectly so.

In order to visualize how far the group scores were above neutrality, we recalibrated each of the scores on a 0 (neutral) to 100 (perfectly happy or satisfied) scale. In other words, we computed, how far each mean score was between the neutral point of the scale and the top of the scale, and converted this to a score that could range from 0 to 100. For the domains, we averaged the 14 satisfaction values

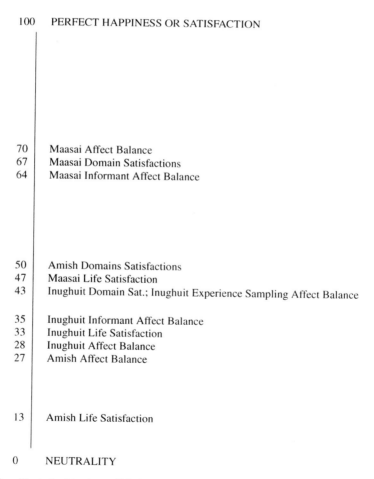

Fig. 1 Recalibrated subjective well-being scores

for each group. The recalibrated scores are shown in Fig. 1. Note that recalibrated scores could not be computed for the memory measure because the top of the scale is unbounded. As can be seen in the figure, all scores were above neutral, but none approached the top of the scale. The scores varied from slightly positive to very positive, with the highest score being only 70 out of 100. Thus, there is substantial room for even happy groups to increase on subjective well-being.

Sex and Age Differences

Women were significantly more satisfied ($p < 0.001$), and had higher affect balance ($p < 0.05$) among the Maasai, but men had higher affect balance among the Inughuit ($p < 0.05$). Age correlated inversely with affect balance among the Maasai ($r = -0.43$, $p < 0.001$). Neither age nor sex produced significant effects among the Amish.

Discussion

The results of the current study strongly support E. Diener and C. Diener's (1996) conclusion that most people are happy. It should be noted that in this study we conceptualized the colloquial term "happiness" to include both the cognitive (life satisfaction) and affective (pleasant and unpleasant emotions) components of SWB rather than a mood state alone. By employing measures of both, we were able to capture a fuller picture of our respondents' well-being. That said, the consistency of our results in terms of demonstrating that most people are happy is impressive. For satisfaction ratings of domains, 42 out of 42 measures (14 domains for each of the three groups) were all significantly positive. Similarly, all six global measures (affect balance and life satisfaction for the three groups) were significantly positive. When we turn to the additional measures—memory, informant, and experience—sampling, they too were all positive. Fifty-three out of the fifty-four measures we employed were significantly above neutral, and at the individual level the majority of people were above neutral on 53 out of 54 measures. Across all measures and all groups, five out of six respondents scored in the positive range. This is a level of data consistency that is virtually unheard of in psychology. Given the extraordinary diversity of our samples, it is clear that there is a broad and consistent phenomenon here.

Although the pattern of findings strongly supports the fact that most people are happy, the data do not indicate that everyone is ecstatic. Instead, most people are mildly happy and satisfied, and only rare individuals approach the tops of the scales. Across the samples in our three studies only one or two percent of respondents tended to score at the peak of the scales, and no respondent out of 358 scored at the top on all such scales. Among those many people who reported moderate happiness, we still found individual variation in satisfaction across life domains. Finally, there were those in our samples, who were either unhappy or dissatisfied. These individuals might be undergoing a set of difficult life events such as the experience of widow-hood, which might make them unhappy for several years (Lucas, Clark, Georgellis, & Diener, 2003), or have a predisposition to depression. The presence of a minority who are dissatisfied or unhappy is consistent with past research showing that a few individuals and groups living in dire circumstances report subjective well-being below the neutral point. For example, we found that homeless people in California are on average dissatisfied with their lives (Biswas-Diener & Diener, 2003, 2006). Thus, our claim is not that there is no societal or individual variation in happiness, but that people living in societies where their current social and physical needs tend to be met, and where no large negative events have recently occurred, will be happy.

To suggest that most people are happy does not mean that we can ignore cultural variations in happiness. For example, Triandis (2000) suggests that cultural factors such as tightness and complexity might influence subjective well-being. The Maasai scored the highest of the three groups on most measures, perhaps due in part to the high regard they have for their own group, as well as the stability of their culture. We also found variations across our three samples in the average levels of specific domain satisfactions, perhaps reflecting differences in local cultural norms or access to social and material resources. For example, the Maasai (Study 1) reported the least amount of satisfaction with domains related to material resources. This could reflect part of a larger cultural phenomenon consistent with a traditional group, whose ability to meet their basic material and social needs can be dramatically affected by ecological change. It could also reflect local expectations and standards for evaluating specific areas of life. The influence of norms on emotions, as discussed in Eid and Diener (2001), also seems apparent in our data. The Inughuit and Amish, for example, both reported low levels of pride. In many cultures, pride is regarded as undesirable (Shimmel, 1992), and this seems to influence how individuals in these groups label their feelings. In Inuit culture, for example, downplaying achievement is an important part of the socializing process (Briggs, 1985). For the Amish humility is an important virtue (Kraybill, 1989), a fact reflected, perhaps, in our sample's low levels of reported satisfaction with domains relating to "Self". Thus, there is cultural variability that is superimposed on the overall pattern of moderate positive subjective well-being.

What are the reasons for the fact that most people experience moderate subjective well-being? E. Diener and C. Diener (1996) suggested that we are pre-wired to experience positive well-being, because this tendency facilitated approach behaviour during our evolutionary history. Although our data are consistent with the idea that people are "built" to be mildly happy, other explanations besides an evolutionarily-based genetic propensity are able to explain our findings. It could be that socialization pressures lead people to report and even experience happiness, at least in western cultures where sociability is prized. Perhaps people are socialized to be happy, or act happy, in order to facilitate smooth social functioning. Another possibility is that people are on average happy, when they live in conditions that are favourable to human needs, and that even the relatively poor, societies we studied are able to meet basic needs for housing, social support, respect, food, and so forth. The idea that positive emotions in many situations are beneficial to successful functioning (see also Fredrickson, 1998; Lyubomirsky et al., 2005) is consistent with an evolutionary argument, but also with socialization and basic need fulfilment explanations as well. Thus, the reason underlying our findings awaits further study.

The finding that most people are happy is consistent with earlier work on the Pollyanna Principle, which was reviewed by Matlin and Stang (1978). These authors proposed that there is a broad tendency for people to be "Pollyannas," able to more accurately and efficiently process pleasant than unpleasant or neutral items. They reviewed evidence showing that this tendency is reflected in language, perception, learning, memory, and cognition. For example, people rate stimuli such as political figures as more positive than negative (Sears & Whitney, 1972), perceive and remember more positive than negative events in their lives, respond with more positive than negative words in a free—association task, and react more quickly to positive words than to negative words. Interestingly, Matlin and Stang note that most people think they are not only happier than the average person, but also are currently happier than they themselves typically are! They also report that people tend to remember events as more pleasant with the passage of time. We suggest that the extensive findings on positivity reviewed by Matlin and Stang are consistent with the argument we make here—that most people are happy. Indeed, the two phenomena—people tending to experience pleasant moods and emotions and evaluations of their lives, and also tending to interpret other stimuli in a positive way—are so closely intertwined that it is impossible at this point to suggest that one is the cause of the other. Instead, cognitive and affective positivity appear to be two sides of the same coin.

Are people truly happier, or do they only avow happiness for self-presentational purposes? Our use of multi-method measurement to some degree supports the former. Not only did our respondents report positive levels of subjective well-being on broad interview items, but their friends also overwhelmingly thought that they were happy. In addition, the Inughuit reported high levels of happiness when contacted at random moments in time. Further, our respondents were able to remember more positive than negative events from their lives. None of these measures is definitive in showing that the respondents were "truly" happy. Nonetheless, taken together they do suggest that the findings are not merely based on self-presentational style in an interview setting. People's friends think they are happy, respondents remember more good than bad events from their lives, they rate the domains of their lives as positive, and they report more positive than negative experiences when contacted in their everyday lives. Although these findings do not conclusively prove that people actually experience a preponderance of happiness, they are certainly suggestive in this regard. If it turns out, however, that most people merely avow happiness to others, this would be an important finding in itself.

How do we reconcile the fact that most people are happy with the idea that losses loom larger than gains (Kahneman & Tversky, 1990). In recent years, a number of scientists have commented on the fact that humans react more strongly to negative stimuli than to positive stimuli (e.g., Rozin & Royzman, 2001). One solution comes from related ideas advanced by Taylor (1991), who proposed that although people react strongly and quickly to negative stimuli, this mobilization is followed by responses that damp down the impact of the event. Taylor also presented evidence that the mobilization-minimization function is stronger for negative than positive stimuli. A similar idea was presented by Ito et al. (1998), who suggested that there is a "positivity offset" in the presence of neutral stimuli, despite the fact that reactions to negative stimuli are stronger than those to positive stimuli. Thus, people appear likely to react strongly to bad events, but over time tend to recover from them. Furthermore, people are likely to feel positive in the presence of positive or neutral stimuli.

There were several limitations to out studies. The internal consistency estimates (Cronbach's alphas) were lower for most measures in our three samples than they typically are in samples in modern societies. This suggests that our participants responded less consistently, perhaps due to their unfamiliarity with surveys or their lack of introspection about their own feelings. Thus, the consistency of the findings is even more impressive, because of the random error introduced by unfamiliarity with surveys.

An important distinction in the emotion literature is between moods and emotions. Unfortunately, our data do not allow us to make this distinction in our respondent's experience. Perhaps the most important limitation is one that points to future research: we do not know the range of conditions and circumstances under which people are happy. Although our current results show that that diverse people are happy, supporting the conclusions of E. Diener and C. Diener that were based on broad surveys of nations from around the globe, we also know that some individuals and a few groups are unhappy. A priority for future research is to determine the conditions that are necessary to make entire groups unhappy.

Finally, there were unexplained differences in our measures in the percentages of the samples that were in the positive range. Although the Maasai (Study 1) were highly positive on most measures, the Amish (Study 2) varied from Affect Balance to Life Satisfaction. On the former 100% of the Amish scored in the positive range, whereas on the latter only 61% did so. The Inughuit (Study 3) scored more consistently across the types of measures. We do not have a ready explanation for why many Amish would be happy in terms of Affect Balance, and yet dissatisfied with their lives. Perhaps their norms for humility are more likely to influence their satisfaction reports. In any event, this discrepancy in the two types of measures, even though both support the general idea that most people have positive SWB, will be important to explore in the future.

If there is a positive offset for happiness, perhaps the affect balance scores are the most direct reflection of this because life satisfaction only indirectly relates to emotions (Suh, Diener, Oishi, & Triandis, 1998; Schimmack, Oishi, Diener, & Suh, 2000), and because life satisfaction can be influenced by many kinds of standards and survey characteristics. It is also interesting to note that all three groups score higher in average domain satisfaction than they do in life satisfaction. Perhaps there are a few negative areas of their lives that carry heavy weight in their overall evaluations. The reason for the higher domain scores than life satisfaction scores is an intriguing avenue for future research.

There are a number of far-reaching implications of our findings. In terms of scholarship on emotions, our findings imply that pleasant emotions must receive equal study with unpleasant emotions. In addition, researchers need to search for the reasons that pleasant emotions seem to predominate in experience. In the field of subjective well-being, the findings are important, because they suggest that the phenomena in this area must be understood against a positive backdrop. People tend to be positive unless there are strong reasons to be negative, and circumstances and personality seem to primarily move people up and down within the positive zone. This framing of the phenomena in this field helps explain why conditions often do not account for substantial amounts of variance in subjective well-being measures. Our findings also indicate that just because well-being scores are positive, whether they be happiness self-ratings or ratings of societal conditions, it does not mean that the targets of the ratings are excellent-people appear predisposed to give positive ratings. Thus, scores perhaps might be high to reflect positive conditions that go beyond the tendency to perceive even neutral things as positive. In other words, positive happiness ratings do not indicate that conditions are excellent or that the society need not be improved.

The findings also point to research in the fields of cross-cultural and developmental psychology. Although our studies used samples from three widely different cultures, we do not fully understand how socialization might influence the positivity of happiness reports, even if there is an evolutionary predisposition toward happiness. Could it be, for instance, that there are socialization practices that can lead to most people being unhappy? Finally, the results are germane to clinical psychology because they imply that perhaps the natural state of people is to be happy, and that deviations from this must result from unusual conditions.

Take-Home Message

E. Diener and C. Diener (1996) reviewed evidence suggesting that most people are happy—they tend over time to be above neutral in their affect and satisfaction. In this paper, we extended this finding to rarely studied groups outside of industrial societies, and we used additional measures beyond global self-reports of happiness with these respondents. The findings were striking in their consistency—53 out of 54 of our measures showed that most people were significantly above neutral in affect balance and life satisfaction. Despite the consistency of the findings, only a handful of our 358 respondents scored at the top of the scale on either affect balance or life satisfaction. People are happy, but not overwhelmingly so. Furthermore, people's satisfaction with various life domains varied depending on life circumstances. Thus, a template for happiness might arise from genetics, socialization, or circumstances, but cultural and individual differences in subjective well-being nevertheless have an influence.

References

Balatsky, G., & Diener, E. (1993). Subjective well-being among Russian students. *Social Indicators Research, 28*, 225–243.

Biswas-Diener, R., & Diener, E. (2006). The subjective well-being of the homeless, and lessons for happiness. *Social Indicators Research, 76,*185–205.

Briggs, J. (1985). Socialization, family conflicts and responses to cultural change among Canadian Inuit. *Arctic Medical Research, 40,* 40–52.

Cronk, L. (1999). *That complex whole: Culture and the evolution of human behavior.* Boulder, CO: Westview Press.

Diener, E., & Diener, C. (1996). Most people are happy. *Psychological Science, 7,* 181–185.

Diener, E., Emmons, R. A. Larsen, R. J. & Griffin, S. (1985). The satisfaction with life scale. *Journal of Personality Assessment, 49,* 71–75.

Diener, E., Scollon, C. K. N. Oishi, S. Dzokoto, V. & Suh, E. M. (2000). Positivity and the construction of life satisfaction judgments: Global happiness is not the sum of its parts. *Journal of Happiness Studies: An Interdisciplinary Periodical on Subjective Well-Being, 1,* 159–176.

Diener, E., Suh, E. M., Lucas, R. E. & Smith, H. (1999). Subjective well-being: Three decades of progress. *Psychological Bulletin, 125,* 276–302.

Eid, M., & Diener, E. (2001). Norms for experiencing emotions in different cultures: Inter- and intranational differences. *Journal of Personality and Social Psychology, 81,* 869–885.

Fredrickson, B. (1998). What good are positive motions?. *Review of General Psychology, 2,* 300–319.

Fredrickson, B. (2001). The role of positive emotions in positive psychology: The broaden-and-build theory of positive emotions. *American Psychologist, 56,* 218–226.

Galaty, J. G. (1986). Introduction. In T. Saitoti (Ed.), *The worlds of Maasai warrior: An autobiography of tepilit Ole Saitoti.* Berkeley and Los Angeles: University of California Press.

Hostetler, J. A. (1993). *Amish society 4.* Baltimore: Johns Hopkins University Press.

Ingold, T. (1986). *The appropriation of nature.* Manchester, UK: Manchester University Press.

Ito, T. A., Cacioppo, J. T. & Lang, P. J. (1998). Eliciting affect using the International Affective Picture System: Trajectories through evaluative space. *Personaility and Social Psychology Bulletin, 24,* 855–879.

Kahneman, D., & Tversky, A. (1990). Prospect theory: An analysis of decision under risk. In P. K. Moser (Ed.), *Rationality in action: Contemporary approaches,* (pp. 140–170).

Kirk, L. (1977). Meaning and context: A study of contextual shifts in meaning of Maasai personality descriptors. *American Ethnologist, 4,* 734–761.

Kraybill, D. B. (1989). *The riddle of Amish culture.* Baltimore: Johns Hopkins University Press.

Lucas, R. E., Clark, A. E., Georgellis, Y. & Diener, E. (2003). Re-examining adaptation and the setpoint model of happiness: Reactions to changes in marital status. *Journal of Personality and Social Psychology, 84,* 527–539.

Lyubomirsky, S., King, L., & Diener, E. (2005). The benefits of frequent positive affect: Does happiness lead to success? *Psychological Bulletin, 131,* 803–855.

Ma, V., & Schoenemann, T. J. (1997). Individualism versus collectivism: A comparison of Kenyan and American self-concepts. *Basic and Applied Social Psychology, 19,* 261–273.

Matlin, M. W., & Stang, D. J. (1978). *The Pollyanna principle: Selectivity, language, memory and thought.* Cambridge, MA: Schenkman.

Myers, D. G. (1992). *The pursuit of happiness.* New York: William Morrow.

Pavot, W., & Diener, E. 1993, 'Review of the Satisfaction with Life Scale. *Psychological Assessment, 5,* 164–172.

Robinson, M. D., & Clore, G. (2002). Episodic and semantic knowledge in, emotional self-report: Evidence for two judgment processes. *Journal of Personality and Social Psychology, 83,* 198–215.

Rozin, P., & Royzman, E. B. (2001). Negativity bias, negativity dominance, and contagion. *Personality and Social Psychology Review, 5,* 296–320.

Sandvik, E., Diener, E., & Seidlitz, L. (1993). Subjective well-being: The convergence and stability of self-report and non-self-report measures. *Journal of Personality, 61*, 317–342.

Schimmack, U., Oishi, S., Diener, E. & Suh, E. (2000). Facets of affective experiences: A framework for investigations of trait affect. *Personality and Social Psychology Bulletin, 26*, 655–288.

Schwarz, N., & Strack, F. (1999). Reports of subjective well-being: Judgmental processes and their methodological implications. In D. Kahneman, E. Diener, & N. Schwarz (Eds.), *Wellbeing: The foundations of alphabet hedonic psychology* (pp. 61–84) New York: Russell Sage Foundation.

Scollon, C. K. N., Diener, E., Oishi, S., & Biswas-Diener, R. (2005). An experience sampling and cross-cultural investigation of the relationship between pleasant and unpleasant affect. *Cognition and Emotion, 19*, 27–52.

Sears, D. O., & Whitney, R. E. (1972). Political persuasion. In Pool (Ed.), *Handbook of communications*. Chicago: Rand McNally.

Shimmel, S. (1992). The seven deadly sins: Jewish, christian, and classical reflections on human nature. New York: Free Press.

Statistical Yearbook for Greenland. (2000). *Gronland, 2000. Statistisk Arbog*. Nuuk, Greenland: The Home Rule Government.

Suh, E., Diener, E., Oishi, S., & Triandis, H. (1998). The shifting basis of life satisfaction judgements across cultures: Emotions versus norms. *Journal of Personality and Social Psychology, 74*, 482–493.

Taylor, S. E. (1991). Asymmetrical effects of positive and negative events: The mobilization— minimization hypothesis. *Psychological Bulletin, 110*, 67–85.

Thomas, D. L., & Diener, E. (1990). Memory accuracy in the recall of emotions. *Journal of Personality and Social Psychology, 59*, 291–297.

Triandis, H. C. (1995). *Individualism and collectivism*. Boulder, CO: Westview Press.

Triandis, H. C. (2000). Cultural syndromes and subjective well-being. In E. Diener & E. M. Suh (Eds.), *Culture and subjective well-being* (pp. 13–36) Cambridge, MA: MIT Press.

Making the Best of a Bad Situation: Satisfaction in the Slums of Calcutta

Robert Biswas-Diener and Ed Diener

Abstract Eighty-three people in the slums of Calcutta, India were interviewed, and responded to several measures of subjective well-being. The respondents came from one of three groups: Those living in slum housing, sex workers (prostitutes) residing in brothels, and homeless individuals living on the streets. They responded to questions about life satisfaction and satisfaction with various life domains, as well as to a memory recall measure of good and bad events in their lives. While the mean rating of general life satisfaction was slightly negative, the mean ratings of satisfaction with specific domains were positive. The conclusion is that the slum dwellers of Calcutta generally experience a lower sense of life satisfaction than more affluent comparison groups, but are more satisfied than one might expect. This could be due, in part, to the strong emphasis on social relationships and the satisfaction derived from them.

There is, perhaps, no city in the world that is so commonly thought of as synonymous with "poverty" than Calcutta, India. By some estimates 40% of India's population and as many as fifty per cent of the children in Calcutta live beneath the poverty line (OFFER 1999). Its notorious nickname, "the black hole of Calcutta" conjures an image in the minds of many westerners of a metropolis full of miserable people. Higher income is associated with many positive outcomes ranging from increased longevity (Wilkenson, 1996) to better health (Salovey, Rothman, Detweiler, & Steward, 2000) to greater overall life satisfaction (Diener & Oishi, 2000). Conversely, low income is often associated with higher crime and poorer health (E. Diener & C. Diener, 1995). Thus, because of the dire poverty in Calcutta, it is possible that it is, in fact, the pit of misery envisioned in the popular imagination. Unfortunately, little research has been conducted with people living in poverty to determine the effects of severe material deprivation on

E. Diener (✉)
Department of Psychology, University of Illinois, Champaign, IL 61820, USA
e-mail: ediener@uiuc.edu

E. Diener (ed.), *Culture and Well-Being: The Collected Works of Ed Diener*, Social
Indicators Research Series 38, DOI 10.1007/978-90-481-2352-0_13,
© Springer Science+Business Media B.V. 2009

subjective well-being (SWB). Do higher crime rates and poorer health, to the extent they exist in a community, necessarily produce a lower sense of well-being? At a more fundamental level, are the extremely poor of the world miserable, and if not, why not?

The characters in Dominique La Pierre's (1983) popular novel set in Calcutta, *The City of Joy*, provide a courageous and hopeful counterpoint to the "black hole" stereotype. Far from exhibiting the despondency normally attributed to extreme poverty, they struggle courageously in the face of dire circumstances, finding joy wherever they can. La Pierre (1983) presented a fictional model of strengths and positive psychology, whereas much of the existing research on poverty has focused on deficits. Is the stereotype of Calcutta's poverty too bleak, or are the characters in *City of Joy* too romantic? The present study attempts to answer these questions by interviewing members of Calcutta's poorest communities—slum dwellers, sex workers, and pavement dwellers—in order to assess their life satisfaction, and suggest explanations of the results.

Maslow (1954) advanced the theory that basic physiological needs such as food and water need to be fulfilled before one can attain self-actualization. We hypothesize then that individuals with greater income, and therefore greater access to basic need fulfillment, will experience a greater sense of well-being. Income has been shown to be a moderate predictor of individual well-being (Diener & Biswas-Diener, 2002; E. Diener, Sandvik, Seidlitz, & M. Diener, 1993) and a reliable predictor of SWB at the national level (E. Diener et al., 1993; Veenhoven, 1991). Veenhoven (1991) proposed that income has the largest effect on SWB for those at the lowest economic levels. That is, the ability to fulfill basic needs such as food, shelter, and sanitation could have a more dramatic impact on an individual's well-being than the ability to vacation or maintain a private vehicle. Veenhoven's theory gains support from Lane (1991), who reported that negative affect (NA) decreased as people's income rose, but that this occurred only at the lowest economic levels. In an analysis of international data provided by Veenhoven (1993) and Michalos (1991), E. Diener, M. Diener, and C. Diener (1995) found a clear curvilinear relation between purchasing power and SWB. Oswald (1997, p. 1827), referring to income beyond the basic need fulfillment level, concluded, "Economic progress buys only a small amount of extra happiness." We therefore predict that the correlation between income and life satisfaction will be greater among the very poor than the correlations that have been consistently reported in richer, western nations (Diener & Lucas, 2000; Diener & Biswas-Diener, 2002).

Theories of adaptation provide a theoretical basis for understanding how people, including people in adverse circumstances, might enjoy relatively high levels of well-being even in adverse circumstances. Research on adaptation suggests that adjustment, in the form of diminished responsiveness to repeated stimuli, is an important piece in understanding SWB (Loewenstein & Frederick, 1999). For example, Silver (1982) found that both quadriplegics and paraplegics exhibited more positive than negative affect as soon as eight weeks after their spinal cord injury. But adaptation might occur more slowly for some stimuli than others. W. Stroebe, M. Stroebe, Abakoumkin, and Schut (1996) report that even after two years widows showed higher average levels of depression than the non-bereaved. Similarly, E. Diener et al. (1995) found lower levels of overall SWB in poor nations (including India), suggesting that poverty is one such stimulus. Thus, the question is whether people living in dire poverty might experience positive well-being if they have been poor for a long period of time.

Most of our information on poverty stricken communities has historically come from anthropologists in the form of descriptive ethnographies (Edgerton, 1992). Scant empirical data exists on the full range of well-being of members of these communities. However, a small body of literature suggests that certain communities and cultures, although poor, enjoy a relatively high level of quality of life, including SWB (e.g. E. Diener & C. Diener, 1995). Unfortunately, most studies were conducted in the West with moderately poor persons, as opposed to extremely impoverished individuals. Banerjee (1997) did conduct an assessment of strengths of 40 slum dwellers in Calcutta and concluded that while all of the research participants had varying degrees of strengths (skills, resources, etc.), these strengths were not sufficient in themselves to explain material success. Rather, the availability of support from the extended family appeared to be a key element of thriving among the slum dwellers. Unfortunately, the Banerjee article largely confines discussion of strengths to their impact on economic, rather than psychological well-being.

The present study provides much needed information about the overall well-being of slum dwellers in Calcutta and proposes a model to explain the findings. In addition, the current study was designed with increased attention to cultural issues that have frequently plagued international studies. Christopher (1999) criticized SWB research because of its foundation in subjective, and therefore individual, judgments. The predominantly western concept of self-esteem, for example, is correlated highly with both SWB and individualsim (E. Diener et al., 1995).

Beside these culturally based criticisms of SWB, it has been shown that a variety of measurement artifacts are produced by self-report measures (Schwarz & Strack, 1999). By using multiple measures in the current study, rather than self-report alone, we can look at the convergent validity between our measures and be more confident of our findings. The current study utilized a measure of life satisfaction (LS), ratings of satisfaction with life domains such as housing and recreation, and a memory recall listing for positive and negative events.

In addition to the multiple measures approach, the current study employed a strategy of "cultural contextualism" as well as "cultural fairness." In the first, the authors gained a better understanding of local cultural values and ideals relevant to the research by conducting interviews in two locations in India (Bhubaneswar, Orissa, and Calcutta, West Bengal). These interviews provide anecdotal evidence that despite differences people in these locations are concerned with many of the same ideals as non-Indians (e.g. positive family relationships and job security). Regardless of similarities, it seems likely that Christopher (1999) is correct in his assertion that members of different cultures weight these ideals differently. However, these differences should be looked at as indicators to help explain variation within the research results. By using domain satisfaction measures as well as global satisfaction measures the current study can illuminate specific domains that underlie global life satisfaction.

Our second strategy, "cultural fairness," reflects our attempt to guard against academic imperialism. We cannot pretend that respondents participating in this study will personally benefit from the new information it produces. Therefore, in an effort to compensate them one of the authors (Robert Biswas-Diener) gave a public lecture on well-being at the slum location in Belgachia and allowed subjects the opportunity to ask questions after the completion of each interview. Also, a monetary donation was made to agencies conducting community betterment projects within the slum areas and red light districts.

Another important aspect of the current study is the use of three separate groups of poverty stricken individuals. The three groups—slum dwellers, sex workers, and pavement dwellers—were selected because they provide rich variation in the experience of poverty. The slum dwellers, while poor, live in well-established communities. Sex workers, on the other hand, live in adequate housing but face relative social isolation because of the stigma attached to their trade. Last, the pavement dwellers, owing to their extreme deprivation, are burdened by an almost complete lack of financial and social security. Because of sensitivity about the circumstances of their lives, access to both the sex workers and pavement dweller communities is limited to foreigners. When contact has been established, it is often by journalists and rarely by researchers. This study begins to fill a crucial gap in our understanding of these overlooked segments of the population and provides us with the opportunity to understand how people make the best of a bad situation.

Methods

Overview

Eighty-three participants were interviewed on a measure of life satisfaction, domain satisfaction, and recall for positive and negative life events. Each participant fell into one of three categories: (1) slum dwellers, (2) sex workers, or (3) pavement dwellers. The interviews for group one and two were conducted in private rooms in or near the home of the respondent. The interviews with group 3, the pavement dwellers, were conducted on public sidewalks at or near the place where the respondent slept.

Respondents

In an effort to sample a broad spectrum of the experience of poverty three distinct groups were selected for the current study. All of the respondents were located through either local contacts, local political organizations, or non-governmental organizations (NGO's) working for public welfare. Participation in the study was voluntary and we received no refusals from any of the slum dwellers or sex workers. A small number of pavement dwellers refused to participate. Respondents did not receive financial compensation for participation in the study, although, unbeknownst to them, monetary contributions were made to organizations conducting community betterment work in their areas. The interviews were conducted with the participant, the researcher, a translator, and, in the case of the sex workers, a social worker present. The social workers, when present, were instructed not to converse with the participant during the interview. Unfortunately, privacy was an impossible condition for the pavement dweller interviews and the respondent was often observed by one or more bystanders. As with the social workers, the bystanders were instructed not to interact with the research participant.

(1) Slum dwellers: Sabera is a 38 year-old woman and occupies a single concrete room in a slum tenement with her husband and five other family members. The room has a bed, a television, cookware, clothes, and a Muslim shrine. Running water is available from a nearby pump and Sabera must use a public latrine. She had five children, but two of her daughters died when they were very young. Sabera spends her day cooking, cleaning, and sewing. She sometimes socializes as she works but reports that she has no real leisure time.

The word "slum" is a generic term referring to a variety of lower class settlements within the city. These slums can be officially recognized *bustees* (slums), which receive municipal water and are often constructed of stable materials such as concrete. Squatter settlements, also a type of slum, are constructed of *kutcha* (crude) materials such as bamboo, thatch, or mud brick (Thomas, 1999). People living in these locations have limited or no access to public utilities and face the constant threat of eviction. Despite the variation in the homes and communities of the slum dwellers, they are sufficiently similar that westerners would consider them both "abject living conditions." More importantly, the slum dwellers, despite possible in-group variation, differ substantially enough from either the sex workers or pavement dwellers to form a cohesive sample. The current study includes both *bustee* dwellers from Belgachia, in Northern Calcutta, and squatters from Garia, in Southern Calcutta. Our slum sample ($N = 31$) included 12 men and 19 women who ranged in age from 18 to 70. Sabera is typical of the slum dwellers.

(2) Sex workers: Kalpana is a thirty-five year old woman who has engaged in prostitution for 20 years. She entered the profession after the death of her mother forced her to help provide for her siblings. Although Kalpana's father is now dead she maintains contact with her brother and sister and visits them once a month in their village. She has a daughter but is only able to visit her once a month. Kalpana had an affair with a married man who she tended to for a year before he died. Currently, Kalpana lives alone in a small rented, concrete room. She practices her profession in this room that is furnished only with a bed, a mirror, a small collection of dishes, and a shrine to the Hindu Gods.

"Sex workers" are prostitutes; men and women who earn money by trading sexual acts for cash. There are more than 40,000 sex workers in West Bengal, the state in which Calcutta is located, most of whom work and reside in the city (Jana, 1999). As with the slum dwellers the sex workers vary considerably in income and relative standard of living. Bengali NGO's who work with this population categorize the sex workers into "A", "B", and "C" grade sex workers. These gradings are structured around the amount of income per customer (e.g. "A" category workers always make more than 100 rupees per customer, or roughly two and a half USD) with "A" category sex workers receiving the highest wages and "C" category workers receiving the lowest. Sex workers in Calcutta frequently do not fit the stereotype of prostitutes in the West. For example, few of the sex workers, particularly the "A" category workers, reported using drugs or alcohol. Similarly, the majority of the sex workers interviewed reported that they felt physically safe and did not fear becoming a victim of violence. It is also important to note that sex workers enter the profession for a variety of reasons ranging from being sold into sexwork (tantamount to sexual slavery) to financial desperation. In addition, sex workers differ widely in how many customers they see each day and for how long they have practiced the profession. Kalpana is typical of a sex worker.

Our sex worker sample ($N = 32$) included 31 women and only 1 man, and ranged in age from 18 to 50. Sex workers were drawn from the Calcutta red light districts of Khalighat, Sonagachi, and Bo Bazar ("A" category = 8, "B" category = 2, "C" category = 12, and ratings were unavailable for 10). The participants had entered the profession for a variety of reasons and had been working anywhere between 3 months and decades.

(3) Pavement dwellers: Rana is fifty-five years old and comes from the neighboring state of Bihar. After being evicted from a rented room he moved to a sidewalk just off of Calcutta's major shopping thoroughfare. He sleeps on a cot with a blanket and covers himself with a tarp during the monsoon. He earns about a hundred rupees a day driving a rented taxi, of which half goes toward food. He returns to Bihar every 6–8 months to see his wife and children.

The term "pavement dwellers" refers to those individuals and families who reside on the sidewalks, street medians, train platforms, or other public spaces of urban Calcutta. There might be more than 200,000 pavement dwellers in Calcutta (Thomas, 1999). There is a range of quality of living conditions even among this group. Pavement dwellers often sleep on sacks or blankets, but some possess a tarpaulin or mosquito net. While many pavement dwellers beg for a living, many are employed (e.g. taxi drivers or rickshaw pullers) and some own rural land or have a small business (e.g. tea stall). It is unclear exactly why people come to live on the streets but anecdotal evidence suggests a range of reasons including cognitive or physical disabilities, financial hardship, and personal choice. Rana is typical of a pavement dweller.

Our sample ($N = 20$) consisted of 16 men and 4 women ranging in age from 18 to 75. Some of the interviewees had lived on the street their entire lives while others had been there only a year. Some of the respondents elected to live on the street voluntarily, citing physical safety and better social environment, while others were forced to live on the street by conditions, such as leprosy and alcoholism, which affect their functioning.

Measures

Each of the respondents participated in a thirty minute structured interview. The interview was conducted through a translator fluent in English, Hindi, and Bengali. The translator was given specific training in interview techniques and participated in role-plays prior to the study. In addition, the translator was required to write a translation of each interview item and important words, such as "satisfaction," "positive," and "negative," were back-translated by a separate native speaker.

The respondents were informed that their participation was voluntary and that their identities would be kept confidential by the researchers. The interview began with questions concerning the respondent's age, housing situation, income, and leisure time. The interview included a measure of life satisfaction, the Satisfaction With Life Scale (SWLS, Diener, Emmons, Larsen, & Griffin, 1985). The SWLS is a five-item questionnaire that asks respondents to make a cognitive assessment of their overall life satisfaction using a 1–7 rating. The SWLS has been shown to possess good psychometric properties (Pavot & Diener, 1993). The one-to-seven rating in this study was depicted on a piece of paper both by numerals and by a corresponding series of faces ranging from an extreme frown (1) to an extreme smile (7). The faces were tested for comprehension prior to the study and each interview conducted only after the participant reported that they understood the scale.

Following the SWLS the subjects were asked to rate their satisfaction with 12 life domains (material resources, friendship, morality, intelligence, food, romantic relationship, family, physical appearance, self, income, housing, and social life). The domains were presented in the same order to all respondents. The respondents were asked to rate their degree of satisfaction with each of the twelve domains on a 1 (extremely dissatisfied) to 7 (extremely satisfied) scale. This scale was accompanied by the same series of response faces as the SWLS. The domains were each categorized as either "broad" (self, material resources, and social life) or "specific" (morality, physical appearance, intelligence, housing, food, income, friends, family, and romantic relationship). Diener et al. (2000) found that these categories showed differential sensitivity in picking up variation in life satisfaction. Broad categories are sensitive to positivity and self-presentation biases while narrow categories are more constrained by concrete detail. For example, Caucasian American college students scored higher on satisfaction with broad domains than with specific ones. Japanese-American college students, on the other hand, showed consistent scoring between the two. This suggests that highly acculturated Americans exhibit a "positivity bias" when evaluating global satisfaction. While the mechanisms underlying this bias are not well understood, it is likely that those individuals from cultures (e.g. American) that exhibit it focus primarily on the best aspects of each domain while neglecting the worst. Furthermore, broad categories are, by definition, sufficiently abstract to allow for this type of heuristic judgment.

Some subjects were unable to answer either the SWLS or domain satisfaction items on a 1–7 scale. These individuals were administered the same items using a simpler, 1–3 scale—with negative, neutral, and positive responses. When inputting the data the researchers converted those answers that used the 1–7 scale into three point answers where 1,2, and 3 were scored as a 1; 4 was scored as a 2; and 5, 6, and 7 were scored as a three. In this way the two types of responses were calibrated for equivalence. In addition, the simpler positive, neutral, and negative format is less likely to weight extremity bias in reporting that might otherwise influence the 1–7 scores.

The interview ended with a memory measure for positive and negative events. The participants were instructed to list as many positive events, and then as many negative events, as they could remember as having occurred during the previous day (called "memory for daily events," or "daily memory"). Following this, they were asked to repeat the task for positive and then negative events occurring during the previous year (called "memory for yearly events," or "yearly memory"). The order of positive and negative recall was counterbalanced among the respondents to control for order effects. Each listing (e.g. "my aunt came to visit") was coded as "1" and a total score given for the number of events remembered. A "memory balance" score for both daily and yearly memories was computed by subtracting the total negative memory score from the total positive memory score. Memory measures, such as the one used in the current study have been shown to converge well with self-report satisfaction measures (Balatsky & Diener, 1993; Sandvik, Diener, & Seidlitz, 1993). Including a memory measure is helpful when conducting SWB research because it provides a SWB score that is not tied to the use of numbers, and that is a direct report of satisfaction. Thus, the memory scores provide a methodological compliment to the standard scales in assessing SWB. A few participants were not administered the memory measure because of time constraints in the interview.

Conditions: Income and Housing

Income and housing scores were assigned by the senior author to each of the participants. These scores should be differentiated from the Income Satisfaction and Housing Satisfaction ratings given by the respondent during the interview. The Objective Income ratings were based on reported household income or, in the case of the sex workers, their professional category. Sex workers for whom we did not know their category received no Income Score. Scores were assigned on a scale that ranged from 1 (under 1,000 rupees per month; approximately 23 USD) to 5 (4,001 rupees per month or above; approximately 93+ USD). Objective Housing scores were assigned to each of the participants based on the overall quality of the housing situation. Factors considered for this rating included quality of construction of the living quarters, overcrowding, availability of public utilities, and amenities such as sewing machines. Scores were assigned on a 1 (meager bedding on the street, exposed to the elements in a crowded location) to 5 (Permanent structure with private or semi-private quarters; running water and electricity available at the location; possibly with private bathroom facilities; and luxury items such as a television, stereo, or telephone present). All income and housing scores were assigned to participants without knowledge of satisfaction scores.

Results

Descriptor Variables

The means and standard deviations for important variables are presented for each of the three groups in Table 1. The means are presented in the left-hand column and the standard deviations appear in parentheses on the right. Sixty-five percent of the respondents were female and the average age was thirty-five. As can be seen, women and men did not differ significantly on the major variables (e.g. women: LS = 1.94 and men: LS = 1.90, *ns*). Age, however, did produce a significant inverse correlation with global domain satisfaction ($r = -0.40$, $p < 0.05$) and for housing satisfaction ($r = -0.42$, $p < 0.05$) but not for LS ($r = -0.18$, *ns*). Thus, older persons were less satisfied. It is likely that this finding is due to the fact that the pavement dweller group, the members of which experienced the greatest material deprivation, contained a large number of older individuals. This conclusion was supported by a regression analysis predicting LS, in which age had a non-significant effect when group membership was controlled. The average Objective Housing ($N = 83$) score was 3.02 and the Objective Income ($N = 64$) rating was 2.46. Thus, the mean family income for our respondents was approximately 60 USD per month.

Table 1 Descriptive statistics

Variable	Slum dwellers	Sex workers	Pavement dwellers	Total
Demographics:				
N	31	32	20	83
Mean age	31.90[A]	30.80[A]	43.20[B]	35.40
Percent women	61[A]	97[B]	20[C]	65
Mean income	2.57[A]	2.28[A]	2.53[A]	2.47
Mean housing rating	3.25[A]	3.68[B]	1.57[C]	3.01
Satisfaction with life:				
Satisfaction with life	2.23[A]	1.81[B]	1.60[B]	1.93
Memory balance	0.00[A]	0.15[A]	-0.88[A]	-0.14
Material satisfaction	2.48[A]	2.07[A]	1.69[B]	2.16
Income satisfaction	2.03[A]	2.04[A]	2.40[A]	2.12
Housing satisfaction	2.14[A]	2.32[A]	1.88[A]	2.15
Food satisfaction	2.60[A]	2.61[A]	2.37[A]	2.56
Social satisfaction	2.41[A]	2.31[A]	2.46[A]	2.38
Family satisfaction	2.73[A]	2.46[B]	2.17[B]	2.50
Romantic satisfaction	2.44[A]	2.41[A]	2.69[A]	2.48
Friendship satisfaction	2.37[A]	2.41[A]	2.23[A]	2.36
Satisfaction with self	2.67[A]	2.31[A]	2.23[A]	2.43
Morality satisfaction	2.80[A]	2.41[A]	2.50[A]	2.58
Intelligence satisfaction	2.59[A]	2.48[A]	2.54[A]	2.54
Satisfaction with physical appearance	2.26[A]	2.31[A]	2.31[A]	2.29

Note. Different letters indicate means that differ by $p < 0.05$ or less.

A one-way ANOVA was conducted to ascertain whether or not the three groups differed from one another on LS. A significant difference was found: $F (2, 77) = 8.39$, $p < 0.001$. A Bonferroni post hoc comparison was conducted to individually compare the groups, and it was found that the slum dwellers differed significantly from the other two groups, but that the sex workers and pavement dwellers did not differ significantly from one another. The slum dwellers scored the highest on measures of LS ($M = 2.23$), the sex workers in the middle ($M = 1.81$), and the pavement dwellers the lowest ($M = 1.60$). Thus, the slum dwellers appeared to be most satisfied. This could be because they rate their satisfaction with specific domains more highly than the other groups (see the discussion of Domain Satisfaction below).

Global Life Satisfaction

The SWLS shows good psychometric properties (Pavot & Diener, 1993) and has been used extensively in the measurement of SWB (e.g. Pavot & Diener, 1993). We conducted an analysis of the instrument's internal reliability with this sample. The Cronbach's alpha was 0.80. The alphas, if any individual item was deleted, range from 0.73 (item #1) to 0.76 (item #3). Item five, "If I could live my life over again I would change almost nothing," showed the lowest overall mean ($M = 1.72$) and did not converge with the other items (alpha = 0.82). This could be because a large number of sex workers gave this item the lowest rating possible, often adding, "I would change everything".

Further support for the convergent validity of the measures comes from the strong loadings of the major measures shown by a principal components analysis, which produced a single strong factor. The component loadings are: SWLS = 0.71; mean specific domain satisfaction = 0.80; global domains satisfaction = 0.77; daily memory = 0.59; and yearly memory = 0.51. The strong single factor underlying all of the measures accounted for 47% of the variance in the measures, with the second and third factors having much smaller eigenvalues. This is very encouraging because subjective well-being measures of very different types converged in their conclusions, and heavily load on a single underlying latent trait of well-being.

The mean score for the three groups on global life satisfaction was 1.93 (on the negative side just under the neutral point of 2). This score is lower than the mean score ($M = 2.43$) reported by a control group consisting of 29 university students in Calcutta. The fact that the three groups in the current study appeared to be neutral, or slightly dissatisfied, overall, suggests that poverty is a condition to which people do not completely adapt. However, scores were not as low as one might expect based on living conditions. In fact, the slum dwellers showed a nonsignificant difference on global LS from the control group. The relatively positive scores for those living in poverty could be because the respondents find satisfaction in specific life domains other than material resources.

Domain Satisfaction

The mean ratings for all twelve ratings of domain satisfaction fell on the positive (satisfied) side, with morality being the highest (2.58) and the lowest being satisfaction with income (2.12). Both global and specific domains predicted LS with standardized beta weights of 0.35 (global) and 0.34 (specific). Material Resources (0.46), friends (0.32), morality (0.29), romantic relationships (0.35), food (0.33), physical appearance (0.36), self (0.39), and family (0.31) all showed significant (at $p < 0.05$ or smaller) correlations with overall life satisfaction (Table 2).

When analyzing the frequency distribution of the nine specific domains only 16% of respondents scored in the negative direction whereas half scored in the negative direction for general life satisfaction. This could be because heavily weighted negative events, such as the death of a child, dampen overall LS but have relatively little effect on specific areas of life such as romantic relationship or satisfaction with food. The relatively high ratings of specific domains, such as family (2.50), friends (2.40), morality (2.58), and food (2.55) are important in understanding the factors that contribute to the subjective quality of life among the poor in Calcutta.

Memory Measure

The mean memory balance score for memory of daily events was slightly positive ($M = 0.11$) while the mean memory balance score for memory of yearly events was slightly negative ($M = -0.26$). This discrepancy is similar to that found between reports of global and specific domain satisfactions. In both cases the narrower, more concrete scale was a better predictor of SWB than the broader, more global scale. This could be because the narrower scale, in this case the daily memory ratings, are more sensitive to small daily pleasures and hassles, such as a visit from a friend or a bad day of business, whereas yearly ratings are more sensitive to larger events. Because of this, large negative events, such as the death of a spouse or a hospitalization, stand out more in the yearly judgements than daily pleasures and this produces lower overall SWB scores. It is logical to assume that large positive events, such as the birth of a child, should also stand out more in yearly memory but that these events are less frequent in the current sample than negative events such as illness. Interestingly, daily and yearly memory measures were differently related to global LS compared to the specific domains. In a regression analysis some satisfaction with specific domains was strongly predicted by the events recalled from yesterday ($p < 0.001$), whereas in the prediction of global LS only events from the year enter into the regression equation ($p < 0.06$). This suggests that some domain satisfactions might result largely from a series of small pleasant or unpleasant experiences in those domains, whereas life satisfaction might be more strongly influenced by certain large life events.

Table 2 Correlations of key variables

Variables	Memory balance	Objective housing	Housing satisfaction	Objective income	Income satisfaction	Family satisfaction	Age
Satisfaction with life	0.27*	0.30*	0.30*	0.45*	0.22	0.33*	-0.18
Memory balance		0.12	0.11	0.04	0.28*	0.25*	-0.22
Objective housing	0.12		0.31*	0.23	-0.10	0.26*	-0.42*
Housing satisfaction	0.11	0.31*		-0.04	0.25*	0.17	-0.10
Objective income	0.04	0.23	0.04		0.10	0.02	-0.10
Income satisfaction	0.28*	-0.10	0.25*	0.10		0.12	0.20
Family satisfaction	0.25*	0.26*	0.20	0.02	0.12		-0.12
Age	-0.22	-0.42*	-0.10	-0.10	0.20	-0.12	

* Significant at the $p < 0.05$ level.

Variables Associated with Basic Needs

The high average rating of food satisfaction (2.56) is a particularly interesting finding because it relates directly to the fulfillment of basic needs. The other two basic needs related variables, housing satisfaction and income satisfaction, were relatively lower average ratings (2.15 and 2.11, respectively) but still positive. Income satisfaction and food satisfaction correlate significantly ($r = 0.33$, $p < 0.05$) suggesting that higher income, as a resource, can be related to possible standards for food satisfaction. For example, more money might enable an individual to acquire greater amounts, better tasting, or a greater variety of food.

Objective Income did not significantly correlate with income satisfaction (0.09, ns). The discrepancy between objective income and income satisfaction could be because factors such as social comparison could influence income satisfaction but not affect ways in which income helps respondents meet basic needs. That is, the respondents may benefit from money as a resource even though they do not strongly desire it. However, Objective Income did correlate strongly and significantly with overall LS ($r = 0.45$, $p < 0.05$) suggesting that, regardless of the personal level of satisfaction associated with income, it can help to buffer the negative effects of poverty. The positive relation between Objective Income and LS also lends support to Veenhoven's (1991) theory of a curvilinear model of income and SWB in that income has the strongest influence on SWB at the poorest levels. Given the strong correlation between objective income and life satisfaction in this study, we examined whether this relation would survive controlling other key variables. The sample was smaller in these analyses because we could examine only those persons with all relevant variables, and the zero-order correlation between income and life satisfaction was even higher in this reduced sample. The zero order correlation was 0.53 ($N = 54$, $p < 0.001$) between income and life satisfaction, and only dropped to 0.52 when self, family, and friendship satisfaction were controlled. When material and income satisfactions were also controlled, the correlation dropped only slightly to a robust 0.48 ($p < 0.001$).

Last, Objective Housing correlated significantly with housing satisfaction ($r = 0.31$). It is likely that this relation is influenced in part by the extremely poor quality of housing possessed by the pavement dwellers. When satisfaction with housing was predictd by group membership the difference between groups disappeared when objective housing was controlled. The three groups differed significantly from one another on objective housing: $F (2, 73) = 4.86$, $p < 0.001$. The sex workers scored the highest on Objective Housing (3.68 compared with 3.25 for slum dwellers and 1.57 for pavement dwellers) and Housing Satisfaction (2.32 compared with 2.14 for slum dwellers and 1.88 for pavement dwellers).

Discussion

Common sense and stereotypes of poverty would lead us to believe that Calcutta's poor are largely dissatisfied. On average the respondents scored slightly negatively on measures of life satisfaction. This is lower than the scores reported by middle class students at a Calcutta university. In addition, life satisfaction was strongly correlated with income. This is consistent with the view that income can have a large impact on SWB at the lowest levels. Differences were found between the three sample groups, with the slum dwellers scoring the highest on life satisfaction, the sex workers in the middle, and the pavement dwellers lowest. In the case of the pavement dwellers it is likely that both quality of living conditions (housing and income) and age influenced their low score (there is evidence to suggest that age and well-being may be correlated in India; Menon & Schweder, 1998). Also, objective health may be a variable correlated with age, and which might lower the LS of older persons in this sample (Diener, Suh, Lucas, & Smith, 1999).

Income satisfaction and objective income did not correlate. It could be that this is a reflection of moderate rather than strong economic aspirations. However, the very high correlation of objective income and life satisfaction is noteworthy. It indicates that economic aspirations might only affect income satisfaction while objective income can influence overall satisfaction. Not only was the relation between income and life satisfaction very strong in this study, but this correlation remained strong even when other variables such as family and financial satisfaction were controlled. The effects of income on life satisfaction seem to be direct effects, not mediated strongly by satisfaction with finances and other domains. Unlike other samples where income and life satisfaction seem to be correlated at low levels, and the correlation is reduced even further when other variables are controlled, in this study the relation remained strong even after controlling relevant variables. Clearly, income has a strong relation to life satisfaction among these very poor individuals.

Despite the low overall life satisfaction scores, the respondents fell into the positive (satisfied) range with all nine of the specific life domains. The participants reported being fairly satisfied with domains concerned with "self" (e.g. morality, physical appearance) and "social relationships" (e.g. friends, family). Of these, satisfaction with morality, self, physical appearance, family, romantic relationships, and friends were all significant predictors of global life satisfaction. In addition, satisfaction with two domains related to basic needs, food and material resources, were also predictors of life satisfaction. Despite the positive degree of satisfaction reported for specific areas of their lives, the respondents scored fairly low on global life satisfaction. Because the Indian respondents do not rate global areas higher than specific, it appears they do not exhibit a "positivity bias." It may be the Indians evaluate areas in a more evenhanded way without focusing primarily on their best areas as Americans seem to do. This discrepancy could also be due to differences in the sensitivity of the various measures. The SWLS, for example, is probably affected more by major positive and negative events than are the domain satisfaction measures. The domain ratings, on the other hand, likely reflect day-to-day experience. In fact, the daily memory measures showed correlations with satisfaction in the nine specific domains, whereas yearly memories were correlated with global LS.

Together, the multiple measures approach to SWB research produced a picture of Calcutta's poor as a group that, while living in sub-standard conditions, are satisfied with many areas of their lives. Social relationships, in particular, appear to be important in understanding our respondents' well-being. It is possible that a strong cultural value placed on family relationships helps provide people in Calcutta with support during hard times. However, for those who often cannot benefit from this social support, as in the case of sex workers and pavement dwellers who have been estranged or separated from their families, these same social relationships are likely a major cause of dissatisfaction as well. So, to the extent the poor can utilize their strong social relationships, the negative effects of poverty are counterbalanced.

Clearly, members of these communities are living in extremely adverse conditions. They suffer from poor health and sanitation, live in crowded conditions, and occupy dwellings of poor quality. Examples of the negative memories reported were "I did not eat yesterday," "I had to have an operation," and "a relative died." In fact, of the 73 respondents who completed the memory measure, 20 mentioned poor health and 10 mentioned a friend or relative dying within the past year. How, then, can they be happy? The very fact that we ask this question is indicative of our heavy prejudice against poverty and our stereotypes of the poor. Perhaps we should be asking why we assume they are miserable.

To help us answer the question of why we believe disadvantaged people are miserable, Kahneman and Schkade (1997) propose the idea of the "focusing illusion." The idea is that people judge the standards of the lives of others based on a few focal attributes, such as a personal deficit or material wealth. For example, we might perceive a newly divorced person as depressed or a lottery winner as happy, but if we expand the scope of focus to include many aspects of these individuals' lives, we may see a different picture. In the case of Calcutta, much of our attention remains focused on the image of poverty and its related ills. However, broader examination reveals a richer picture with positive life aspects. The participants in this study do not report the kind of suffering we expect. Rather, they believe they are good (moral) people, they often are religious (and religion has been shown to be associated with SWB, Diener et al., 1999), and, they have rewarding families (marriage is associated also, Diener et al., 1999). They have satisfactory social lives and enjoy their food. So the complete picture requires not just focus on the deficits of poverty and poor health but includes the positive aspects of the respondents' lives. In this way we can see that broadening the focus of attention provides us with more information and a more positive picture. To illustrate this, we return to our case vignettes:

(1) Slum dwellers: Despite the fact that two of Sabera's daughters died she states "my son gives me the most joy" and eagerly anticipates him getting a job at a nearby bakery. She was married at the age of fifteen and indicates that her husband, a tailor, is a major source of happiness in her life. Among her daily goals Sabera rates *namaz* (daily prayer) as the most important. When she is asked about the most challenging aspect of her life she does not mention overcrowding or low income. Rather, she says that it will take work to marry off her daughters.

(2) Sex workers: While Kalpana is afraid that her old village friends will look down on her because of her profession, her family members do not. She manages to visit them once a month and enjoys the visits. She has an eight year-old

daughter and is thankful that she earns enough to keep her in boarding and provide a nanny for her. Kalpana says that she is happy having a daughter.

(3) Pavement dwellers: Rana has enough money saved up so that he could, if he chose, rent a room. However, he prefers living on the street, citing a better social environment and increased personal safety. He notes that the place where he sleeps does not flood during the monsoon. He remains dissatisfied that he spends so much time away from his family, but eagerly anticipates his visits home. Rana is a deeply religious man and has set a personal goal for himself: He would like to save enough money to build a small temple [shrine] in his native village.

We can see that much of poverty in Calcutta is a case of there being "more to the story than meets the eye." The findings presented in this study tell us that we have overlooked a deep well of understanding that could be provided by the marginalized members of societies around the world. It should be apparent that while the poor of Calcutta do not lead enviable lives, they do lead meaningful lives. They capitalize on the non-material resources available to them and find satisfaction in many areas of their lives. Perhaps it is time we turned from an overused deficits model of understanding poverty to a more positive strengths model.

More research needs to be conducted before we fully understand the relation between poverty and well-being. This study was conducted in a single geographical area with relative cultural homogeneity. Future research, designed with an emphasis on the strengths and resources of those living in poverty, should be conducted in other locations and, ideally, with larger samples. Current researchers have documented the effects of poverty on well-being, but little attention has been paid to the effects of well-being on the effects of poverty. Last, the reason for the discrepancy in our data between general LS and specific domain satisfaction remains uncertain and further research should be conducted to address this issue.

In the end, our instincts serve us well when we condemn poverty as a social ill. People who live in poverty appear to suffer a lower sense of well-being than those who do not. But even in the face of adverse circumstances these people find much in their lives that is satisfying. A better understanding of the complex processes that underlie the relationship between poverty and well-being will help us make policy recommendations and design interventions aimed at promoting economic and psychological improvement in poverty stricken areas.

Acknowledgments The authors would like to thank Dr. Ahalya Hejmadi, Avirupa Bhaduri, Mr. Sur and the DSMC for their assistance in Calcutta.

References

Balatsky, G., & Diener, E. (1993). Subjective well-being among Russian students. *Social Indicators Research, 28*, 225–243.
Banerjee, M. M. (1997). Strengths in a slum: A paradox? *Journal of Applied Social Sciences, 22*, 45–58.

Christopher, J. C. (1999). Situating psychological well-being: Exploring the cultural roots of its theory and research. *Journal of Counseling and Development, 77*, 141–152.

Diener, E., & Biswas-Diener, R. (2002). Will money increase subjective well-being? A literature review and guide to needed research. *Social Indicators Research, 57*, 119–169.

Diener, E., & Diener, C. (1996). Most people are happy. *Psychological Science, 7*, 181–185.

Diener, E., & Diener, C. (1995). The wealth of nations revisited: Income and quality of life. *Social Indicators Research, 36*, 275–286.

Diener, E., Diener, M., & Diener, C. (1995). Factors predicting the subjective well-being of nations. *Journal of Personality and Social Psychology, 69*, 851–864.

Diener, E., Emmons, R. A., Larsen, R.J., & Griffin, S. (1985). The satisfaction with life scale. *Journal of Personality Assessment, 49*, 71–75.

Diener, E., & Lucas, R. E. (2000). Explaining differences in societal levels of happiness: Relative standards, need fulfillment, culture, and evaluation theory. *Journal of Happiness Studies: An Interdisciplinary Periodical on Subjective Well-Being, 1*, 41–78.

Diener, E., & Oishi, S. (2000). Money and happiness: Income and subjective well-being across nations. In E. Diener & E. M. Suh (Eds.), Subjective well-being across cultures. Cambridge, MA: MIT Press.

Diener, E., Sandvik, E., Seidlitz, L., & Diener, M. (1993). The relationship between income and subjective well-being: Relative or absolute? *Social Indicators Research, 28*, 195–223.

Diener, E., Scollon, C. K. N., Oishi, S., Dzokoto, V., & Suh, E. M. (2000). Positivity and the construction of life satisfaction judgements: Global happiness is not the sum of its parts. *Journal of Happiness Studies: An Interdisciplinary Periodical on Subjective Well-Being, 1*, 159–176.

Diener, E., Suh, E. M., Lucas, R. E. & Smith, H. E. (1999). Subjective well-being: Three decades of progress. *Psychological Bulletin, 125*, 276–302.

Edgerton, R. B. (1992) *Sick societies: Challenging the myth of primitive harmony.* New York: The Free Press.

Jana, S. (1999). *Namaskar.* Calcutta: Canvas Advertising Agency.

Lane, R. E. (1991). *The market experience.* Cambridge, UK: Cambridge University Press.

LaPierre, D. (1985). *The city of joy.* Garden City, New York: Doubleday & Company, Inc.

Loewenstein, G., & Frederick, S. (1999). Hedonic adaptation: From the bright side to the dark side. In D. Kahneman, E. Diener, & N. Schwarz (Eds.), *Understanding quality of life: Scientific perspectives on enjoyment and suffering* New York: Russell-Sage.

Maslow, A. H. (1954). *Motivation and personality.* New York: Harper & Row.

Menon, U., & Schweder, R. A. (1998). The return of the "White man's burden": The moral discourse of anthropology and the domestic life of Hindu women. In R. A. Schweder (Ed.), *Welcome to middle age! (and other cultural fictions)* (pp. 139–187). Chicago: The University of Chicago Press.

Michalos, A. C. (1991). *Global report on student well-being.* New York: Springer-Verlag.

OFFER. (1998–1999). *A reading between the lines.* Calcutta, India: Teamwork.

Oswald, A. J. (1997). Happiness and economic performance. *The Economic Journal, 107*, 1815–1831.

Pavot, W., & Diener, E. (1993). Review of the Satisfaction with Life Scale. *Personality Assessment, 5*, 164–172.

Salovey, P., Rothman, A. J., Detweiler, J. B., & Steward, W. T. (2000). Emotional states and physical health. *American Psychologist, 55*, 110–121.

Sandvik, E., Diener, E. & Seidlitz, L. (1993). Subjective well-being: The convergence and stability of self-report and non-self-report measures. *Journal of Personality, 61*, 317–342.

Schkade, D. A., & Kahneman, D. (1997). *Would you be happier in California: A focusing illusion in judgments of well-being.* Working paper, Princeton University.

Schwarz, N., & Strack, F. (1999). Reports of subjective well-being: Judgemental processes and their methodological implications. In D. Kahneman, E. Diener, & N. Schwarz (Eds.), Well-being: The foundations of hedonic psychology (pp. 61–84). New York: Russell Sage Foundation.

Silver, R. L. (1982). *Coping with an undesirable life event: A study of early reactions to physical disability*. Doctoral dissertation, Northwestern University, Evanston, IL.

Stroebe, W., Stroebe, M., Abakoumkin, G., & Schut, H. (1996). The role of loneliness and social support in adjustment to loss: A test of attachment versus stress theory. *Journal of Personality and Social Psychology, 70*, 1241–1249.

Thomas, F. C. (1999). *Calcutta: The human face of poverty*. Calcutta, India: Penguin Books.

Veenhoven, R. (1993). *Happiness in nations: Subjective appreciation of life in 56 nations* (pp. 1946–1992). Rotterdam: Risbo.

Veenhoven, R. (1991). Is happiness relative?. *Social Indicators Research, 24*, 1–34.

Wilkeson, R. G. (1996). *Unhealthy societies: The afflictions of inequality*. London: Routledge.

Conclusion: What We Have Learned and Where We Go Next

Ed Diener

What We Have Learned

Several broad conclusions can be drawn from the articles presented in this volume. First, there are some universals or near universals in terms of the causes of happiness, but there are also influences that seem specific to different cultures. Second, it appears that for emotional well-being, people around the globe tend to be above neutral unless they live in dire circumstances. Third, the measures of well-being are valid across cultures, but there are biases that can lower the validity of measures, and these biases can vary in different cultures. In the following, I review several conclusions that I draw from the literature on well-being and culture.

Differences in Well-Being Across Cultures

We have learned much about the mean-level differences in well-being between cultures and nations. In general, rich nations, or those with democratic governance, high levels of human rights, and high levels of "social capital" (including factors such as interpersonal trust), have higher levels of well-being on average. We also know that some cultures have higher levels of well-being than others, holding objective conditions such as income equal. For example, Latin Americans report high levels of positive emotions, especially when conditions such as income in the region are controlled statistically. Although Latin Americans score very high on positive emotions, they do not score quite as high on other types of well-being, such as Cantril's Ladder. We also have initial information on the well-being of smaller, more homogeneous cultures such as the Maasai, where levels of well-being are sometimes high.

We have little information on how cultures score on various methods of measuring well-being, for example on experience-sampling versus survey measures.

E. Diener (✉)
Department of Psychology, University of Illinois, Champaign, IL 61820, USA
e-mail: ediener@uiuc.edu

E. Diener (ed.), *Culture and Well-Being: The Collected Works of Ed Diener*, Social
Indicators Research Series 38, DOI 10.1007/978-90-481-2352-0_14,
© Springer Science+Business Media B.V. 2009

Such knowledge would give us a deeper understanding of cultural differences in well-being. An issue that needs to be studied more is the variability in well-being within cultures and what causes such variability.

Do cultures differ in well-being because of cultural factors such as norms, values, and the form of social relationships? We know that factors such as national income can relate strongly to some forms of well-being, such as the types of well-being captured by Cantril's Ladder scores. We know that other conditions like social trust relate more strongly to other types of well-being, such as positive emotions. It also appears that cultural norms governing the experience and display of emotions can influence the reporting of well-being in cultures. We have much less knowledge about how culturally prescribed activities, norms about social relationships, and the virtues that are valued in a culture influence feelings of well-being. Thus, we have discovered important things about the correlates of well-being across cultures, but there is much more to learn.

The Structure of Well-Being Across Cultures

We know that there are consistent structural patterns of well-being across cultures. For example, positive and negative emotions form separable factors, and, in turn, they are distinct from judgments of well-being. The separate factors seem to persist across all cultures, although the degree of independence varies. However, there are also patterns or structures, the way certain feelings of well-being covary, that vary across cultures. Although factor analysis and cluster analysis are often used to compare structures across cultures, latent class analysis (LCA) is an emerging method that can delve into structural differences of groups within cultures. We are just beginning to analyze latent classes within cultures and to compare these classes across cultures. The statistics of latent classes give recognition to the fact that the structures of well-being within a culture can vary across individuals. Furthermore, there might be latent classes, or groups of individuals, in different cultures that are similar to one another and other latent classes that are unique to a culture.

The Value Placed on Subjective Well-Being Across Cultures

Shigehiro Oishi and Jeanne Tsai have both been leaders in exploring how people differentially value specific feelings, and how these values can, in turn, influence the moods they report and experience. For example, devaluing pride or aroused positive emotions could lead to socialization practices that diminish these feelings. It might be that some feelings are more susceptible to cultural molding than are other feelings, which are perhaps more strongly influenced by temperament. For instance, in the Eid and Diener article in this volume we found that norms for positive emotions were more strongly associated with the experience of them than was true for negative emotions and those respective norms.

We also know that people's priorities can lead them to sacrifice current feelings of well-being in order to achieve other goals, such as mastery. This is a very important finding because it suggests that cultures may differ in their pursuit of positive feelings, and may differ in the likelihood to which people will sacrifice good feelings to pursue other goals. We have enough findings in this area to know that there are very promising associations to explore, but we also need much more study to fully map the ways that cultural values influence feelings of well-being.

Measurement Validity Across Cultures

There are indications that our measures have some degree of validity across cultures. For instance, mean average values of nations often correlate highly with societal characteristics of nations. The correlations are often considerable within each culture as well. For example, Canril's Ladder has correlated over 0.80 with national income, clearly indicating that there is a substantial degree of agreement in what the scale means in different societies. Furthermore, Ladder scores correlate with income in all societies, again indicating some common factor in what the scale assesses in different cultures. These types of findings indicate that cultural comparisons can be made validly in many cases. However, there is also evidence that measurement error is greater in some societies than in others, for example in places where the respondents have had little experience answering surveys, or where they have thought less about their well-being. For instance, it might be that in societies where people have fewer options in life they have given less thought to whether they are "happy," and, therefore, their answers are less reliable.

We also know from the validity evidence that measurement artifacts or errors are not so serious across cultures that they negate any substantive interpretation of the findings. The studies on measurement artifact differences across cultures suggests that they do exist and can make some differences in the findings, but typically are not so large that they can explain all the cultural differences that are uncovered. Nonetheless, we need more research on factors such as the effects of translation and other artifacts on well-being scores. However, as described later, the issue of measurement artifacts can be more conceptually complex than many people recognize.

Differences in Correlates and Causes of Well-Being Within Cultures

Table 1 presents the correlations between two well-being variables—Cantril's Ladder and Affect Balance—and income and psychological needs for selected nations. There were about 1,000 respondents selected in a representative way from each nation. The psychological needs score is the average of four needs that are based on Self-Determination Theory (Deci & Ryan, 2002), which suggests there are three universal human needs—for relationships, autonomy, and mastery. In the Gallup World Poll, we assessed these needs from four aspects: (1) Being able to count on others in an emergency; (2) Freedom to choose how to spend one's time yesterday; (3) Learning something new yesterday; and (4) Doing what one does best yesterday.

Table 1 Correlations within nations

Nation	Ladder-income	Ladder-needs	PA-income	PA-needs
Norway	23	21	02	15
Netherlands	26	11	04	17
Germany	32	11	09	19
Finland	27	15	14	19
Switzerland	22	16	03	25
Sweden	21	15	06	27
China	22	14	00	27
UK	18	21	04	28
France	24	18	14	28
Indonesia	15	15	09	29
Poland	26	14	06	29
Singapore	29	12	03	30
Uganda	19	09	02	33
Senegal	21	10	07	34
South Korea	29	30	11	34
Guatemala	21	12	06	34
Russia	28	16	14	34
Argentina	22	15	08	34
Nigeria	14	10	02	35
Italy	21	14	05	36
Hungary	38	22	18	36
Japan	09	18	01	36
Botswana	27	12	07	36
Mexico	16	21	16	37
Thailand	19	12	08	37
Panama	34	14	06	37
India	17	19	12	38
Vietnam	13	23	00	38
Brazil	11	19	05	39
South Africa	35	21	04	41
Bangladesh	18	19	07	42
Israel	16	31	08	42
US	24	26	12	43
Chile	29	26	10	45
Macedonia	29	27	05	47
Venezuela	19	17	05	50
Cuba	16	21	06	51
Honduras	31	16	04	51
Albania	39	32	26	59
Over all respondents	35	24	12	40

We created a needs score by averaging these four items. The Positive Affect score was the mean of two positive affect items (smiling/laughing and enjoyment).

Table 1 reveals several facts about the correlates of well-being across cultures. First, it can be seen that income correlates much more strongly with the Ladder score than with Positive Affect (PA). Across all respondents in the Gallup World Poll, the correlation was almost three times as strong for the Ladder as for PA. This means that people's global judgments of their lives are much more associated with income than is their positive affect. In most nations, there is hardly any correlation between income and PA. In contrast, the Deci and Ryan Needs are more strongly associated with PA than with the Ladder score. Thus, different predictors are associated with different well-being variables, indicating the absolute requirement of including a range of well-being measures in cross-cultural studies.

Table 1 also shows that there are cross-cultural universals. Global judgments of life as reflected in the Ladder are correlated significantly with income in every nation. Similarly, the needs are significantly associated with PA in every nation. However, differences between nations are also evident in the table. For instance, the association between needs and PA varies from a low of 0.15 in Norway to a high of 0.59 in Albania. Perhaps because conditions are generally better, the meeting of psychological needs is less predictive of PA in Northern Europe, as more people have their needs met. Similarly, income is associated only 0.09 with the Ladder in Japan, but by 0.39 in Albania, and 0.35 in South Africa. Whereas income usually predicts the Ladder better than needs do, in some nations this pattern is reversed, for example in Vietnam and Israel.

Thus, Table 1 reveals that there can be both universals and particulars in the correlates of well-being across societies. Several of the articles in this book present data with similar patterns, where a variable such as self-esteem correlates more highly with life satisfaction in some nations than in others, for example. It is evident that we very much need cross-cultural research to understand well-being.

Personality and Culture

Personality shows average differences across nations (McCrae & Allik, 2002), and personality is related to well-being, which, in turn, also differs across nations. We do not know whether personality differences cause well-being differences across cultures, whether emotional differences cause personality differences, or whether the two are, in fact, aspects of the same systems. Research that examines personality change in cultures and the socialization of personality could help us to better understand the cultural differences in well-being and personality. Furthermore, we need to give more attention to cultural differences in the way that personality is associated with well-being. For example, Lucas, Diener, Grob, Suh, and Shao (2000) examined the degree to which extroversion correlates with well-being across cultures and found that the correlation was positive in all nations they studied, but the size of the association varied substantially. Is this perhaps because there are person–culture fit effects such that some personality types are more valued in some cultures, or are more successful in certain cultures? Clearly, much more work is needed on the interaction of personality and culture on well-being.

Do National Boundaries Capture Culture?

One criticism that often arises in cross-cultural work is that nations are often used as proxies for cultural comparisons. And yet, the critique continues, nations are often made up of heterogeneous individuals who do not all share the same culture. For example, the USA includes not only European-Americans, but other ethnic groups such as Hispanics and Asians. Within the Hispanic group there are Cuban-Americans, Mexican-Americans, and so forth. Thus, a reasonable question is whether it is valid to treat the USA and other nations as "cultures." In addition, cultural influences may spread beyond national borders to many countries in a region, for example, the Latin culture which to some extent spreads across the continent of South America. Thus, a major issue is whether national comparisons are, in fact, valid when it comes to making inquiries about cultures.

The objections to considering nations as cultures often come from an ideological perspective by researchers who want to claim cultural uniqueness for a group within a nation and who want to recognize the individual ethnic groups for their important contributions and lifestyle differences. Of course, we must recognize that every cultural group is to some degree unique and special, but the degree of similarity of groups is also important. In some sense the question of nations and cultures is an empirical one, but it should be recognized that it is also a matter of degrees of similarity. All people in a nation such as the USA might share some cultural values and beliefs that on average separate them from other nations, but there are also unique cultural factors that characterize smaller groups within larger cultures. It is a mistake to think of culture as an entity, rather than as a dynamic set of beliefs and values, which can vary to some degree across groups and yet also have some similarities even across very large groups. Thus, nations can capture cultural effects even if there are distinct cultural groups within them.

Some beliefs, values, and practices are consistent across small groups such as communities, and others can be consistent across world regions. Thus, "culture" is not something that occurs exactly in some specified groups that we must study at that level, but instead is a more flexible concept that can vary at different levels of inclusiveness. In this sense, we can analyze cultural differences in well-being at the level of world regions and geopolitical areas, in nations, and in smaller groups and regions within nations. For example, the USA might share cultural characteristics with other Northern European countries, and yet within the USA there might be regional differences between the South and West, and between Hispanics who are of Cuban versus Guatemalan origin. Culture can be parsed at different levels, and the strength of the cultural effects at each level must be discovered empirically. The fact that correlations across nations between well-being and other variables, such as income, are extremely high suggests that at times nations serve as a useful level of analysis.

The Consequences of Well-Being Across Cultures

It is fitting that this question comes last because we have virtually no empirical knowledge of answers to the question of whether the outcomes of feelings of well-being differ across cultures. Even within the westernized cultures of North America and Europe, there are not yet substantial data on how happy versus unhappy people behave and succeed. Whether it be life satisfaction or positive emotions, we are only just beginning to understand the results on future behavior and success of having a high level of well-being; and we have only a little information about optimal levels of well-being. In other cultures around the globe, we have even less knowledge. It is not a foregone conclusion that we can extrapolate the existing findings to other regions of the world because culture might have a large impact on what levels of well-being produce the most success in life. Thus, this area is a priority for future research. In addition to broad surveys, it will require longitudinal and experimental research, and thus requires ambitious scientific undertakings. The knowledge gained will be so important, however, that the effort will be worth it.

General Conclusions

The past decade has seen an explosion of knowledge about culture and well-being. A decade ago we knew little, and we now know a great amount. I am grateful to my students, former students, and others, who have contributed to this burgeoning field. We now know, for example, that it is likely that cultures vary in well-being in part because of objective conditions within each culture, such as income and fulfillment of basic needs. We also know that factors related to the value placed on subjective well-being and the nature of social relationships also influence the average levels of well-being experienced in nations. Moreover, we understand that there are both human universals and cultural particulars when it comes to the causes of happiness. People across cultures differ, for example, on the degree to which reported self-esteem is related to life satisfaction, but a deep feeling that one is living correctly probably predicts well-being in all cultures. Two decades ago we had almost no knowledge in this area.

Where We Need to Go Next

In the sections above, many unknowns are apparent. We have learned about cultural differences in well-being, but there is much more that we do not know. In the following sections, I outline additional promising avenues for research.

Methods

As should be clear, studies that use multiple measures are highly desirable when it comes to studying well-being across cultures. Not only do we need to use multiple methods when possible, such as supplementing survey measures with experience-sampling and informant reports, but we also need to assess the various types of well-being such as life satisfaction, positive affect, and negative affect. We know that various methods and different types of well-being together can show different patterns when comparisons are made across cultures, and, therefore, it is no longer justifiable to make general conclusions about well-being based on a single type of measure. For instance, we cannot make statements about the "happiest nation" unless we have used several types of methods and assessed the major forms of well-being.

What Is an Artifact?

The issue of measurement artifacts raises a number of intriguing and challenging questions about the nature of the processes leading to well-being. Because each artifact can also usually be an actual influence on well-being, the question is raised as to whether it is a measurement problem or a process that gives us insight into the composition of well-being. For example, take the following potential measurement artifacts:

> Language translation
> Socially desirable responding
> Scale number use
> Humility in responding
> Positivity biases
> Memory biases

When we measure well-being across cultures, we inevitably face the challenge of translating the scales into multiple languages, and finding words with the identical connotative meaning can be difficult. For example, in some languages an exact equivalent of the word "happy" does not exist. Furthermore, there are different meanings of "happy" in the English language, and the question arises as to which meaning is appropriate in the question. Thus, researchers often use multiple items and words in order to try to focus on the specific concept. But note that it is possible that the words available in a language shape the way people think in that culture, and frequently-used words might prime the ideas that are most salient to people. Thus, language differences might reflect differences in experience.

Although it is important to try to find equivalent meaning when translating scales across cultures, the pattern of meaning of words might not be identical, as the structure of concepts varies across cultures. This means that translation is more than just a technical exercise; it ultimately also involves a mapping of concepts. This does not necessarily imply that comparisons are hopeless because there might be many concepts for which the structure of meaning is somewhat uniform across cultures. At the same time, it does mean that there is plenty of opportunity for researchers to study the relation of concepts in different cultures and see how these structures influence reports and feelings of well-being.

Socially desirable responding was initially thought to be merely a measurement response bias that interfered with scale validity, but it was soon realized that the propensity to give socially desirable responses was related to the respondent's personality; and this tendency, in turn, was sometimes related to the concept being measured. In these cases, controlling for "social desirability," which was viewed by some later researchers as the desire to please others, leads to lower validity of the well-being scores. A forced-choice measure of well-being created in my laboratory showed validity scores lower than comparable scales that did not control this response tendency. Thus, although there is obviously some tendency for people to give answers that appear desirable to others, individual differences in this tendency (as opposed to situational factors in the interview that might influence desirable responding) appear to be related to well-being and inversely related to neuroticism. Thus, viewing response-biases as mere errors is a mistake.

Number use is yet another area where at first a response tendency seems to be a simple methodological problem but with deeper analysis turns out to be possibly related to psychological processes that are linked to the actual experience of well-being. For example, a tendency to avoid the ends of scales could result from a mindset of not wanting to stand out or be unusual and a wish to appear average and part of the group. In contrast, attraction to using the extremes of the scale might follow from an individualistic mindset in which the person wants to stand out and be unique. These two mindsets, however, could be related to the way that well-being is experienced. Thus, sometimes a measurement "artifact" might be just an artifact, and sometimes it could be more. It is both an empirical and theoretical challenge to understand when response predispositions are merely measurement problems and when they are related to the nature of the phenomenon being assessed. However, it is possible that a tendency to respond with either the middle numbers of a response scale, or with extreme numbers, lowers the validity of measures. In several studies, we have controlled for extremity response and it made no difference; but in one study, it did alter the standing of groups. Thus, response tendencies should be examined, but they should not automatically be controlled for without careful analysis.

The other possible artifacts I list are subject to the same conceptual issues. Humility might alter a person's responses, but it might also alter a person's feelings of well-being. The same can be said of positivity and memory biases. I am not saying that each of the response tendencies will necessarily be related to feelings of well-being, but I am suggesting that this is a possibility that must be explored. We cannot automatically assume that artifacts are just measurement problems, but need to also explore whether these predispositions relate in interesting ways to the dynamics of well-being. This is a wonderful opportunity for important research.

Statistical Approaches

Although standard statistical approaches such as correlations, T-tests, and linear regression remain the mainstays of statistical approaches in this area, investigators should also familiarize themselves with the newer statistics being used in the field. These approaches often allow the more accurate analyses of questions, and at times allow new questions to be asked. An example of an approach that is relatively new to the field is Hierarchical Linear Modeling (HLM). This method allows us to examine whether the effects of specific variables are consistent across cultures, and if not, what factors might moderate the differences. Another useful statistical method is Item Response Theory (IRT), which allows researchers to adjust responses to scale items depending on how people use the response categories. Yet another useful approach is Latent Class Analysis, which can be employed to examine different groups within a culture that have different patterns of responding. These and other new approaches can be quite helpful in achieving more valid conclusions, although it should be warned that many of these statistics require large numbers of respondents for accurate estimates.

Theoretical Questions

Earlier in the chapter, I have alluded to many of the theoretical issues that are only partially resolved. For example, how do culturally-prescribed activities affect well-being? Are there person-culture fit factors that influence the well-being of individuals in different cultures? There are additional cross-cultural questions such as whether social comparison effects differ across cultures and the issue of what factors influence adaptation to conditions across cultures. One of the most interesting questions is why some cultures, such as those in Latin America, show higher overall levels of well-being than other regions. Another missing question is about the relative impact of culturally unique goals and values on well-being versus the influence of cross-cultural universals. This question is likely to vary with the type of well-being measured. In this same vein, more research is needed on which influences on well-being are universal across cultures and why.

Another area for in-depth study is the influence of values on feelings of well-being. If people value certain types of well-being more than those in other cultures, does this lead to higher levels of that type of well-being? And further, what are the processes explaining how this occurs? If people value a type of well-being, does this influence the optimal level of it?

As mentioned earlier, perhaps the biggest question in the field is the issue of optimal levels of well-being for effective functioning, and this question is particularly acute in the cross-cultural area where there are virtually no studies. If people value other feelings such as mastery over positive emotions, does this moderate the effects of various positive feelings on achieving success? Are there universals across cultures in how certain feelings of well-being, such as joy, influence sociability, creativity, or feelings of energy? In order to delve into these questions, experimental studies will be helpful – for example, studies in which moods are induced and behavior is compared between the experimental and the control group. In addition, longitudinal studies will be essential so that we can disentangle the direction of influence between well-being and outcomes. The endeavor that explores the outcomes of well-being on future success is one of the most important remaining issues in the field, if not the most important, and, therefore, it fully deserves the intense kinds of studies that can yield solid results.

Because of television, international travel, and the print media, the world in many ways is becoming more homogeneous. Therefore, it is of utmost importance to understand the strengths of the various cultures, including the well-being they produce. Although there is now an enormous worldwide focus on economic development, we would do well to also understand the societal and cultural conditions that lead to high well-being.

References

Deci, E. L., & Ryan, R. M. (Eds.) (2002). *Handbook of self-determination research*. Rochester, New York: University of Rochester Press.

Lucas, R. I., Diener, E., Grob, A., Suh, E. M., & Shao, L. (2000). Cross-cultural evidence for the fundamental features of extraversion. *Journal of Personality and Social Psychology, 79*, 452–468.

McCrae, R. R., & Allik, J. (2002). *The five-factor model of personality across cultures*. New York: Springer.

Printed in the United States
218406BV00001B/4/P